W0230657

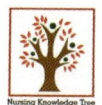

Understanding
Pathophysiology
of Diseases
(System-wise disorders as per INC Syllabus)

Kanika Rai

BSc (N), Gold Medalist in MSc (N), PhD (N)

Professor and Head of Department (Medical Surgical Nursing)
Maharishi Markandeshwar College of Nursing
Maharishi Markandeshwar (Deemed to be University)
Mullana, Ambala, Haryana

Founder
Kanika's Nursing Academy
Chandigarh

Foreword
Sukhpal Kaur

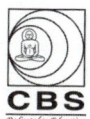

CBS
Dedicated to Education

CBS Publishers & Distributors Pvt Ltd

• New Delhi • Bengaluru • Chennai • Kochi • Kolkata • Lucknow
• Mumbai • Hyderabad • Nagpur • Patna • Pune • Vijayawada

Understanding
Pathophysiology
of Diseases
(System-wise disorders as per INC Syllabus)

ISBN: 978-93-90619-11-5

Copyright © Publishers

First Edition: 2022

Published by **Satish Kumar Jain** and produced by **Varun Jain** for

CBS Publishers & Distributors Pvt Ltd

4819/XI Prahlad Street, 24 Ansari Road, Daryaganj, New Delhi 110 002, India.
Ph: +91-11-23289259, 23266861, 23266867   Website: www.cbspd.com
Fax: 011-23243014
e-mail: delhi@cbspd.com; cbspubs@airtelmail.in.

Corporate Office: 204 FIE, Industrial Area, Patparganj, Delhi 110 092
Ph: +91-11-4934 4934   Fax: 4934 4935
e-mail: feedback@cbspd.com; bhupesharora@cbspd.com

Branches

- **Bengaluru:** Seema House 2975, 17th Cross, K.R. Road, Banasankari 2nd Stage, Bengaluru 560 070, Karnataka
  Ph: +91-80-26771678/79   Fax: +91-80-26771680
  e-mail: bangalore@cbspd.com

- **Chennai:** 7, Subbaraya Street, Shenoy Nagar, Chennai 600 030, Tamil Nadu
  Ph: +91-44-26680620, 26681266   Fax: +91-44-42032115
  e-mail: chennai@cbspd.com

- **Kochi:** 68/1534, 35, 36-Power House Road, Opp. KSEB, Cochin-682018, Kochi, Kerala
  Ph: +91-484-4059061-65   Fax: +91-484-4059065
  e-mail: kochi@cbspd.com

- **Kolkata:** 6/B, Ground Floor, Rameswar Shaw Road, Kolkata-700 014, West Bengal
  Ph: +91-33-22891126, 22891127, 22891128
  e-mail: kolkata@cbspd.com

- **Lucknow:** Basement, Khushnuma Complex, 7-Meerabai Ma Rg, (Behind Jawahar Bhawan), Lucknow-226001, Uttar Pradesh
  Ph: +0522-4000032
  e-mail: tiwari.lucknow@cbspd.com

- **Mumbai:** PWD Shed, Gala No. 25/26, Ramchandra Bhatt Marg, Next to J.J. Hospital Gate No. 2, Opp. Union Bank of India, Noor Baug, Mumbai-400009
  Ph: +91-22-66661880/89   Fax: +91-22-24902342
  e-mail: mumbai@cbspd.com

Representatives

• **Hyderabad**	+91-9885175004	• **Patna**	+91-9334159340
• **Pune**	+91-9623451994	• **Vijayawada**	+91-9000660880

Printed at: Magic International Pvt. Ltd., Greater Noida, UP, India

Foreword

It gives me immense pleasure to write the foreword for the book, *Understanding Pathophysiology of Diseases* authored by Dr Kanika Rai. The book is designed as per the curriculum laid down by Indian Nursing Council and is correlated with the chapters of Medical Surgical Nursing. The content of the book is straightforward having a detailed overview of the sequence of changes that occur as a result of various disease conditions. This 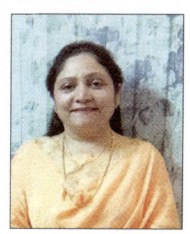 book will provide the nursing students with clear and simple explanations about the deviation from healthy state to illness and also will encourage the students to develop a detailed understanding of specific disorders and their main causes. As I reviewed the book prior to writing this foreword, I was impressed by the salient features of this book that include colorful illustrations, figures and flowcharts throughout the content for an easy grasp of the pathophysiological concepts. I am happy to announce that this book will definitely serve the purposes of the students and enrich them with a thorough understanding of the disease conditions.

I congratulate the author for bringing out this idea of writing a book on the topic which is most frequently searched by students.

Sukhpal Kaur

Lecturer
National Institute of Nursing Education (NINE)
Postgraduate Institute of Medical Education and Research (PGIMER)
Chandigarh

Contributor and Reviewers

Contributor

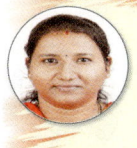

Bindu Joseph
RN, RM, MSc(N), CTVS
Ex-Faculty
MM College of Nursing
Maharishi Markandeshwar (DU)
Mullana, Ambala (Haryana)

Reviewers

Alka Saxena
MSc (MSN)
Principal
KS Nursing College
Gwalior, Madhya Pradesh

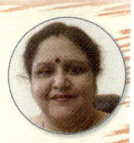

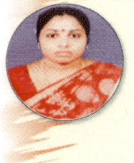

G Dhanalakshmi
RN, RM, MSc(N), MSc(Psy), MBA, PhD
Professor cum Vice Principal
Head of Department
Medical Surgical Nursing
Billroth College of Nursing
Chennai, Tamil Nadu

Jasinder Pal Kaur
RN, RM, MSc(N), CTVS
Professor cum Head of Department
Medical Surgical Nursing
Dasmesh College of Nursing
Faridkot, Punjab

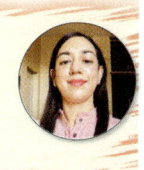

Reviewers' names are arranged in alphabetical order

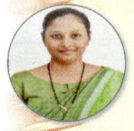

Manu Nagra
RN, RM, MSc(N), CTVS
Associate Professor
SPHE College of Nursing
Gharuan, Mohali, Punjab

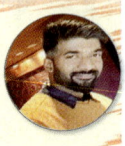

Sembian N
RN, RM, MSc(N), Ortho
Associate Professor
Nursing College
Uttar Pradesh University of Medical Sciences
Saifai, Etawah, Uttar Pradesh

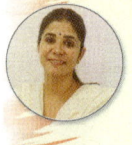

Simaranjit Kaur
RN, RM, MSc(N), CTVS
Associate Professor
College of Nursing
Adesh University
Bathinda, Punjab

Reviewers' names are arranged in alphabetical order

Preface

Pathophysiology is an essential topic for the nurses to understand. The essence of critical thinking is the ability of nurses to act according to their knowledge and understanding. Because of this reason, the nursing students as well as nurses should understand the pathophysiological changes that take place in any disease. This helps them to think critically and apply that knowledge while taking care of the patients. Considering the importance of learning and understanding the concepts related to pathophysiology, it is an honest effort to bring out a compact but an enriched content for making the nursing students well-versed with the changes that occur in various disease conditions.

Pathophysiology helps build a strong foundation of nursing practice enabling nurses to provide quality care. The book has been organized into 17 chapters divided in accordance with the curriculum given by Indian Nursing Council, parallel to the chapters of Medical Surgical Nursing. The content has been designed in an interesting manner with the help of illustrations, flowcharts and figures for a better understanding of pathophysiological concepts.

The motivation behind writing this book is my own interest in the pathophysiological concepts as I am specialized in Medical Surgical Nursing. Moreover, I have observed the students facing issues regarding an organized content related to pathophysiology and searching from multiple sources. I am pretty confident that not only the nursing students and nurses, but the undergraduate students of other medical disciplines will also be benefitted from the content presented in this book.

I sincerely thank the Almighty for His blessings and all near and dear ones for their constant support and motivation at the time of writing this book.

Kanika Rai

Acknowledgments

I am thankful to all the individuals who have helped me and put their time and efforts towards publication of this book.

I want to thank **Mr Satish Kumar Jain** (Chairman) and **Mr Varun Jain** (Managing Director), M/s CBS Publishers and Distributors Pvt Ltd for their immense support and guidance in the publication of this book. One more person who has acted like the backbone, as far as the publication of this book is concerned, is **Mr Bhupesh Aarora** [Sr. Vice President – Health Science Division (Publishing and Marketing)], without whom this book wouldn't have been what it is today.

I would also like to convey my special thanks to the entire team of CBS Publishers and Distributors for their extreme hard work at every stage. I extend my special thanks to Ms Nitasha Arora (Publishing Head & Content Strategist), and Dr Anju Dhir (Product Manager cum Commissioning Editor-Medical) for their editorial support. I would also extend my thanks to Mr Shivendu Bhushan Pandey (Sr. Manager & Team Lead), Mr Manoj K Yadav (Production Manager), Mr Ashutosh Pathak (Sr. Proofreader cum Team Coordinator) for putting their hard work and efforts to bring out this handbook on time.

Nursing Knowledge Tree

An Initiative by CBS Nursing Division

"Coming together is a beginning. Keeping together is progress. Working together is success."

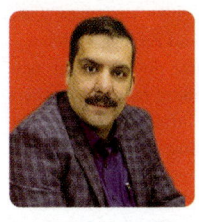

It gives us immense pleasure to share with you that the Nursing Knowledge Tree—An Initiative by CBS Nursing Division, has successfully established itself in the field of nursing as we have been able to stand as a strong contender by sharing approximately 50% of the market share. This growth could not have been possible without your invaluable contribution as our reader, author, reviewer, contributor and recommender, and your outstanding support for the growth of our titles as a whole. You people are the pillars of our series and we are so glad that you all have strengthened our basic foundation.

Nursing Knowledge Tree has been a pioneer and specialist in publishing best quality books for nursing education. Keeping in mind the changing trends in nursing education, we, at Nursing Knowledge Tree, have taken up a mission to bring student-friendly and syllabus-based books written by Subject Experts PAN India.

Our Noteworthy Achievements:

- Our nationally-acclaimed titles
  - *PGIMER NINE Clinical Nursing Procedures*—**Sandhya Ghai**
  - *Target High Staff Nurse Entrance Examination*—**Muthuvenkatachalam S, Ambili M Venugopal**
  - *CBS Nursing Drug Guide*—**Yogesh Gulati/Rakesh Sharma**
  - *Textbook of Nursing Foundations*—**Harindarjeet Goyal**
  - *Essentials of Biochemistry*—**Harbans Lal**
  - *Textbook of Nursing Education*—**Ratna Prakash**
  - *Nursing Research in 21st Century*—**Sukhpal Kaur and Amarjeet Singh**
  - *Essentials of Applied Microbiology*—**D R Arora and Brij Bala Arora**
  - *Textbook of Pediatric Nursing*—**Meharban Singh and Raman Kalia**
- Liaised with the topmost institutes of the country, like **AIIMS, NIMHANS, PGIMER NINE, CMC-Vellore, Manipal University, JIPMER, RAK-Delhi**, etc.
- Published **100+ Quality Nursing Books** and more than **50 New Books** on various subjects for Nursing Undergraduates, Postgraduates and Nursing superspecialty are under process and will be releasing in 2021.

- Increased our social presence by participating in more than **200+ National Conferences, CME's, College Exhibitions & Webinars** in previous years.
- We have come out with **Nursing Next Live**, an EdTech platform, the Next Level of Nursing Education, where we bring learning to people, instead of people going for learning. Through NNL App we are providing various study modules/plans covering All Subjects/All Topics, Video Lectures, Question Banks, E-notes and a Variety of Tests. Students can choose the plan as per their needs and requirements.
- We are excited to announce that we are coming out with our new initiative—**Nursing Next Live Social**, where nursing faculty members can share as well as gain knowledge, with the aim to revolutionize the way the nursing segment connects. It's going to be India's first networking platform for Nursing Segment.

Our Journey towards providing Quality Nursing Education is Incomplete without YOU ! Join Us Now !

We specialize in publishing nursing books of superior quality, going ahead we see us publishing more and more quality content and it will only be possible when intellectuals from across the nation come together. Keeping pace with the advancements, we want to strengthen the nursing sector, which was long neglected, and establish a strong foundation when it comes to quality content for the segment.

We are determined to bring about changes in the Nursing Education System and will do it for sure with your support and contribution. We will be delighted if you join hands with us as Author, Contributor or Reviewer and take the vision of quality education for nursing students ahead.

Let's join hands together and share our ideas and knowledge. Be the part of this Revolution. We are looking forward to your cooperation in future as well. Share your CVs at **bhupesharora@nursingnextlive.in** or scan the given QR code and fill the form or you can talk to me directly at +9555353330.

With Best Wishes!
Mr Bhupesh Aarora
Sr. Vice President – Health Science Division
(Publishing and Marketing)

Special Features of the Book

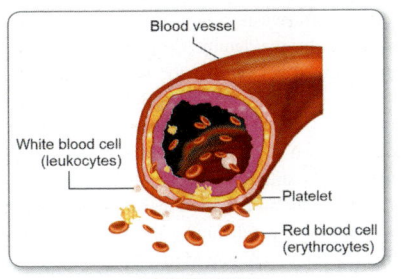

Fig. 1: Components of blood

Self-explanatory **images** included to enhance understanding of topic

Contains **flowcharts** to make the pathophysiological concepts more clear and easy to grasp

Flowchart

| Inflammatory lesions |
| Blood from aorta returns to left ventricle during diastole |
| Left ventricle dilates and thickens |
| Arteries attempt to compensate for higher pressures by reflex vasodilation |
| Peripheral arterioles relax, reducing peripheral resistance and diastolic blood pressure |

Table 1: Differences between rheumatoid arthritis and osteoarthritis

Parameter	Rheumatoid arthritis	Osteoarthritis
Age at onset	Young to middle age	Usually >40 years of age
Nodules	Present, especially on extensor surfaces	Heberden's (DIPs) and Bouchard's (PIPs) nodes

Useful **tables** are included from clinical and diagnosis Point of View

SARS CORONAVIRUS-2

A highly relevant topic on **SARS CORONAVIRUS-2** Pathophysiology has been included to keep the readers abreast of the various aspects of this deadly disease

The Severe Acute Respiratory Syndrome (SARS) coronavirus-2 is a novel coronavirus belonging to the family Coronaviridae. It is known to be responsible for the outbreak of a series of recent acute atypical respiratory infections originating in Wuhan, China. The disease caused by this virus, termed coronavirus disease 19 or simply COVID-19, rapidly spread throughout the world at an alarming pace and was declared a pandemic by the World Health Organization (WHO) on March 11, 2020. Let us discuss the pathophysiology of Covid-19 and its different stages.

Also Know

If the fibrous cap is **thick**, it can resist the stress from blood flow and vessel movement. If the fibrous cap is thin, lipid core may grow causing it to rupture and hemorrhage into plaque allowing a thrombus to form. This is called atherothrombosis.

Also Know boxes have been included in between the text to enhance the knowledge of the readers

Contents

Contents

Contents

Contents

SARS Coronavirus-2

The Severe Acute Respiratory Syndrome (SARS) Coronavirus-2 is a novel coronavirus belonging to the family Coronaviridae. It is known to be responsible for the outbreak of a series of recent acute atypical respiratory infections originating in Wuhan, China. The disease caused by this virus, termed coronavirus disease 19 or simply COVID-19, rapidly spread throughout the world at an alarming pace and was declared a pandemic by the World Health Organization (WHO) on March 11, 2020. Let us discuss the pathophysiology of Covid-19 and its different stages.

In the asymptomatic phase, SARS-CoV-2, received via respiratory aerosols, binds to the nasal epithelial cells in the upper respiratory tract. Local replication and propagation of virus occur in the conducting airways along with an infection of the ciliated cells. The duration of this stage is around two days with a limited immune response. The individuals tend to be highly infectious at this stage despite having a low viral load.

In the next stage, the virus migrates to the upper respiratory tract from the nasal epithelium through the conducting airways. With the involvement of upper airways, manifestations, like fever, dry cough and malaise appear. The immune response in this stage is very high involving the release of C-X-C motif chemokine ligand 10 (CXCL-10) and interferons (IFN-β and IFN-λ) from the cells infected by the virus. This mounted immune response is enough to contain the spread of infection.

About 1/5th of infected patients progress to the next stage in which there occurs an involvement of lower respiratory tract with an onset of acute respiratory distress syndrome (ARDS). The virus is able to invade the type-2 alveolar epithelial cells and starts replicating. The virus-laden pneumocytes start releasing different cytokines and inflammatory markers such as interleukins (IL-1, IL-6, IL-8, IL-120 and IL-12), tumor necrosis factor-α (TNF-α), IFN-λ and IFN-β, CXCL-10, monocyte chemoattractant protein-1 (MCP-1) and macrophage inflammatory protein-1α (MIP-1α). Owing to this cytokine storm, neutrophils, CD4 helper T cells and CD8 cytotoxic T cells begin to get sequestered in the lung tissues, leading to inflammation and injury to lung tissues. The persistent injury caused by the sequestered inflammatory cells and viral replication lead to loss of both types 1 and 2 pneumocytis. This diffuses alveolar damage ultimately culminated into ARDS.

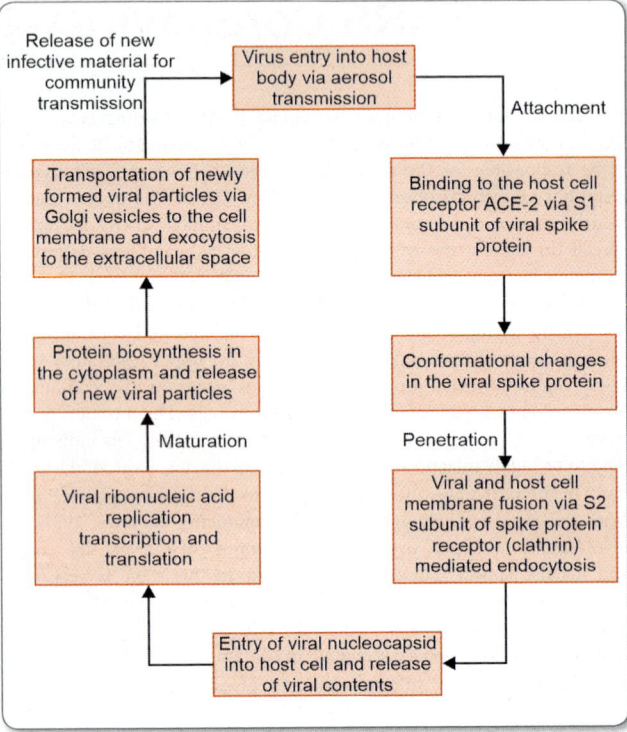

Fig. 1: The severe acute respiratory syndrome coronavirus-2 life cycle

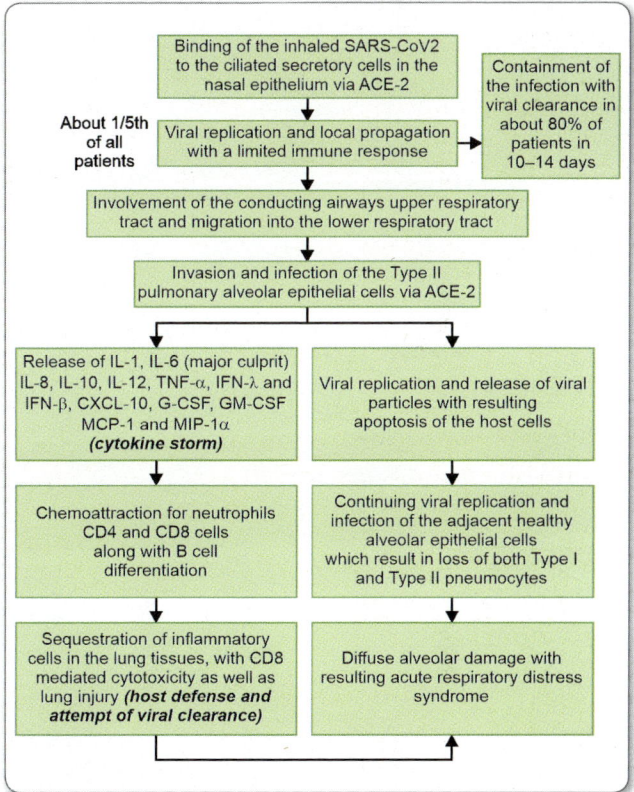

Fig. 2: Pathophysiology of COVID-19

Abbreviations: CXCL-10, C-X-C motif chemokine ligand 10; G-CSF, granulocyte colony-stimulating factor; GM-CSF, granulocyte-macrophage colony-stimulating factor; IFN, interferon; IL, interleukin; MCP-1, monocyte chemoattractant protein-1; MIP-1α, macrophage inflammatory protein-1α; SARS-CoV-2, severe acute respiratory syndrome coronavirus-2; TNF-α, tumor necrosis factor-α

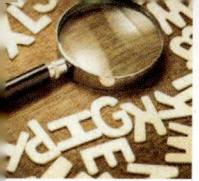

Glossary

- **Abscess:** Painful collection of pus caused by bacterial infection.
- **Alkalosis:** Excessive blood alkalinity caused by overabundance of bicarbonates in blood or loss of acids from blood.
- **Anaerobic:** Living, occurring or existing in the absence of free oxygen.
- **Anastomosis:** Surgical connection between two structures.
- **Androgen:** Steroid hormone that stimulates male characteristics (The two main androgens are androsterone and testosterone).
- **Anemia:** Reduction in the number and volume of red blood cells and the amount of hemoglobin.
- **Aneurysm:** Sac formed by the dilation of the wall of an artery, a vein, or the heart.
- **Angiogenesis:** Formation of new blood vessels.
- **Angiography:** Radiographic visualization of blood vessels after injection of radiopaque contrast material.
- **Antigen:** Foreign substances such as bacteria or toxins that induce antibody formation.
- **Apoptosis:** Process of programmed cell death.
- **Atrophy:** Decrease in size of a cell, tissue, organ, or body part.
- **Autoimmune:** Disease that is caused by substances that usually prevent illness.
- **Autosome:** Any chromosome other than the sex chromosomes.
- **Benign:** Not malignant or recurrent; favorable for recovery.
- **Biopsy:** Process of removing tissue from living patients for diagnostic examination.
- **Bone marrow:** Soft organic material filling the cavities of bones.
- **Bursa:** Fluid-filled sac or cavity found in connecting tissue in the vicinity of joints; acts as a cushion.
- **Calcification:** Process of calcium build-up in the body tissue causing it to harden.

- **Calculus:** Any abnormal concentration, usually made up of mineral salts, within the body; for example, gallstones and renal calculi.
- **Carcinogen:** Substance that causes cancer.
- **Carcinogenesis:** The origin, production, or development of cancer.
- **Carcinoma:** Malignant growth of epithelial cells that tend to infiltrate the surrounding tissues and metastasize.
- **Cell:** Smallest living component of an organism; the body's basic building block.
- **Chymotrypsin:** Digestive enzyme that breaks down protein in small intestine (Duodenum).
- **Collateral:** A subordinate or accessory part.
- **Colonization:** Presence of bacteria on a body surface.
- **Convalescent:** Period of recovery from serious illness or surgery.
- **Cortisol:** Steroid hormone.
- **Cytokines:** Cell signalling molecules.
- **Cytoplasm:** Aqueous mass within a cell that contains organelles, is surrounded by the cell membrane, and excludes the nucleus.
- **Demyelination:** Destruction of a nerve's myelin sheath, which interferes with normal nerve conduction.
- **Deoxyribonucleic acid (DNA):** Complex protein in the cell's nucleus that carries genetic material and is responsible for cellular reproduction.
- **Diastolic:** Pressure of blood during relaxation of heart.
- **Disease:** Pathologic condition that occurs when the body cannot maintain homeostasis.
- **Diuresis:** Condition in which too much filtration of body fluids is done by the kidneys.
- **Dysplasia:** Abnormal development of tissue.
- **Effusion:** An outpouring of fluid.
- **Embolism:** Sudden obstruction of a blood vessel by foreign substances or a blood clot.
- **Empyema:** Collection of pus in the pleural space.
- **Encephalopathy:** Damage or disease affecting the brain.
- **Endocrine:** Pertaining to internal hormone secretion by glands (Endocrine glands, including the pineal gland, the islets of Langerhans in the pancreas, the gonads, the thymus, and the adrenal, pituitary, thyroid, and parathyroid glands that secrete hormones directly into circulation).
- **Endogenous:** Occurring inside the body.
- **Engorgement:** State of a body part that becomes swollen or filled with fluid.

- **Erythropoiesis:** Production of red blood cells or erythrocytes.
- **Eventration:** Protrusion of contents of abdomen through a defect or weakness in the abdominal wall.
- **Exacerbation:** Increase in the severity of a disease or any of its symptoms.
- **Exocrine:** External or outward secretion of a gland (Exocrine glands discharge through ducts opening on an external or internal surface of the body; they include the liver, the pancreas, the prostate, and the salivary, sebaceous, sweat, gastric, intestinal, mammary, and lacrimal glands).
- **Exogenous:** Occurring outside the body.
- **Exudation:** Process of fluid emission by an organism through pores or wound.
- **Fibrinolysis:** Breakdown of fibrin by the enzymes in the blood clots.
- **Fibrotic:** Thickening and scarring of tissue.
- **Fissures:** Long, deep crack in the lining of body organs.
- **Fistulas:** Abnormal connection between two body parts.
- **Gangrene:** Death of body tissue caused by lack of blood flow or serious bacterial infection.
- **Glucagon:** Hormone released during the fasting state that increases blood glucose concentration.
- **Hartmann's pouch:** Diverticulum occurring at the neck of gall bladder.
- **Homeostasis:** Dynamic, steady state of internal balance in the body.
- **Hyperemia:** An excess of blood in the vessels supplying an organ or other body part.
- **Hyperplasia:** Excessive growth of normal cells that cause an increase in the volume of a tissue or organ.
- **Hypoxia:** Reduction of oxygen in body tissues below normal levels.
- **Immunocompetence:** Ability of cells to distinguish antigens from substances that belong to the body and to launch an immune response.
- **Incubation:** Process of keeping something in the right condition at right temperature so that it can develop.
- **Insufficiency:** Inability of organ to perform its normal function.
- **Insulin:** Hormone secreted into the blood by the islets of Langerhans located in the pancreas; promotes the storage of glucose, among other functions.

- **Lesion:** Damage caused to the part of body tissue due to an injury or illness.
- **Lymphoma:** Cancer of lymphatic system.
- **Malabsorption:** Insufficient intestinal absorption of nutrients.
- **Malignant:** Condition that becomes progressively worse and results in death.
- **Megakaryocytes:** Cells in the bone marrow making platelets.
- **Meiosis:** Process of cell division by which gametes (egg or sperm) are formed.
- **Metaplasia:** Process of cell replacement.
- **Metastasis:** Transfer of malignant cells via pathogenic microorganisms or vascular system from one organ or body part to another not directly connected with it.
- **Mitosis:** Ordinary process of cell division in which each chromosome with all its genes reproduces itself exactly.
- **Mucosa:** Moist, inner lining of body organs and cavities.
- **Mutation:** Change in the sequence of DNA.
- **Myelin:** A lipid-like substance surrounding the axon of myelinated nerve fibers that permits normal neurologic conduction.
- **Myelitis:** Inflammation of the spinal cord or bone marrow.
- **Myeloma:** Cancer that forms in the white blood cell.
- **Myosin:** Fibrous protein which forms the contractile filaments of muscle cells.
- **Necrosis:** Cell or tissue death.
- **Neoplasm:** Abnormal growth in which cell replication is uncontrolled and progressive.
- **Neuritic plaques:** Areas of nerve inflammation; found on autopsy examination of the brain tissue of people with Alzheimer's disease.
- **Neuron:** Highly specialized conductor cell that receives and transmits electrochemical nerve impulses.
- **Nutrient:** Substance used by an organism for growth, survival and reproduction.
- **Occlusion:** Closure or blockage of any body organ or blood vessel.
- **Omphalocele:** Birth defect of the abdominal wall.
- **Oncotic Pressure:** Pressure induced by albumin on plasma in blood vessels that displaces the water molecules.
- **Organelle:** Structure of a cell found in the cytoplasm that performs a specific function; for example, the nucleus, mitochondria, and lysosomes.
- **Osmolality:** Concentration of a solution expressed in terms of osmoles of solute per kilogram of solvent.

- **Osmoreceptors:** Specialized neurons located in the thalamus that are stimulated by increased extracellular fluid osmolality to cause release of antidiuretic hormone, thereby helping to control fluid balance.
- **Osteoblasts:** Bone-forming cells whose activity results in bone formation.
- **Osteoclasts:** Giant, multinuclear cells that reabsorb material from previously formed bones, tear down old or excess bone structure, and allow osteoblasts to rebuild new bone.
- **Paroxysm:** A sudden recurrence or attack of a disease.
- **Pepsin:** Stomach enzyme that breaks down proteins into smaller peptides.
- **Perforation:** Hole that develops through the wall of a body organ
- **Perfusion:** Passage of blood through the blood vessels or other channels.
- **Peripheral Resistance:** Resistance of arteries to the flow of blood.
- **Peristalsis:** Intestinal contractions, or waves, that propel food toward the stomach and into and through the intestine.
- **Phagocyte:** Cell that ingests microorganisms, other cells, and foreign particles.
- **Phagocytosis:** Engulfing of microorganisms, other cells, and foreign particles by a phagocyte.
- **Plaque:** A deposit of fat, cholesterol, calcium or waste product that builds up in the arteries.
- **Plasma:** Liquid part of the blood that carries antibodies and nutrients to tissues and carries away wastes from tissues.
- **Pneumonitis:** Inflammation of lung tissue.
- **Pneumothorax:** Collapsed lung.
- **Prodromal:** Period between initial appearance of symptoms till the full development of fever.
- **Prolapse:** Displacement of part or organ of the body from its normal position resulting in its protrusion from the orifice.
- **Proliferation:** Growth by rapid production of new parts.
- **Proximal:** Nearest to.
- **Pulmonary alveoli:** Grapelike clusters found at the ends of the respiratory passages in the lungs; sites for the exchange of carbon dioxide and oxygen.
- **Pulsus paradoxus:** Pulse marked by a drop in systolic blood pressure greater than 10 mm Hg during inspiration.
- **Pyrosis:** Heartburn.
- **Regurgitation:** Backflow of swallowed food to the mouth.

- **Renin:** Enzyme produced by the kidneys in response to an actual or perceived decline in extracellular fluid volume; an important part of blood pressure regulation.
- **Replication:** Biological process of producing two identical replicas of DNA from one original molecule of DNA.
- **Sarcoma:** Connective tissue neoplasm formed by proliferation of mesodermal cells.
- **Scarring:** Process of repairing of wound.
- **Sepsis:** Pathologic state resulting from microorganisms or their poisonous products in the bloodstream.
- **Sigmoidoscopy:** Inspection of the rectum and sigmoid colon through a sigmoidoscope.
- **Stasis:** Stagnation of the normal flow of fluids, such as blood and urine, or within the intestinal mechanism.
- **Stenosis:** Constriction or narrowing of a passage or orifice.
- **Stomatitis:** Inflammation of the mucous membrane of the mouth
- **Stricture:** Narrowing of urethra.
- **Subacute:** A condition between acute and chronic.
- **Surfactant:** Lipid-type substance that coats the alveoli, allowing them to expand uniformly during inspiration and preventing them from collapsing during expiration.
- **Synovial fluid:** Viscous, lubricating substance secreted by the synovial membrane, which lines the cavity between the bones of free moving joints.
- **Synovitis:** Inflammation of the synovial membrane.
- **Systemic:** Affecting or connected with the whole of something.
- **Systolic:** Pressure of blood during contraction of heart.
- **Tendon:** Fibrous cord of connective tissue that attaches the muscle to bone or cartilage and enables bones to move when skeletal muscles contract.
- **Thalassemia:** An inherited blood disorder causing body to have less hemoglobin than normal.
- **Tissue:** Large group of individual cells that perform a certain function.
- **Translocation:** Change in location of chromosomes.
- **Trypsin:** Digestive enzyme that breaks down protein.
- **Tubules:** Small tubes in the kidney; minute, reabsorptive canals that secrete, collect, and conduct urine.
- **Uremia:** Abnormally high level of waste products in the blood.
- **Vasospasm:** Narrowing of arteries that is caused by persistent contraction of blood vessels.

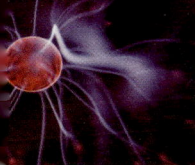

Basics of Pathophysiology

CELL

Cells are the basic structural units of all living things. There are different cells that function for sustaining a life. Homeostasis is considered to be one of the hallmarks of all living beings and the cells have the ability to maintain this function. **Homeostasis** is the ability to maintain a relatively stable internal state that persists despite changes in the world outside. The various types of cells are shown in Figure 1.

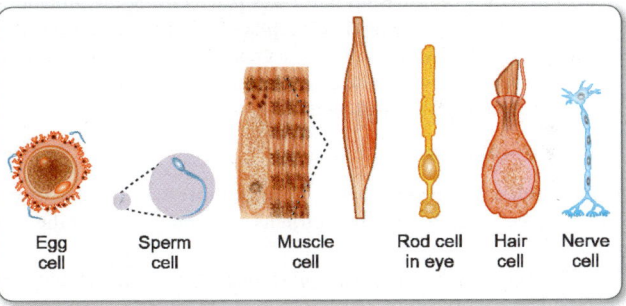

Fig. 1: Types of cells

On the other hand, the tissue is a group of cells that perform specific functions and include muscles, bones and blood. Two or more than two types of tissues form an organ like heart, liver, brain, etc. These organs further are integrated into the systems like cardiovascular, gastrointestinal, central nervous system, etc.

Components of Cell

There are three main basic components of every cell including:

1. **Cell membrane** that surrounds and protects the cell.
2. **Cytoplasm**, a watery substance containing ions, proteins and organelles.

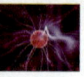

3. **Organelles**, responsible for carrying out certain activities for the growth and reproduction of cells.

Organelles further include endoplasmic reticulum, Golgi apparatus, lysosomes and mitochondria:

- Endoplasmic reticulum provides mechanical support and synthesizes protein.
- Golgi complex synthesizes phospholipids and produces lysosomes.
- Lysosomes cause destruction of damaged cells and digestion of phagocytosed material.
- Mitochondria is responsible for production of adenosine triphosphate (ATP).

Cell Division

The division of cells is a means of reproduction in the unicellular organisms whereas it is required for growth and maintenance of tissues in case of multicellular organisms.

Mitosis is a cell division that takes place during the growth of animals and helps the tissues to get replaced or repaired. A single cell divides into two cells, which are exact copy of each other and have same number of chromosomes. In meiosis, division of a single cell occurs into four cells having half number of chromosomes.

Cell Cycle—Mitosis

Before a cell starts dividing, it is in the **interphase**, which is the period when the cell is gathering the nutrients and energy to start the cell cycle.

The phases of the cell division through mitosis are depicted in Figures 2 and 3.

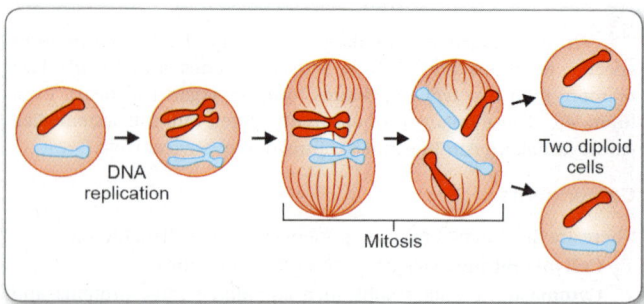

Fig. 2: Mitosis

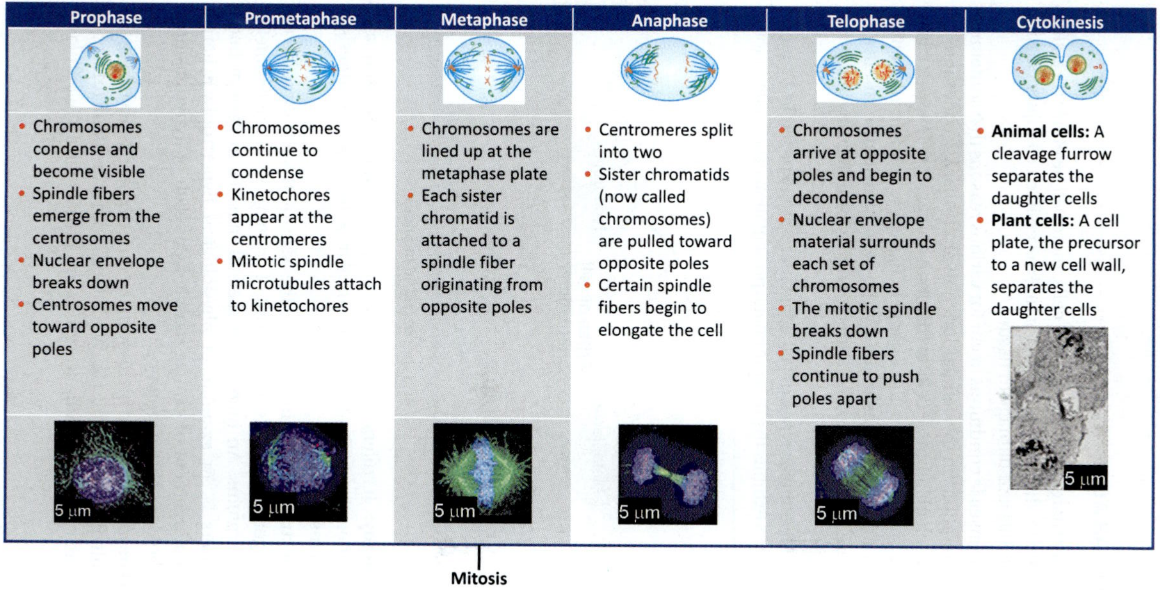

Prophase	Prometaphase	Metaphase	Anaphase	Telophase	Cytokinesis
• Chromosomes condense and become visible • Spindle fibers emerge from the centrosomes • Nuclear envelope breaks down • Centrosomes move toward opposite poles	• Chromosomes continue to condense • Kinetochores appear at the centromeres • Mitotic spindle microtubules attach to kinetochores	• Chromosomes are lined up at the metaphase plate • Each sister chromatid is attached to a spindle fiber originating from opposite poles	• Centromeres split into two • Sister chromatids (now called chromosomes) are pulled toward opposite poles • Certain spindle fibers begin to elongate the cell	• Chromosomes arrive at opposite poles and begin to decondense • Nuclear envelope material surrounds each set of chromosomes • The mitotic spindle breaks down • Spindle fibers continue to push poles apart	• **Animal cells:** A cleavage furrow separates the daughter cells • **Plant cells:** A cell plate, the precursor to a new cell wall, separates the daughter cells

Mitosis

Fig. 3: Phases of mitosis

CELLULAR ADAPTATION

Whenever there is an injury to the cells, there will be either reversible cell injury leading to adaptation or an irreversible cell injury causing death of cells and damage to tissues.

The disease conditions occur for various reasons that sometimes cause alterations in the cellular function or the disease condition can be the result of failure of cells to maintain homeostasis. In such cases, the cells must adapt to the changes. Basically, cellular adaptation refers to all the changes made by the cells in response to adverse environmental changes. The adaptation may be either physiologic or pathologic.

The five major types of cell adaptations are depicted in Figures 4 and Figure 5 exhibits the diagrammatic presentation of cell adaptations.

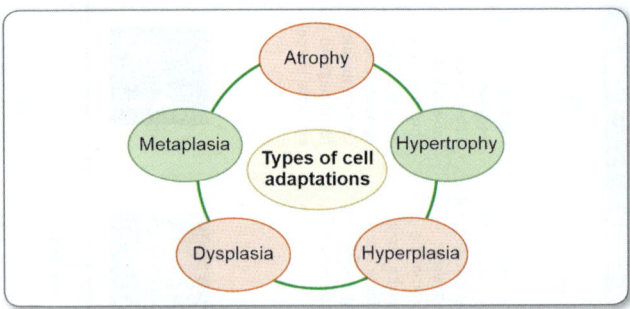

Fig. 4: Types of cell adaptations

1. **Atrophy:** It refers to decrease in size of the cells and also degeneration of tissues that is caused by a decrease in synthesis of proteins.

2. **Hypertrophy:** An increase in the size of tissues through the enlargement of cells is the result of an increase in the organelles and proteins. An increase in skeletal muscles in case of body-builders is an example of physiological hypertrophy whereas an enlargement of cardiac muscle as a result of hypertension is pathological hypertrophy.

3. **Hyperplasia:** It is an increase in the number of cells occurring as a result of increased mitosis. When there is an increase in functional capacity as required, it results in physiological hyperplasia.

Pathologic hyperplasia is the result of an excessive stimulation of hormones or growth factors.

4. **Dysplasia:** A disordered growth of epithelium leads to dysplasia. It is not considered to be true adaptation and is related to hyperplasia.

5. **Metaplasia:** It is a reversible change in which one cell type is replaced by another. For example, in case of chronic smokers, ciliated columnar epithelium lining the trachea and bronchi is transformed into stratified squamous epithelial cells.

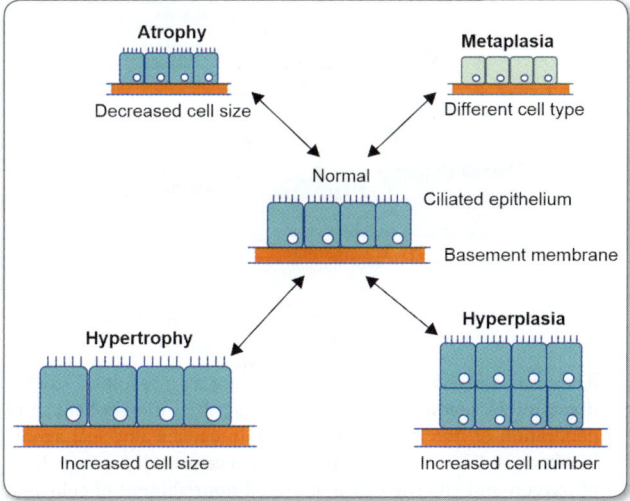

Fig. 5: Diagrammatic representation of different types of cell adaptations

Types of Cell Injury

Damage to the cells results from changes in either internal or external environments, and this damage can be reversible or irreversible. Homeostasis is restored based upon the extent of injury or damage. Hypoxia is known to be the most common cause of cell injury. Reversible cell injury leads to adaptation whereas irreversible injury causes death of cells.

Two broad categories of cell injury involve the acquired and genetic causes.

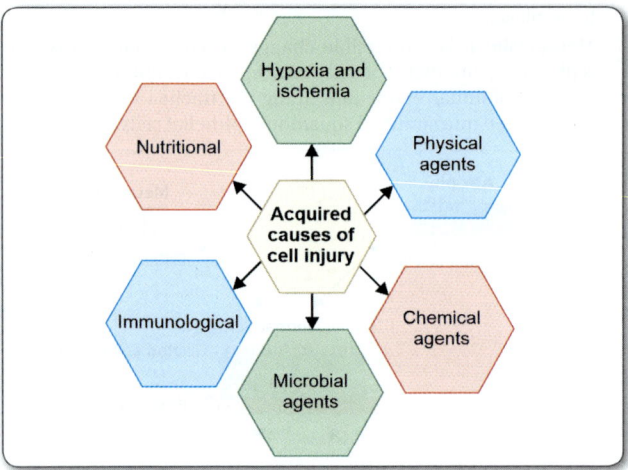

Fig. 6: Acquired causes of cell injury

- **Acquired causes:** Hypoxia and ischemia as a result of oxygen deprivation leading to failure of aerobic metabolism and generation of free radicals are the main causes. Physical agents like heat, radiation or direct trauma also cause cell damage. Lack of oxygen and glucose cause impaired nourishment of cells that results in cell injury (Fig. 6).
- **Genetic causes:** About 50% of total mortality in infancy and childhood in Western countries and 95% of that in developing countries are contributed by genetic defects. Examples include Down's syndrome and sickle cell anemia.

REPAIR OF CELLS

The body tries to repair or replace the cells in case of a cellular injury so as to continue the normal functions. In case of cell death, it is removed and replaced so as to provide structural support to the remaining cells through the attachment with connective tissues.

Normal cells try to regenerate the damaged cells, which is not always possible, so the purpose of repair process is to fill the gap caused by the damaged cells so as to maintain structural continuity.

HOMEOSTASIS

Homeostasis refers to the ability of body to regulate its internal environment in response to changes or fluctuations in the internal or external environment. The brain, kidneys, liver and pancreas are involved in maintaining homeostasis.

The regulation of body temperature, heart rate, blood pressure, and circadian rhythms is done by the hypothalamus. The kidneys regulate the blood-water level, reabsorption of substances in blood, maintenance of electrolyte levels, regulation of pH, and removal of toxic products. The metabolization of toxic substances and maintenance of carbohydrate and lipid metabolism is done by the liver.

Homeostasis can be influenced by internal (intrinsic) or external (environmental) conditions. A receptor or sensor, integrating center and effector are the basic components of every homeostatic response. Positive and negative feedback mechanisms enable these three components to maintain homeostasis (Figs 7 to 9).

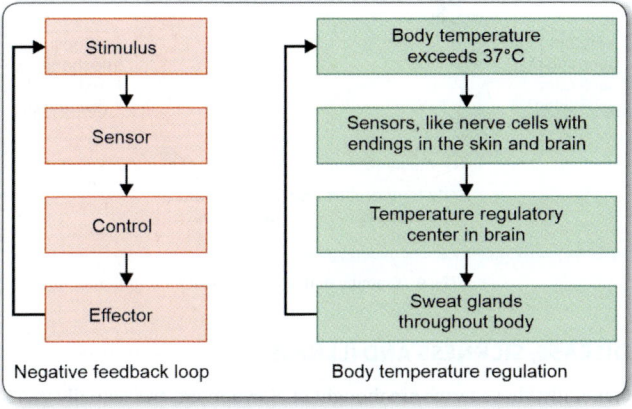

Fig. 7: Maintenance of homeostasis

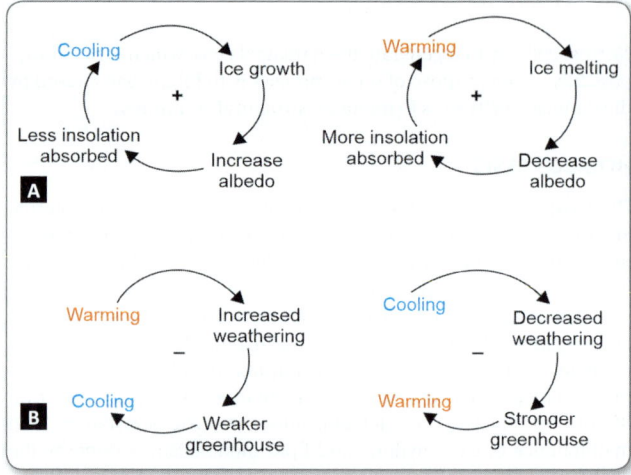

Figs 8A and B: A. Positive feedback mechanism; **B.** Negative feedback mechanism

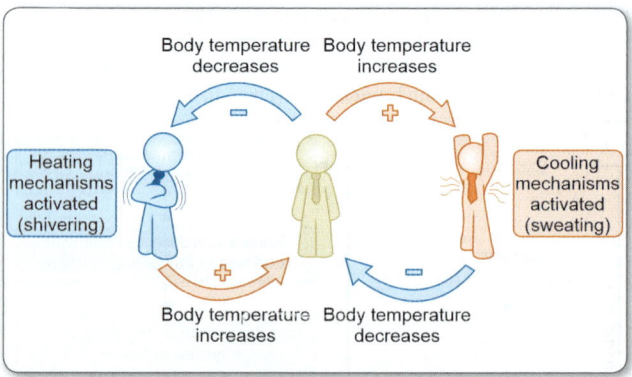

Fig. 9: Example of negative feedback

DISEASE, SICKNESS AND ILLNESS

Generally, these terms are thought of as synonyms but actually there is a difference between these. Diseases are to be cured while illness can be managed. Sickness is a reaction the patient shows when acquires a disease condition. The patient's experience can be well described through these three terms (Fig. 10).

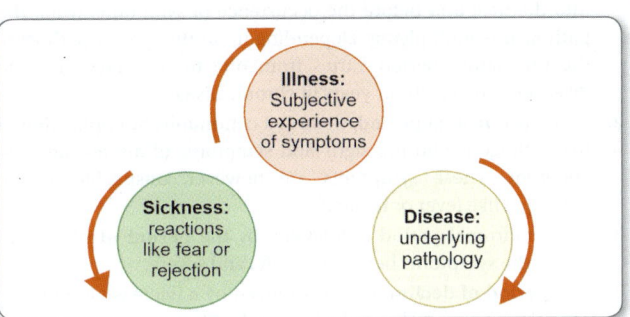

Fig. 10: Disease, illness and sickness

PATHOPHYSIOLOGY AND DISEASE

Pathophysiology, the concurrence of pathology and physiology, is the study of deranged physiological processes that are associated with a disease condition or an injury. Pathology describes the abnormal condition or state whereas pathophysiology explains about the changes in functions that take place in an individual as a result of disease or pathologic condition.

Phases of Diseases

Diseases progress through five stages as: (1) incubation period, (2) prodromal phase, (3) period of illness, (4) period of decline and (5) period of convalescence (Fig. 11).

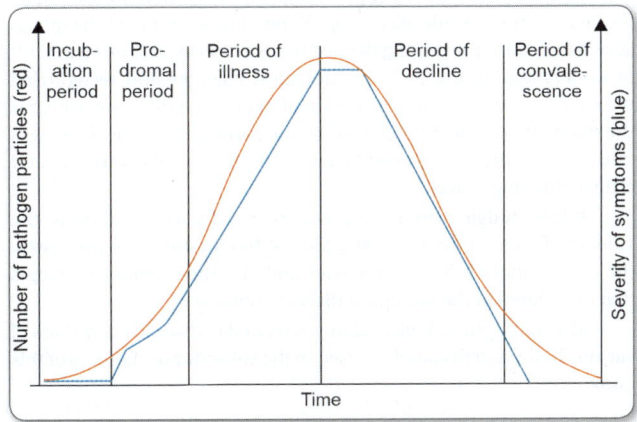

Fig. 11: Phases of disease

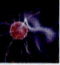

1. The **incubation period** occurs after an initial entry of pathogen into the host and before the occurrence of symptoms when the pathogen is multiplying. Depending upon the type of pathogen, the incubation period varies from one to two days in acute diseases and months or years in chronic diseases.

2. In the **prodromal period**, there is a continuous multiplication of the pathogens and the signs and symptoms of disease become apparent. These symptoms are however, unspecific to the pathogen like fever or headache.

3. The prodromal period is followed by the **period of illness**, in which the symptoms become specific and severe.

4. The **period of decline** is characterized by a decrease in number of pathogens and also a decline in the signs and symptoms of disease. As the immune system is weakened by the primary infection, the patients become susceptible to the development of secondary infections in the decline phase.

5. The last phase is known as **convalescent period** where recovery takes place. The patient generally returns to the normal level of functioning, however, in some cases where a permanent damage occurs, there will not be a full repairing of tissues.

IMPORTANCE OF PATHOPHYSIOLOGY IN NURSING

As discussed, the study of physical and biological disturbances that occur in the body as a result of the disease is termed as pathophysiology. Pathophysiology serves as the basis of nursing practice, as it helps in forming a strong foundation for the major nursing roles and responsibilities like opting for diagnostic examination, managing the acute and chronic illnesses, taking care of patient's health in general and also preventing the occurrence of disease. The end result of understanding the pathophysiological changes and recognizing the signs and symptoms is provision of quality nursing care, which is the main aim of nursing. For putting the pathophysiological changes into practice, the nurses need to have a strong clinical knowledge and critical thinking as well.

While studying the pathophysiology of disease conditions, the students focus on the understanding of biophysiological processes, the disturbances in these processes and also the scientific concepts that are related to the biology of disease conditions.

The pathophysiological changes related to disease conditions of various body systems are discussed in the subsequent chapters of this book.

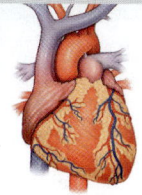

Pathophysiology of Cardiovascular Disorders

INTRODUCTION

The Cardiovascular System performs the main function of supplying the oxygenated blood to the cells and tissues for meeting their demand for oxygen as well as nutrient supply. Whenever, there is an increased demand for oxygen by the cells as in case of exercise, the blood vessels expand to about five times of their actual size to supply blood to the heart so that it is able to meet that demand. But in case, there is an obstruction in the flow of blood through the coronary artery caused by fatty deposits or plaque, imbalance between supply and demand of oxygen occurs, resulting in the increase of the workload of the heart.

The coronary arteries are mainly responsible for supplying oxygenated blood to the heart for maintaining its function. And, whenever any problem occurs in the coronary arteries, there will be an onset of a series of pathophysiological changes starting from deficiency of oxygen supply to ultimately necrosis of myocardial fibers and then failure of heart.

Let us now review one by one; what all changes take place in the major disease conditions of heart that are interrelated.

Firstly, let's talk about the disease of coronary arteries. There can be so many risk factors for the development of heart diseases and these can be categorized as modifiable and non-modifiable risk factors.

- **Modifiable risk factors**: High blood pressure, high blood cholesterol, smoking, obesity, physical inactivity, diabetes mellitus and stress.
- **Non-modifiable risk factors:** Age, gender and heredity.

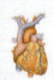

CORONARY ARTERY DISEASE

Pathophysiological Changes

Fats, lipids are deposited in intima of arterial wall

↓

Activation of inflammatory response

↓

T-lymphocytes and monocytes infilterate the area to ingest lipids and then die

↓

Proliferation of smooth muscle cells within the vessel forming a fibrous cap over dead fatty core

↓

Formation of deposits called atheromas or plaque

↓

Protrusion of plaque into lumen of vessels

↓

Narrowing of lumen

↓

Obstruction in blood flow

↓

Leading to damage to an area of the heart

Also Know

If the fibrous cap is **thick**, it can resist the stress from blood flow and vessel movement. If the fibrous cap is thin, lipid core may grow causing it to rupture and hemorrhage into plaque allowing a thrombus to form. This is called atherothrombosis.

To summarize, coronary artery disease is caused by the deposition of cholesterol or plaques in the interior lining of the artery (Fig. 1). The deposition of these compounds causes thickening of the layer of the artery and eventually narrowing the arterial lumen decreasing the flow of blood to the heart. Whenever, an injury occurs to the endothelial layer of the coronary artery, a large number of LDLs start penetrating that area and initiate the chain of inflammatory process. The process of oxidation starts, and large number of leukocytes or macrophages are attracted to the area of damage. These cells start to engulf the lipoproteins forming a complex on the site known as fatty streak.

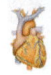

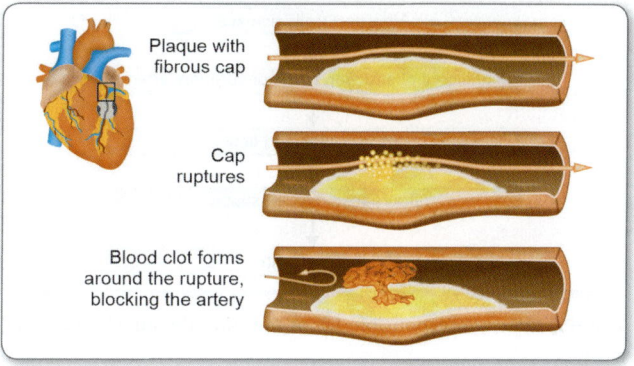

Fig. 1: Blood clot formation blocking the artery

After the formation of fatty streak, smooth muscle cells migrate to the area, multiply and produce an extracellular matrix. With the formation of this extracellular matrix, the fatty streak is converted into an atheromatous plaque. This lesion starts protruding towards the inner lining of the blood vessel causing a significant narrowing of the lumen, leading to decrease in amount of oxygenated blood being supplied to the heart.

ANGINA PECTORIS

Angina pectoris, commonly known as chest pain, is mainly the result of ischemia caused to the myocardium, which is caused by an imbalance between the supply and demand of oxygen to the myocardial cells. In the absence of sufficient amount of oxygen, the cells switch to anaerobic metabolism from the aerobic one. Angina pectoris is presented as the main manifestation of myocardial ischemia (Fig. 2). The pathophysiological changes are depicted in the flowchart as follows:

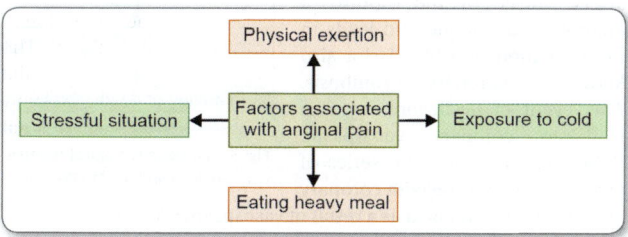

Fig. 2: Factors associated with typical anginal pain

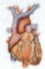

Pathophysiological Changes

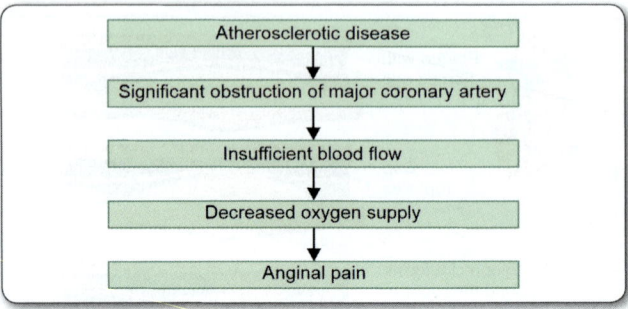

These factors are responsible for aggravating the attack of anginal pain.

- **Physical exertion:** Precipitates an attack by increasing myocardial oxygen demand.
- **Exposure to cold:** Causes vasoconstriction and elevate blood pressure with increased oxygen demand.
- **Eating heavy meal:** Increases blood flow to mesenteric area for digestion, thereby reducing blood supply available to heart muscle.
- **Stress** or any **emotion provoking** situation: Release of adrenaline and increasing blood pressure, which may accelerate heart rate and myocardial workload.

MYOCARDIAL INFARCTION

Myocardial infarction (heart attack) is the result of irreversible damage to the myocardial tissues caused by prolonged level of ischemia and hypoxia. It commonly results when there is an occlusion of coronary artery caused by the rupture of atheromatous plaque and leads to the formation of a blood clot also known as coronary thrombosis. This event of occlusion can also lead to coronary vasospasm. Below, you can find the series of changes, one starting with coronary atherosclerosis and next as a result of vasospasm (Fig. 3).

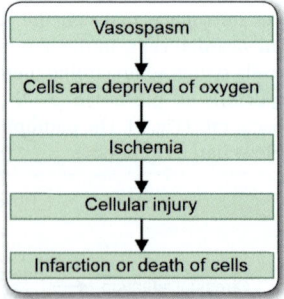

Fig. 3: Pathophysiological changes in myocardial infarction

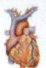

Pathophysiological Changes

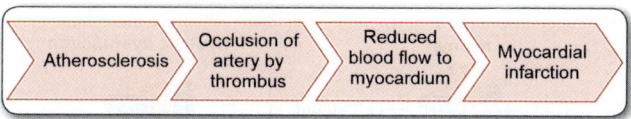

Atherosclerosis › Occlusion of artery by thrombus › Reduced blood flow to myocardium › Myocardial infarction

HEART FAILURE

Heart failure develops when the heart is not able to pump the required amount of blood to the tissues for ensuring that the metabolic demands are met or when the heart is only able to pump the blood with some compensating mechanisms. The dysfunction of myocardium can be defined as systolic or diastolic; left or right sided heart failure. Depending upon the duration of heart failure, several counter regulatory mechanisms are activated. Activation of sympathetic nervous system and Renin-angiotensin mechanism attempt to restore both cardiac output and tissue perfusion leading to exacerbation of the damage.

When an adequate stroke volume cannot be ejected from the left ventricle, whole pressure gets shifted to right side, causing systolic dysfunction. As a result, the heart is not filled with blood properly. Adequate filling cannot be maintained owing to diastolic stiffness, which then increases the diastolic pressure-volume causing diastolic heart failure (Fig. 4). The most dominant type of heart failure occurs in the left side but right side can also lead to serious consequences. All these types are explained here one by one with the help of flowcharts showing the series of changes.

Two types of heart failure:

1. Left-sided heart failure

    There are two types of left-sided heart failure

    (i)   Systolic dysfunction

    (ii) Diastolic dysfunction

2. Right-sided heart failure

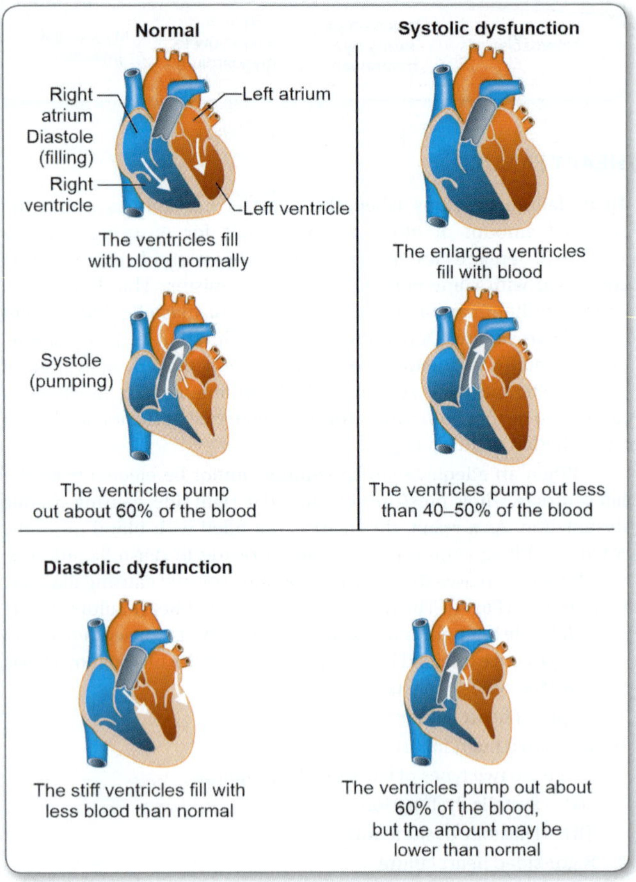

Normal

Right atrium
Diastole (filling)
Right ventricle
Left atrium
Left ventricle

The ventricles fill with blood normally

Systole (pumping)

The ventricles pump out about 60% of the blood

Systolic dysfunction

The enlarged ventricles fill with blood

The ventricles pump out less than 40–50% of the blood

Diastolic dysfunction

The stiff ventricles fill with less blood than normal

The ventricles pump out about 60% of the blood, but the amount may be lower than normal

Fig. 4: Comparison between normal, systolic dysfunction and diastolic dysfunction

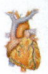

Pathophysiological Changes in Systolic Heart Failure

Atherosclerotic disease (CAD)

↓

Damage to heart muscle cells and tissues

↓

Causes loss of beta-adrenergic receptor sites

↓

Stimulates sympathetic nervous system (SNS) to release epinephrine and norepinephrine

↓

Sympathetic stimulation and decrease in renal perfusion by failing heart causes release of renin by kidney

↓

Renin promotes formation of angiotensin I

↓

Conversion of angiotensin I to II in the presence of angiotensin converting enzyme (ACE)

↓

Causes release of aldosterone

↓

Sodium and fluid retention and stimulation of thirst center

↓

Exacerbation of myocardial fibrosis

↓

Increases stress on ventricular wall

↓

Increases the workload of heart

↓

Contractility of myocardial fibers decreases with an increase in heart's workload

↓

Decrease in amount of blood ejected from ventricle

↓

Systolic heart failure

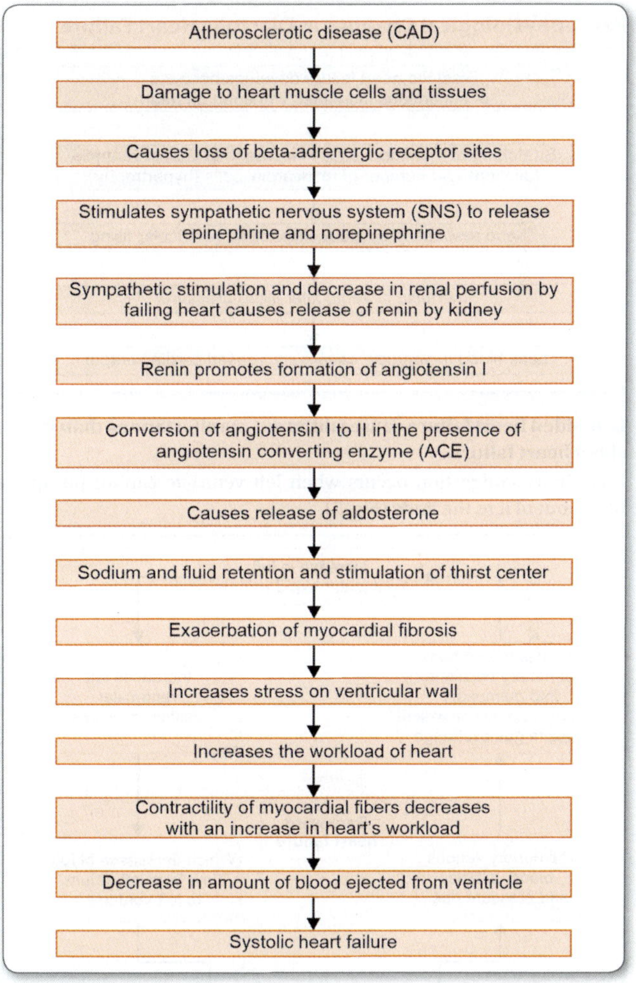

Abbreviation: CAD, coronary artery disease

Pathophysiological Changes in Diastolic Heart Failure

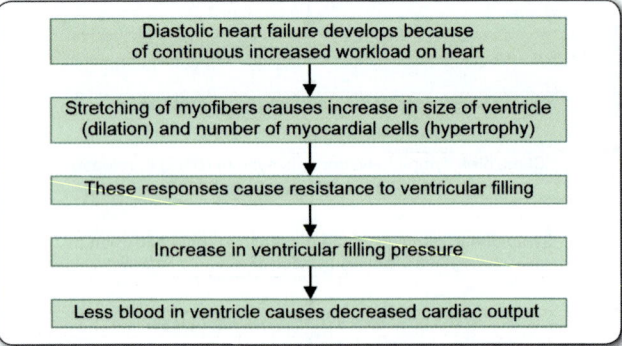

Left-sided heart failure causes different manifestations than right-sided heart failure.

Pulmonary congestion occurs when left ventricle cannot pump its blood out of it to the body (Fig. 5).

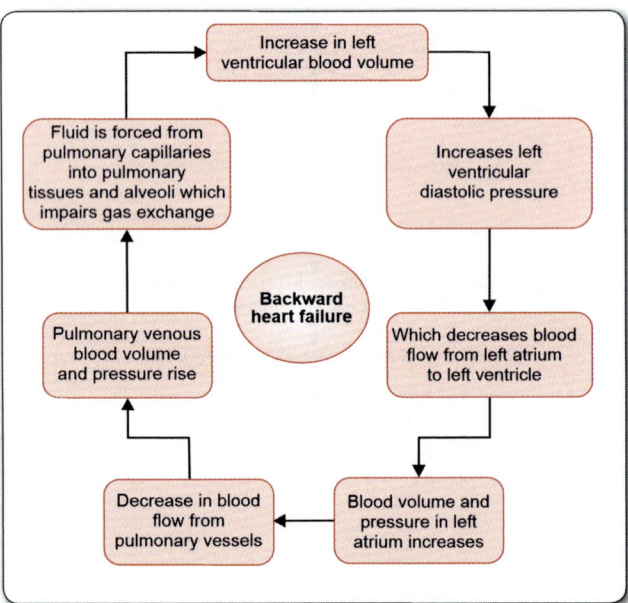

Fig. 5: Backward heart failure

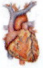
Failure of Right Ventricle

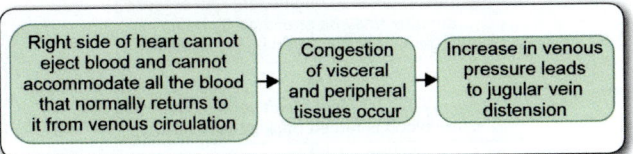

Right side of heart cannot eject blood and cannot accommodate all the blood that normally returns to it from venous circulation → Congestion of visceral and peripheral tissues occur → Increase in venous pressure leads to jugular vein distension

MITRAL VALVE PROLAPSE

Normally, blood flows through the heart across the valves in a single direction. The heart valves are very sensitive to the changes in pressure within the chambers. When the pressure in the chamber proximal to these valves get increased, the valves open whereas when the pressure in the chamber beyond the valves increases, they snap shut. Valvular heart diseases are caused either by insufficiency of valves or valvular stenosis. Valvular insufficiency caused by diseased valve leads to regurgitation or backflow of blood in the atrium or ventricle leading to increased workload on the heart. Valvular stenosis caused by calcium build-up leads to increase in pressure and decreased flow of blood when it attempts to cross through the stenotic area, causing volume overload. The valvular diseases may progress onto cause heart failure resulting from its inability to act as a pump and meet the metabolic demands. The pathophysiological changes of main valvular heart diseases are shown in the flowcharts.

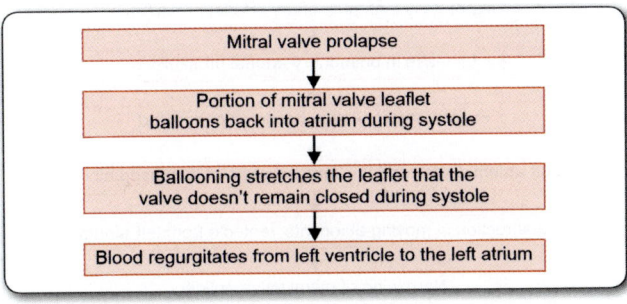

Mitral valve prolapse
↓
Portion of mitral valve leaflet balloons back into atrium during systole
↓
Ballooning stretches the leaflet that the valve doesn't remain closed during systole
↓
Blood regurgitates from left ventricle to the left atrium

MITRAL REGURGITATION

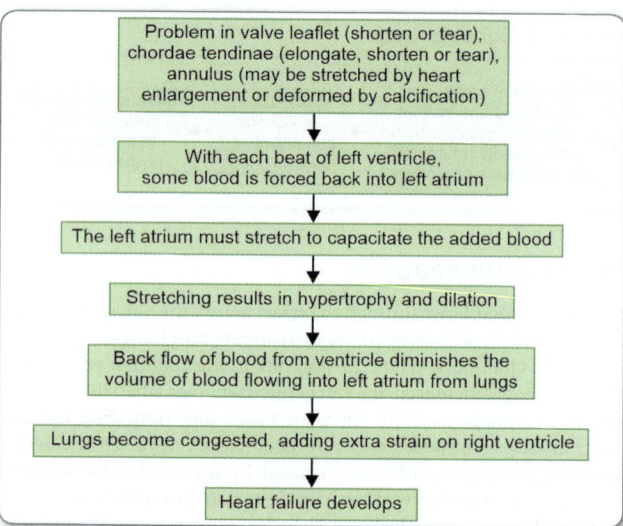

Problem in valve leaflet (shorten or tear), chordae tendinae (elongate, shorten or tear), annulus (may be stretched by heart enlargement or deformed by calcification)

↓

With each beat of left ventricle, some blood is forced back into left atrium

↓

The left atrium must stretch to capacitate the added blood

↓

Stretching results in hypertrophy and dilation

↓

Back flow of blood from ventricle diminishes the volume of blood flowing into left atrium from lungs

↓

Lungs become congested, adding extra strain on right ventricle

↓

Heart failure develops

MITRAL STENOSIS

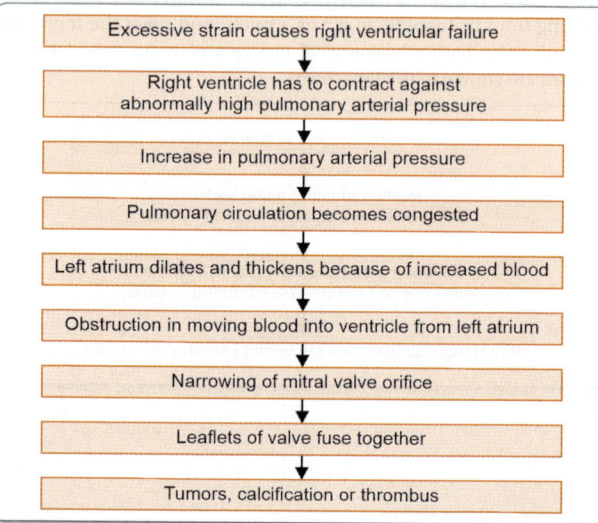

Excessive strain causes right ventricular failure

↓

Right ventricle has to contract against abnormally high pulmonary arterial pressure

↓

Increase in pulmonary arterial pressure

↓

Pulmonary circulation becomes congested

↓

Left atrium dilates and thickens because of increased blood

↓

Obstruction in moving blood into ventricle from left atrium

↓

Narrowing of mitral valve orifice

↓

Leaflets of valve fuse together

↓

Tumors, calcification or thrombus

AORTIC STENOSIS

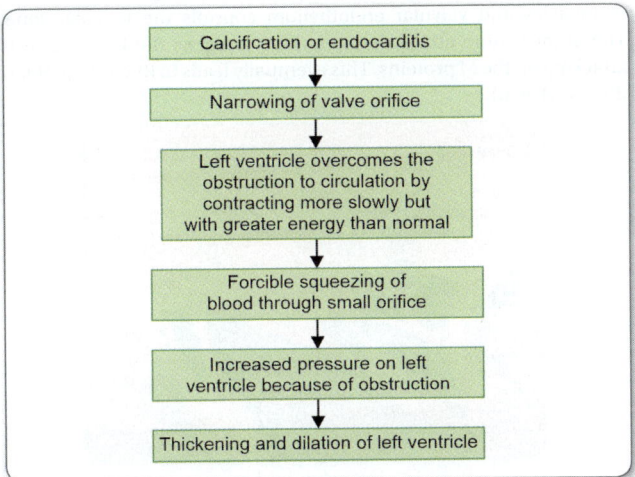

Calcification or endocarditis

↓

Narrowing of valve orifice

↓

Left ventricle overcomes the obstruction to circulation by contracting more slowly but with greater energy than normal

↓

Forcible squeezing of blood through small orifice

↓

Increased pressure on left ventricle because of obstruction

↓

Thickening and dilation of left ventricle

AORTIC REGURGITATION

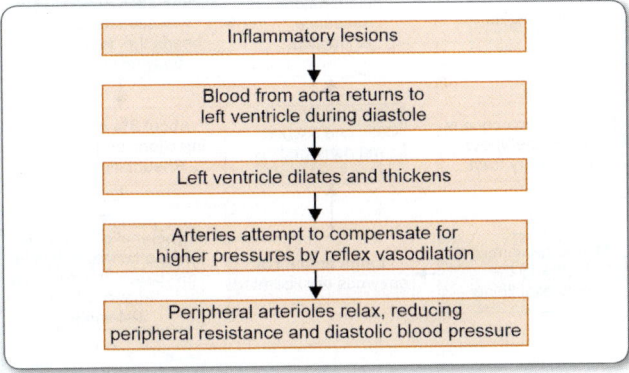

Inflammatory lesions

↓

Blood from aorta returns to left ventricle during diastole

↓

Left ventricle dilates and thickens

↓

Arteries attempt to compensate for higher pressures by reflex vasodilation

↓

Peripheral arterioles relax, reducing peripheral resistance and diastolic blood pressure

RHEUMATIC HEART DISEASE

Rheumatic heart disease is an inflammation and scarring of heart areas triggered by an autoimmune reaction to infection with group A streptococci. This means that the immune system reacts to different parts of the body, thinking it is protecting it from a disease or bacteria.

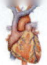

Streptococcal A carries M-proteins that are similar in structure to the cardiac antigens in humans. Myosin and valvular endothelium are those antigens. Myosin is responsible mainly for contraction of muscles and valvular endothelium controls the vascular tone. The autoimmune attack destroys these antigens thinking that it is attacking on the M proteins. This eventually leads to Rheumatic Heart disease (Fig. 6).

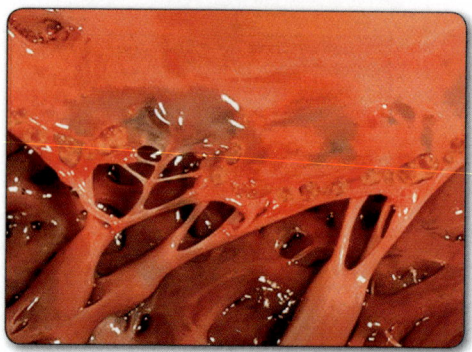

Fig. 6: Rheumatic heart disease

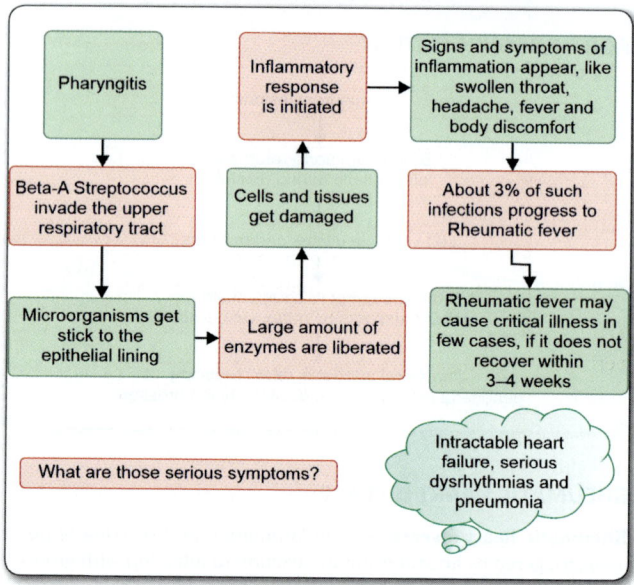

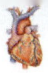

Progression of Rheumatic Fever to Rheumatic Heart Disease

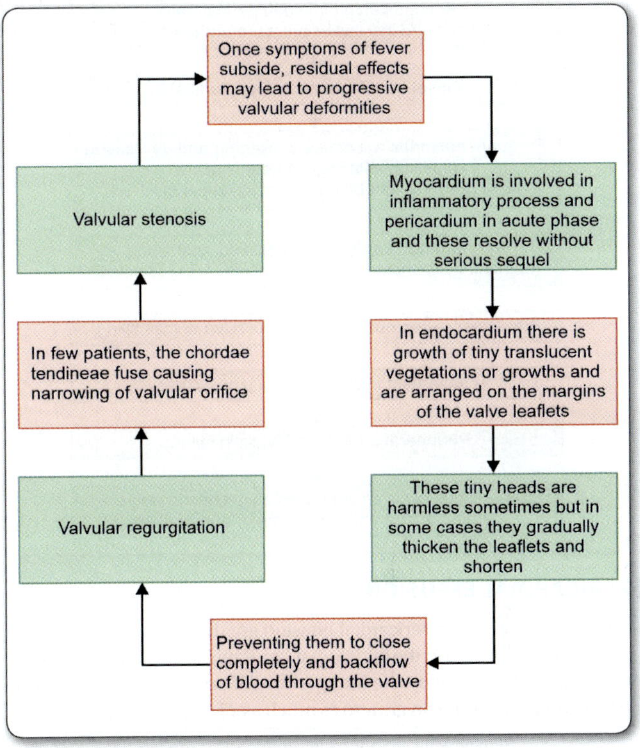

```
┌─────────────────────────────────────────────────────────────┐
│                                                             │
│         ┌──────────────────────┐                            │
│         │ Once symptoms of fever│                           │
│         │ subside, residual     │                           │
│         │ effects may lead to   │                           │
│         │ progressive valvular  │                           │
│         │ deformities           │                           │
│         └──────────────────────┘                            │
│                                                             │
│  ┌──────────────┐      ┌──────────────────────┐             │
│  │              │      │ Myocardium is involved│             │
│  │  Valvular    │      │ in inflammatory process│            │
│  │  stenosis    │      │ and pericardium in    │            │
│  │              │      │ acute phase and these │            │
│  └──────────────┘      │ resolve without       │            │
│                        │ serious sequel        │            │
│                        └──────────────────────┘             │
│  ┌──────────────┐      ┌──────────────────────┐             │
│  │ In few       │      │ In endocardium there  │             │
│  │ patients, the│      │ is growth of tiny     │             │
│  │ chordae      │      │ translucent vegetations│            │
│  │ tendineae    │      │ or growths and are    │             │
│  │ fuse causing │      │ arranged on the margins│            │
│  │ narrowing of │      │ of the valve leaflets │             │
│  │ valvular     │      └──────────────────────┘             │
│  │ orifice      │                                           │
│  └──────────────┘                                           │
│                                                             │
│  ┌──────────────┐      ┌──────────────────────┐             │
│  │              │      │ These tiny heads are  │             │
│  │  Valvular    │      │ harmless sometimes but│             │
│  │  regurgitation│     │ in some cases they    │             │
│  │              │      │ gradually thicken the │             │
│  └──────────────┘      │ leaflets and shorten  │             │
│                        └──────────────────────┘             │
│         ┌──────────────────────┐                            │
│         │ Preventing them to    │                           │
│         │ close completely and  │                           │
│         │ backflow of blood     │                           │
│         │ through the valve     │                           │
│         └──────────────────────┘                            │
│                                                             │
└─────────────────────────────────────────────────────────────┘
```

PERICARDITIS

Acute pericarditis develops quickly causing inflammation of pericardial sac along with pericardial effusion.

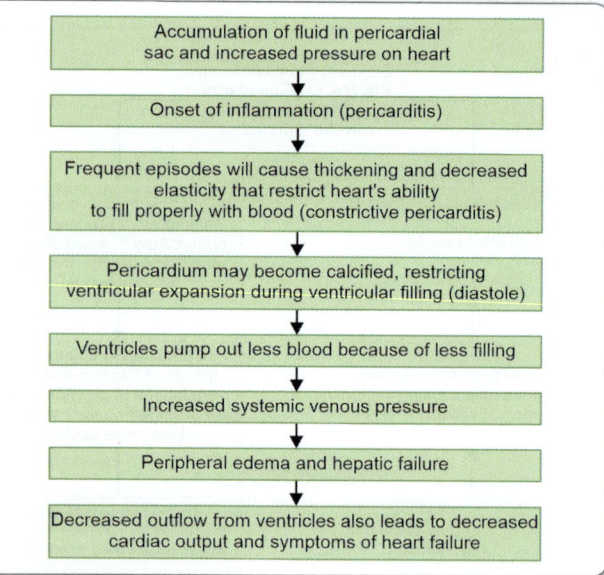

PERICARDIAL EFFUSION

The manifestations of pericardial effusion are dependent on the rate of accumulation of fluid in the pericardial sac. Rapid accumulation of about 80 mL fluid may increase the intrapericardial pressures whereas slowly progressing effusions can grow to as much as 2 L without any symptoms.

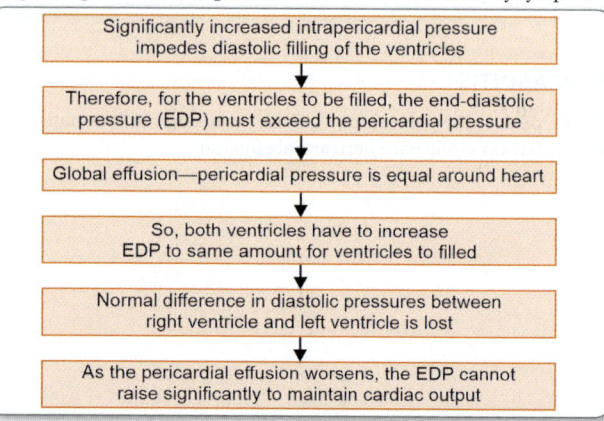

MYOCARDITIS

Inflammation and scarring of myocardium are caused by an infiltrate of myocardium with lymphocytes, neutrophils or granulomas. As a result of which, poor contractility occurs further leading to heart failure.

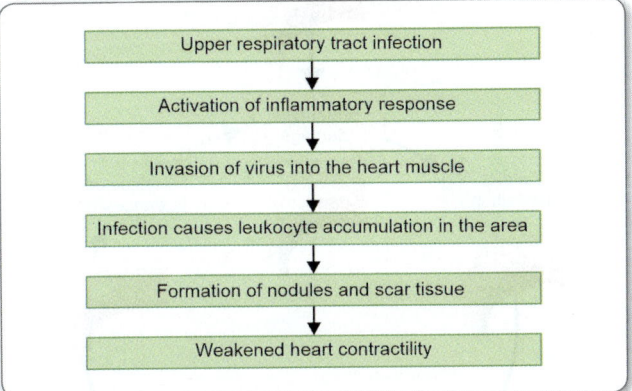

ENDOCARDITIS

Inflammation of endocardial surface of the heart may include valves or mural endocardium. Infective endocarditis involves three critical elements, i.e. preparation of valvular area for adherence of bacteria; then adhesion of bacteria to the surface; and finally bacterial survival onto the surface, further causing infective vegetations. Normally, the circulating bacteria are not able to adhere to the endothelial surface. It is only in the presence of trauma to the valve that the disruption of the endothelial surface occurs. And it poses the surface to the colonization by circulating bacteria (Fig. 7).

Let us review how these changes occur through the flowchart and the cycle given in the figure.

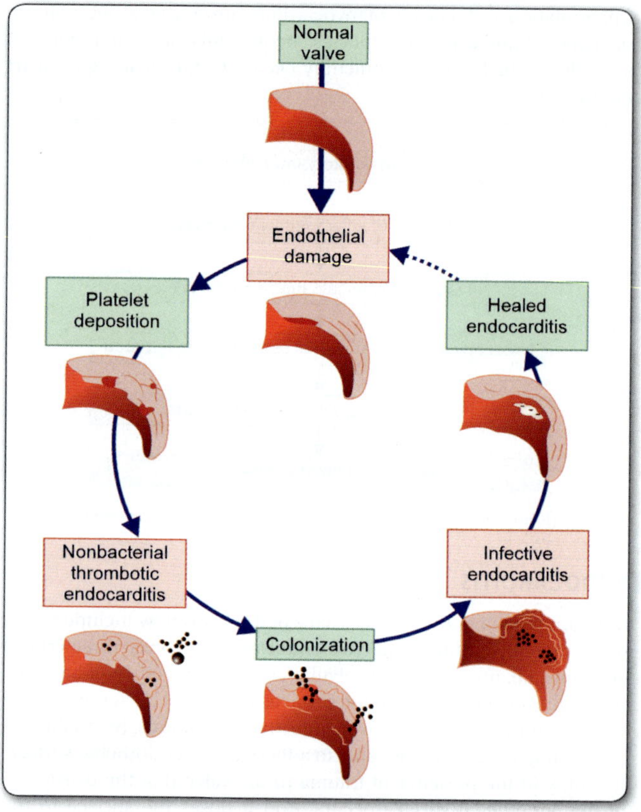

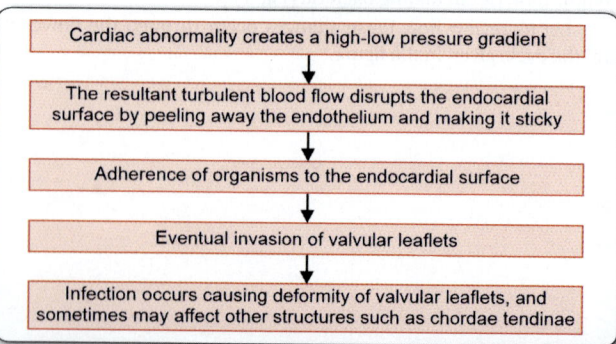

Fig. 7: Cycle of endocarditis

Cardiac abnormality creates a high-low pressure gradient

↓

The resultant turbulent blood flow disrupts the endocardial surface by peeling away the endothelium and making it sticky

↓

Adherence of organisms to the endocardial surface

↓

Eventual invasion of valvular leaflets

↓

Infection occurs causing deformity of valvular leaflets, and sometimes may affect other structures such as chordae tendinae

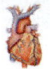

COR PULMONALE

Pulmonary hypertension associated with the disease conditions of the lungs cause an increase in the filling of right side of the heart causing Cor pulmonale.

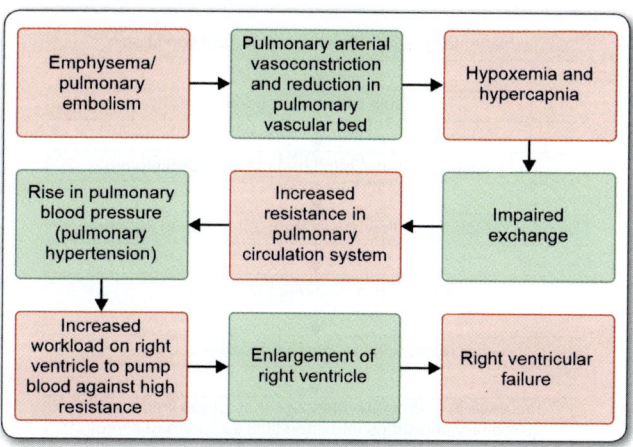

PULMONARY EDEMA

It is often caused by congestive heart failure when the heart is not able to pump blood effectively, fluid backs up into the veins of the lungs. Increased pressure in these veins forces fluid out of the veins and into the air spaces (alveoli). This interferes with the exchange of oxygen and carbon dioxide in the alveoli.

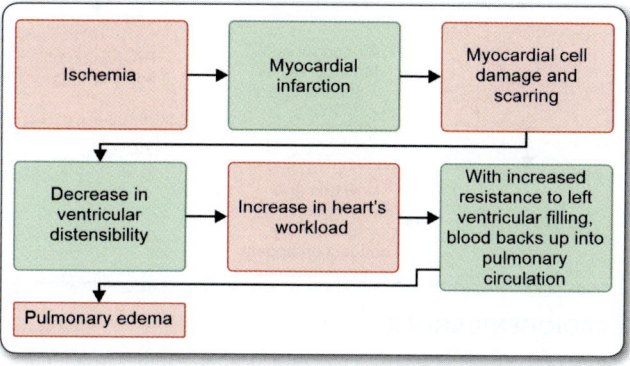

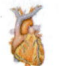

Pulmonary edema can even be the result of non-cardiac conditions such as renal or liver failure, cancer or impaired lymphatic drainage. The changes are mentioned as follows in the flowcharts.

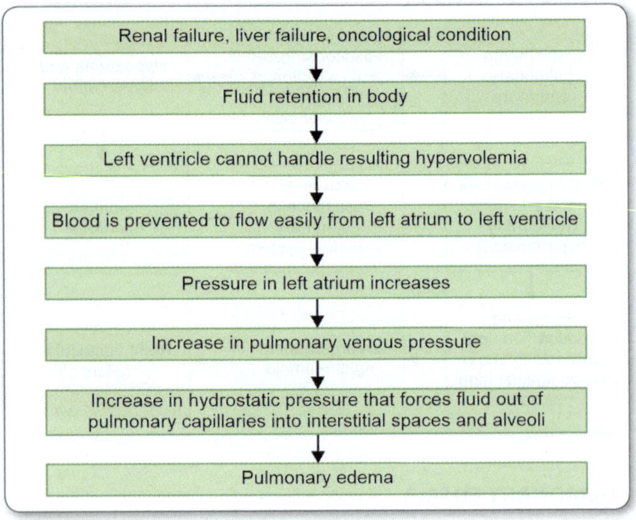

Renal failure, liver failure, oncological condition

↓

Fluid retention in body

↓

Left ventricle cannot handle resulting hypervolemia

↓

Blood is prevented to flow easily from left atrium to left ventricle

↓

Pressure in left atrium increases

↓

Increase in pulmonary venous pressure

↓

Increase in hydrostatic pressure that forces fluid out of pulmonary capillaries into interstitial spaces and alveoli

↓

Pulmonary edema

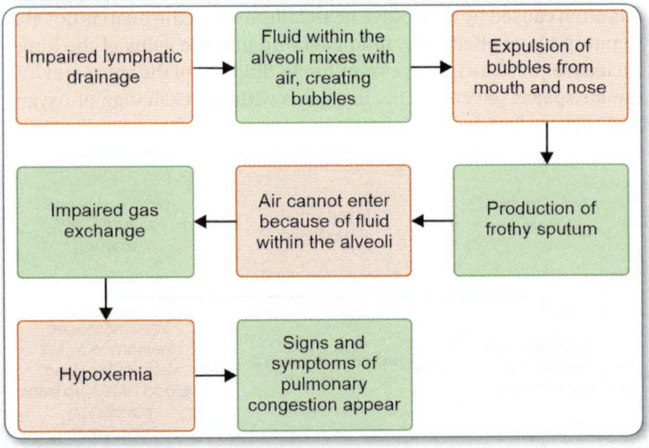

Impaired lymphatic drainage → Fluid within the alveoli mixes with air, creating bubbles → Expulsion of bubbles from mouth and nose

↓

Impaired gas exchange ← Air cannot enter because of fluid within the alveoli ← Production of frothy sputum

↓

Hypoxemia → Signs and symptoms of pulmonary congestion appear

CARDIOGENIC SHOCK

Cardiogenic shock occurs as a low cardiac output state caused due to heart failure. Myocardial ischemia causes alteration both in systolic

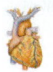

and diastolic functions of the ventricles, resulting in a significant decrease in myocardial contractility. This eventually leads to a spiral of low cardiac output and low blood pressure, thereby exacerbating coronary ischemia and impaired myocardial contractility.

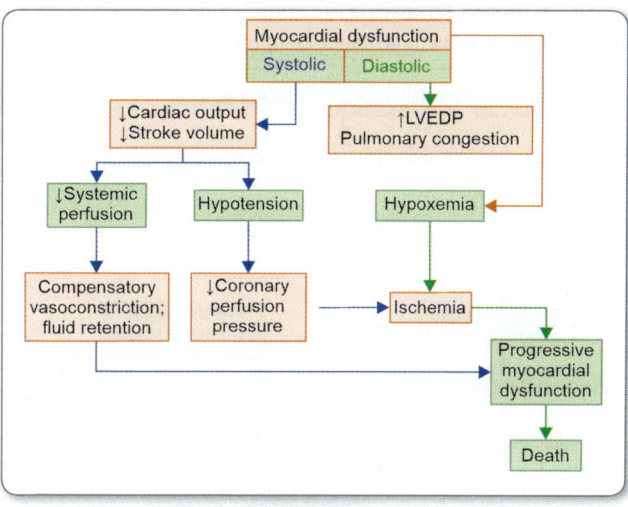

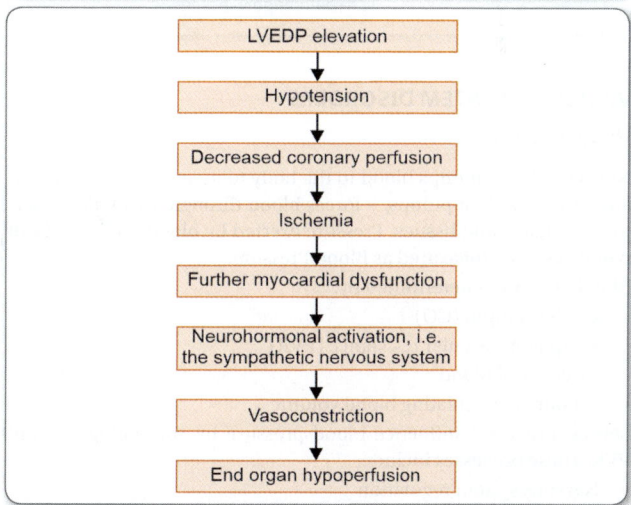

Abbreviation: LVEDP, left ventricular end-diastolic pressure

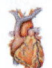
CARDIAC TAMPONADE

A clinical syndrome, cardiac tamponade occurs due to accumulation of fluid in the pericardial space, causing reduction in ventricular filling and eventual hemodynamic compromise.

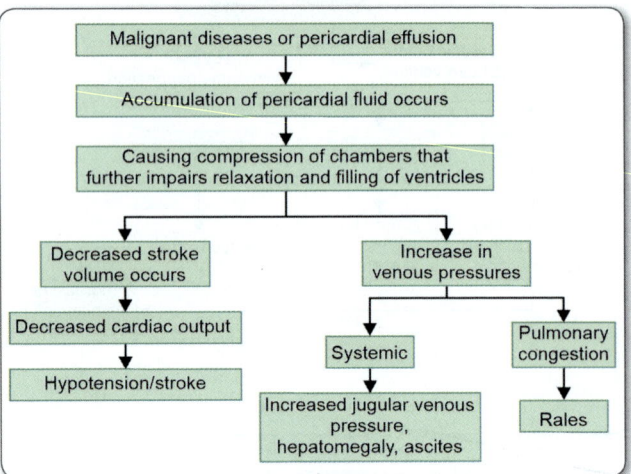

VASCULAR SYSTEM DISORDERS

Hypertension

Normally, heart pumps blood to the body to meet cells' needs for O_2 and nutrients. As it pumps, it forces blood through the blood vessels to vital organs and tissues. Pressure exerted by blood on the walls of blood vessels is measured as Blood Pressure.

Blood pressure is determined by:

- Cardiac output (CO)
- Peripheral vascular resistance (PVR)
- Viscosity of blood
- Amount of circulating blood volume

Several processes influence blood pressure by controlling CO and PVR. These processes include:

- Nervous system regulation
- Arterial baroreceptors and chemoreceptors
- Renin-angiotensin-aldosterone mechanism
- Balancing of body fluids

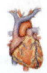

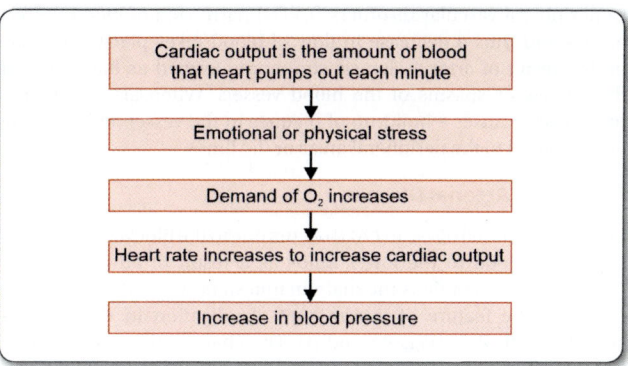

The PVR is the opposition that blood encounters as it flows through the vessels.

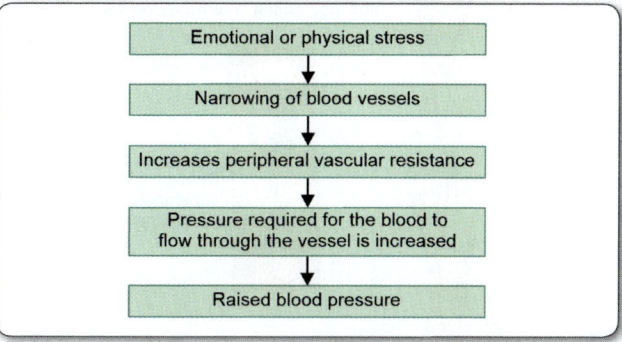

- Factors that hamper normal blood pressure regulation cause hypertension and many of these factors are not well understood.
- Overstimulation of sympathetic nervous system (SNS) leads to vasoconstriction and causes hypertension.
- Alterations in chemoreceptors and baroreceptors may also affect the development of hypertension.

For example, baroreceptors may become less sensitive because of prolonged increase in vessel pressure and subsequently fail to cause vasodilation through vessel stretching.

- Elevation in level of hormones that causes sodium retention such as aldosterone leads to retention of fluid.
- Changes in renal function that alter the fluid excretion also result in an increase in overall body fluid that may cause hypertension.

PERIPHERAL VASCULAR DISORDERS

In peripheral vascular disorders (PVDs) narrowing of blood vessels occurs and thus a decrease in flow of blood takes place. This may be the result of arteriosclerosis commonly termed as hardening of the vessels or spasms of the blood vessels. When arteriosclerosis develops, it causes a build-up of plaques in the vessel, reducing the flow of blood to the peripheral areas or the limbs.

Peripheral Arterial Disease

Peripheral arterial disease (PAD) occurs due to the blockage of arteries supplying blood to the lower limbs as a result of atherosclerosis. Critical limb ischemia is the main manifestation of PAD causing the characteristic feature of intermittent claudication in the patients suffering with PAD (Figs 8A and B). The changes that take place in PAD are shown as follows:

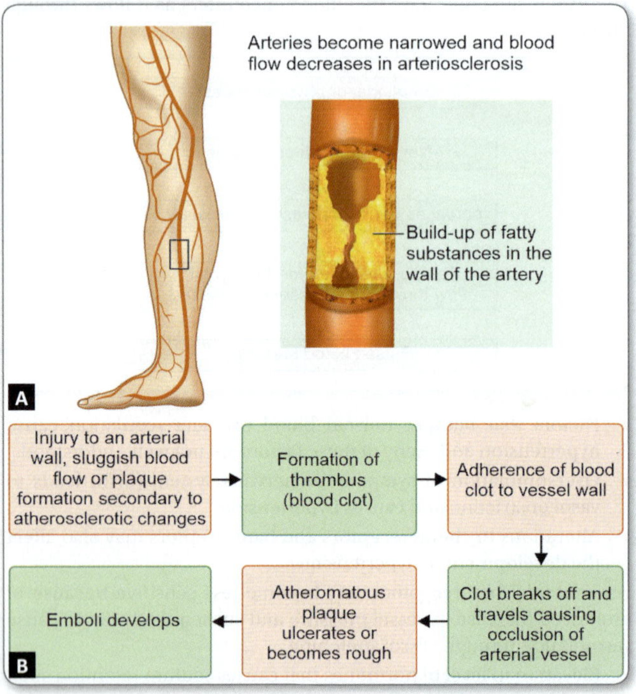

Arteries become narrowed and blood flow decreases in arteriosclerosis

Build-up of fatty substances in the wall of the artery

A

Injury to an arterial wall, sluggish blood flow or plaque formation secondary to atherosclerotic changes → Formation of thrombus (blood clot) → Adherence of blood clot to vessel wall

↓

Emboli develops ← Atheromatous plaque ulcerates or becomes rough ← Clot breaks off and travels causing occlusion of arterial vessel

B

Figs 8A and B: Peripheral arterial disease

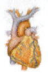

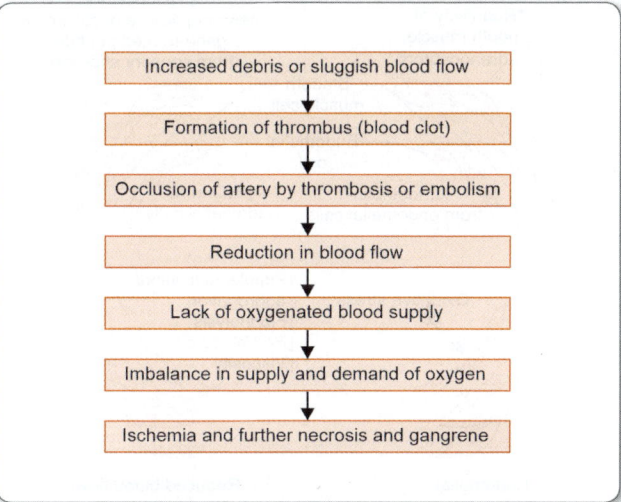

RAYNAUD'S DISEASE

Raynaud's disease is mainly characterized by recurrent and reversible spasms of digital arteries and smaller arterioles, and is triggered by exposure to cold and emotional stress. The affected areas experience intense vasospasm with associated change in color and subsequent hyperemia. A clear distinction occurs between the ischemic and unaffected areas (Figs 9 and 10).

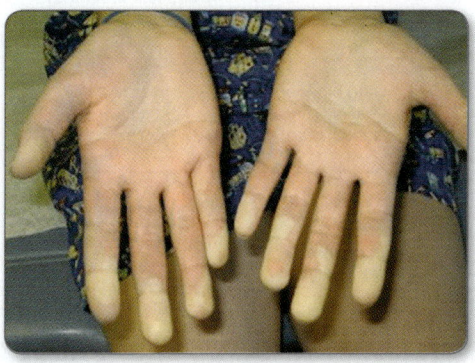

Fig. 9: Raynaud's disease

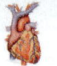

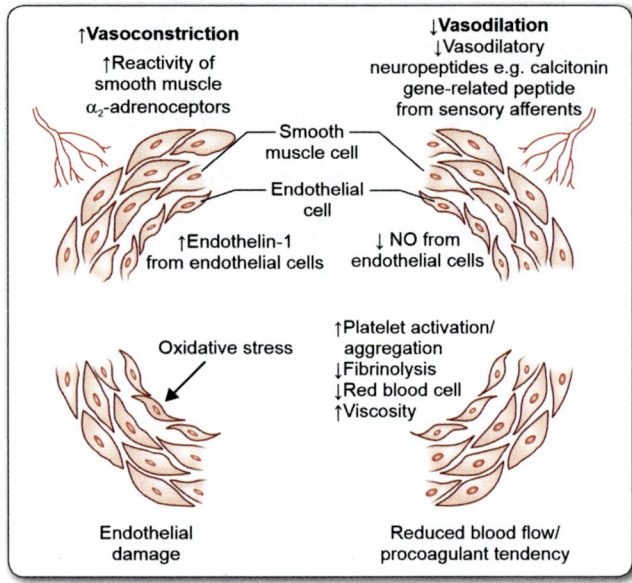

Fig. 10: Effects of vasoconstrictive response

The pathophysiological changes in Raynaud's disease are shown in as follows:

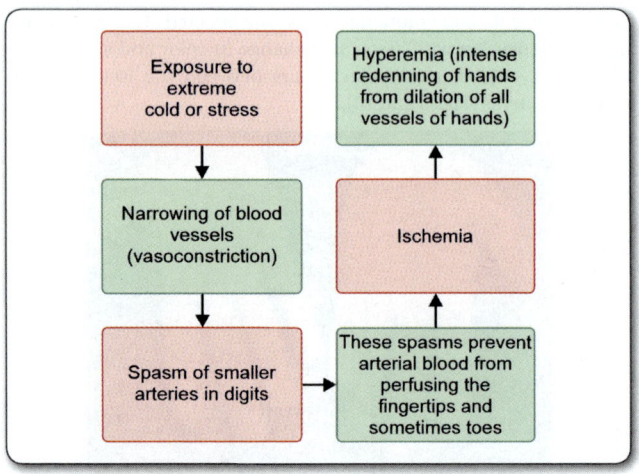

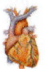

ANEURYSM

Any weakness or destruction of the middle layer of blood vessel leads to the occurrence of aneurysm. It happens as a result of constant pressure exerted by the circulating blood onto the walls of the artery causing enlargement of the weakened part of the artery. The symptoms result from the compression of surrounding structures or eventual rupture of the enlarged artery that causes hemorrhage. Other than atherosclerosis, infection, trauma or congenital defect of the artery may also cause aneurysm. Thoracic and abdominal aneurysms are the common types. The changes are mentioned in the flowchart as follows:

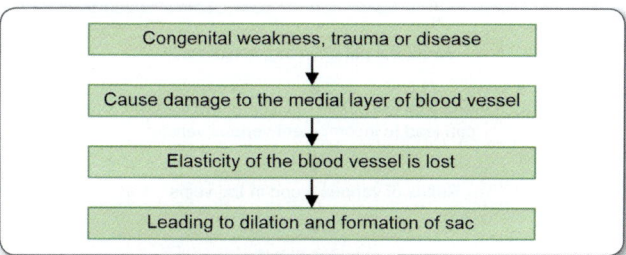

VARICOSE VEINS

Normal and varicose veins are depicted in Figure 11.

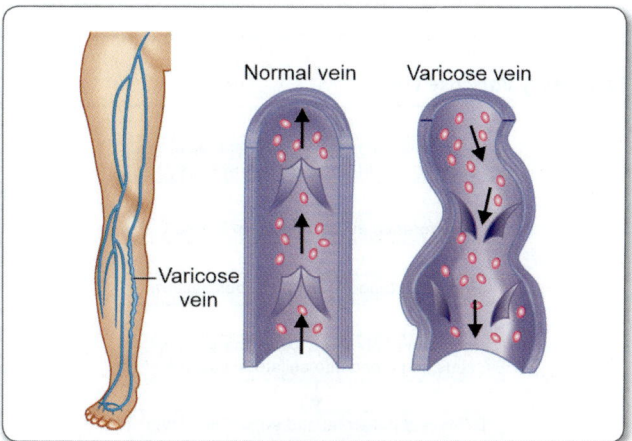

Fig. 11: Normal and varicose veins

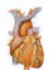

Pathophysiology of Varicose Veins

- Veins are thin-walled vessels that are easily distended by the chronic pooling of blood in the lower extremities (Fig. 11).
- The venous valves work in conjunction with skeletal muscle pumps present in the legs to move blood back to the heart from the extremities.
- Chronic distention of veins can reduce effectiveness of one-way venous valves that are present in the lumen to prevent the back flow of blood and lead to a condition termed valvular incompetence.

Primary Varicose Veins

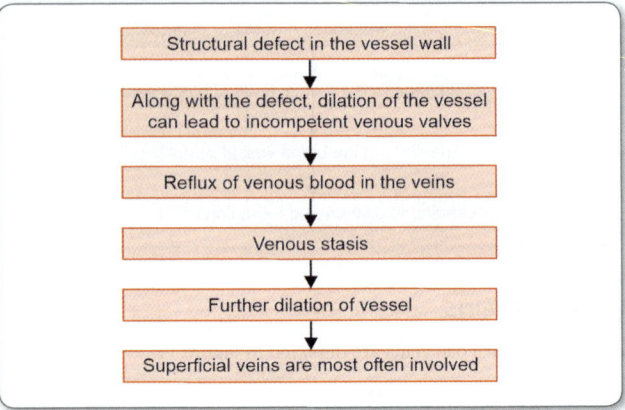

Structural defect in the vessel wall
↓
Along with the defect, dilation of the vessel can lead to incompetent venous valves
↓
Reflux of venous blood in the veins
↓
Venous stasis
↓
Further dilation of vessel
↓
Superficial veins are most often involved

Secondary Varicose Veins

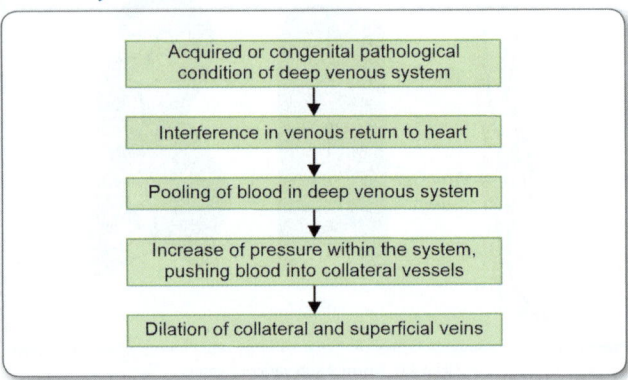

Acquired or congenital pathological condition of deep venous system
↓
Interference in venous return to heart
↓
Pooling of blood in deep venous system
↓
Increase of pressure within the system, pushing blood into collateral vessels
↓
Dilation of collateral and superficial veins

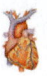

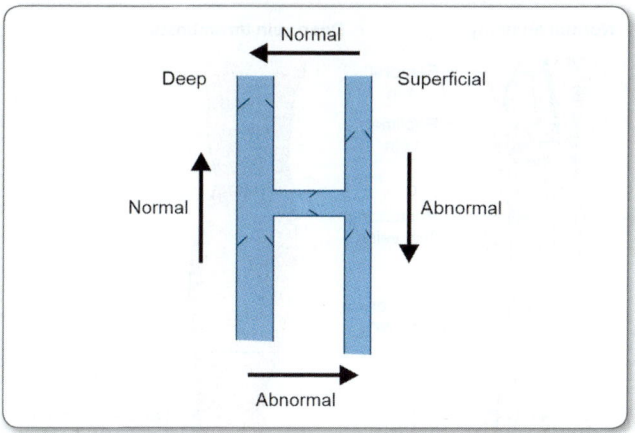

DEEP VENOUS THROMBOSIS

In normal physiology, superficial veins are thick-walled muscular structures that lie just under the skin such as greater saphenous, lesser saphenous, cephalic, basilic and external jugular veins. Deep veins have less muscle in media and thin walled (Figs 12A and B).

Valves lie in the deep and superficial veins, which permit unidirectional flow of blood toward the heart. Valves are present at the base of the segment of vein that is expanded into the sinus. When blood starts to flow backward, this arrangement allows rapid closure of the valves by allowing them open without coming into contact with the wall of the vein.

Another kinds of veins are called perforating veins, which allow one-way blood flow from superficial to deep venous system.

Let us see how the venous stasis occurs.

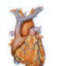

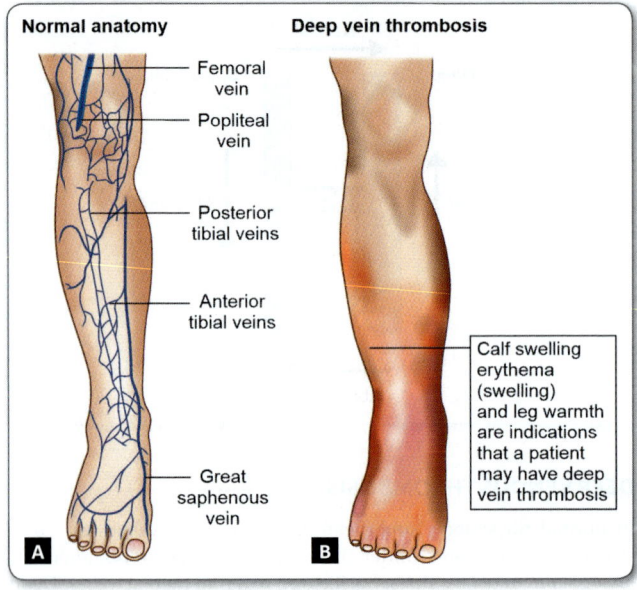

Figs 12A and B: Deep vein thrombosis

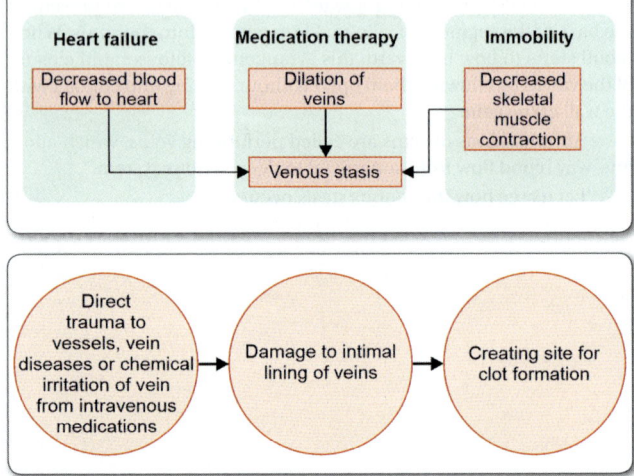

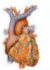

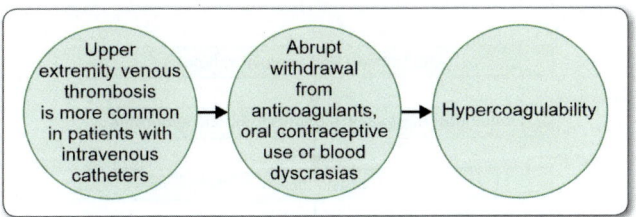

CHRONIC VENOUS INSUFFICIENCY

Venous reflux can be caused by incompetence of venous valves, inflammation of vessel wall and hypertension. Aggravation of these mechanisms occur due to dysfunctional pump mechanisms as in case of immobile patients and stiffness in joints. The sequence of changes is depicted in the flowcharts as follows:

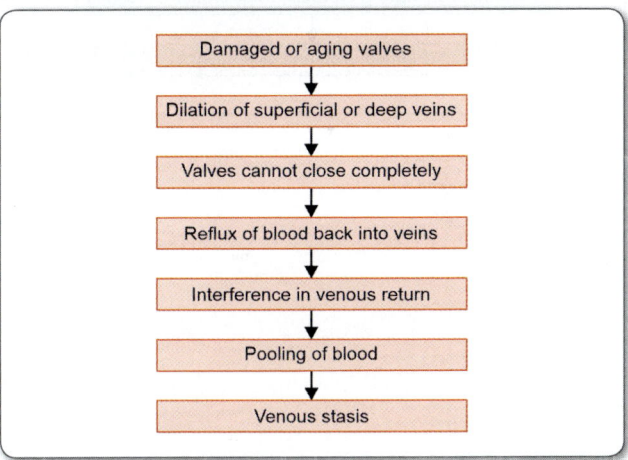

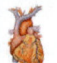

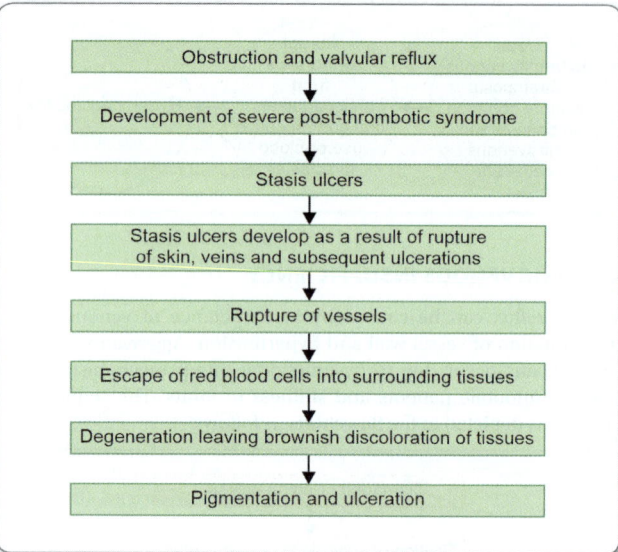

Obstruction and valvular reflux

Development of severe post-thrombotic syndrome

Stasis ulcers

Stasis ulcers develop as a result of rupture of skin, veins and subsequent ulcerations

Rupture of vessels

Escape of red blood cells into surrounding tissues

Degeneration leaving brownish discoloration of tissues

Pigmentation and ulceration

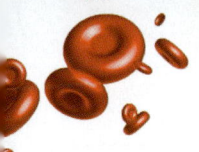

Pathophysiology of Blood Disorders

INTRODUCTION

Blood is composed of many components, such as plasma, platelets, white blood cells (leukocytes) and red blood cells (erythrocytes) (Fig. 1). In a healthy adult, total blood volume is responsible for around 7–8% of the total body weight. An adult has approximately 4–5 L of blood that circulates in an adult human body at a given time. About 55% of the total blood volume is plasma and the rest 45% is made up of different forms of elements or cells (Fig. 2). The critical function of the blood is to transport hormones, gases, nutrients and wastes around the human body. Blood also plays an important role in immunological functions as well as homeostatic regulation of pH and temperature.

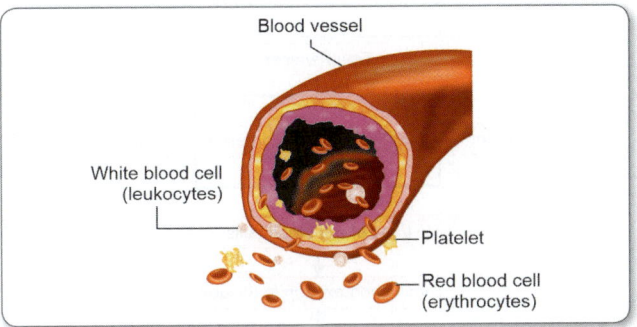

Fig. 1: Components of blood

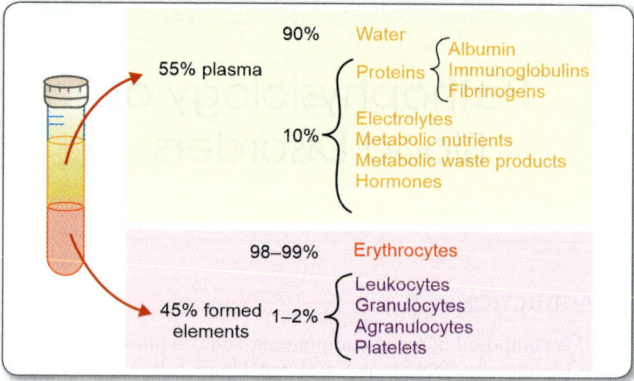

Fig. 2: Composition of blood

ANEMIA

Anemia is the result of imbalance between loss of RBCs and their production. This can occur as a result of nutritional deficiencies and inflammation (leading to ineffective erythropoiesis).

The following stages are involved in the development of anemia.

Loss of RBCs

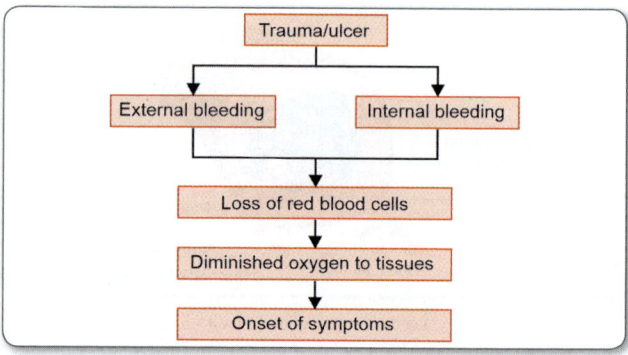

THALASSEMIA

Thalassemia is an inherited blood disorder in which the body synthesizes defective hemoglobin (the protein in red blood cells that carries oxygen), reduces the production of one or more globulin chains within the hemoglobin molecule. The disorder results in excessive destruction of red blood cells, causing anemia.

There are two main types of thalassemia:

1. Alpha thalassemia in which a gene or genes related to the alpha globin protein are mutated.
2. Beta thalassemia in which similar gene defects affect production of the beta globin protein.

Both alpha and beta thalassemias have two subtypes:

1. Thalassemia major in which defective gene is inherited from both the parents.
2. Thalassemia minor in which children receive the defective gene from only one parent and become carrier of the disease and usually do not have symptoms.

> Beta thalassemia major is also called **Cooley's anemia**.

THROMBOCYTOPENIA

Platelets have an important role in clotting and bleeding functions. Like the other cells in the blood, i.e. red blood cells and white blood cells, platelets originate in the bone marrow. Platelets are formed from megakaryocytes that are present in the bone marrow. Two third of the platelets, which are released from the bone marrow are the circulating platelets and the rest one third of the platelets are stored (sequestered) in the spleen.

Decreased production of platelets within the bone marrow, increased destruction of platelets, or increased consumption of platelets can lead to low platelet count. In case of severe Thrombocytopenia, spontaneous bleeding or delay in the normal process of clotting can occur. In case of mild thrombocytopenia, there may not be any adverse effects in the clotting or bleeding pathways.

DISSEMINATED INTRAVASCULAR COAGULATION

In disseminated intravascular coagulation (DIC), excessive thrombin and fibrin are produced in the circulating blood. Platelet aggregation is increased and coagulation factor is consumed during the process. DIC leads to venous thrombotic and embolic manifestations, if occurs slowly over weeks or months.

The DIC causes primarily bleeding, if occurs rapidly over hours or days. Rapidly occurring DIC is characterized by increased partial thromboplastin time and prothrombin time, elevated levels of plasma D-dimers, thrombocytopenia and decreased plasma fibrinogen level. Bleeding is controlled by correcting the cause and replacing platelets, coagulation factors and fibrinogen. For the patients who have or are at risk of getting venous embolism, prophylactic heparin therapy is administered.

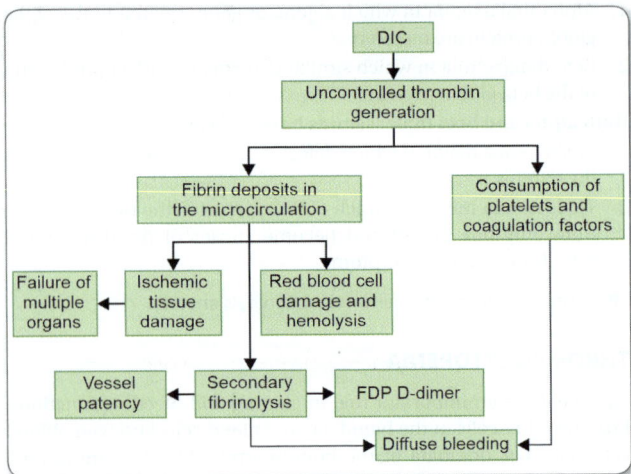

Abbreviations: DIC, disseminated intravascular coagulation; FDP, fibrin degradation product

- **Generation of a hyperthrombinemic state:**
  - During injury, cascade activation of a factor pathway is caused by the exposure of tissue factors thromboplastins and factor III.
  - Formation of endothelial cell tissue factor is triggered by the bacterial endotoxins and cytokines.
  - Clotting cascade can also be initiated by tissue phospholipids in case of severe trauma.

Tissue phospholipids $\xrightarrow{}$ TF + Factor VIII $\xrightarrow{\text{Factor Xa}}$ TF/VII complex

TF/VII complex $\xrightarrow[\text{Activate}]{}$ Factor IX and X $\longrightarrow$ Thrombin
(leading to development of)

Abbreviation: TF, tissue factor

- **Alteration of the physiological anticoagulant levels:**
  Three most common anticoagulants present in the body are:
  (i) Antithrombin
  (ii) Active protein C
  (iii) Tissue factor pathway inhibitor (TFPI)

In case of DIC, antithrombin and active protein C are decreased.

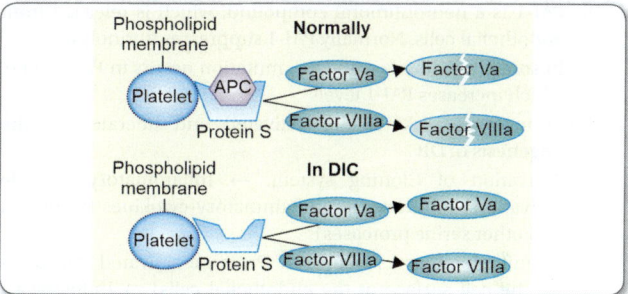

Abbreviations: APC, active protein C; DIC, disseminated intravascular coagulation

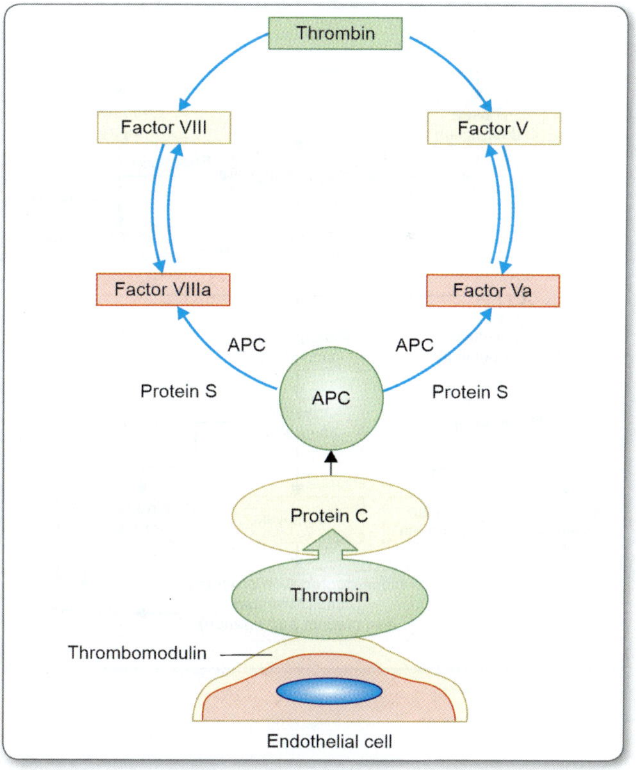

Endothelial cell

Abbreviation: APC, active protein C

- Impaired fibrinolysis at the onset of DIC.
  - PAI-1 is a neurohumoral compound, which is released from endothelial cells. Normally PAI-1 suppresses fibrinolysis.
  - In some individuals with DIC, mutation occurs in PAI-1 gene, which increases PAI-1 levels
- Inflammatory cytokines are activated and liberated in the pathogenesis of DIC.
  - Activation of Clotting system. → Inflammatory cascade activation → Induced proinflammatory cytokines (thrombin and other serine proteases)
  - Proinflammatory cytokines + Protease-activated receptors (of the cell surface of the endothelial cells) → Inducing an inflammatory and clotting reaction.

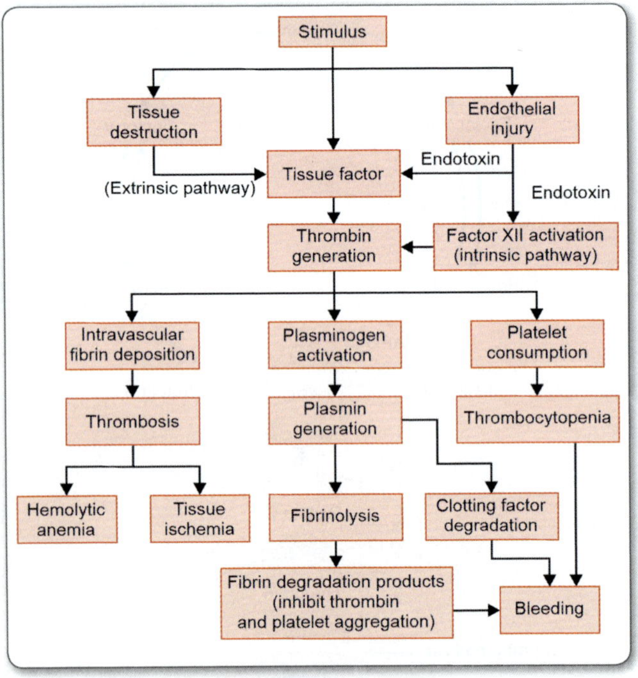

```
                          Stimulus

   Tissue                                      Endothelial
   destruction                                 injury
                                      Endotoxin
                        Tissue factor ◄──────
   (Extrinsic pathway)                         Endotoxin

                        Thrombin        ◄──   Factor XII activation
                        generation            (intrinsic pathway)

   Intravascular        Plasminogen           Platelet
   fibrin deposition    activation            consumption

   Thrombosis           Plasmin               Thrombocytopenia
                        generation

   Hemolytic  Tissue    Fibrinolysis          Clotting factor
   anemia     ischemia                        degradation

              Fibrin degradation products
              (inhibit thrombin          ──►   Bleeding
              and platelet aggregation)
```

LEUKEMIAS

Acute Myeloid Leukemia

- The defect in the hematopoietic stem cell, which differentiates into all myeloid cells, i.e. monocytes, granulocytes, erythrocytes, and platelets, results in acute myeloid leukemia (AML).
- AML can affect any age group, although it occurs rarely before 55 years of age.

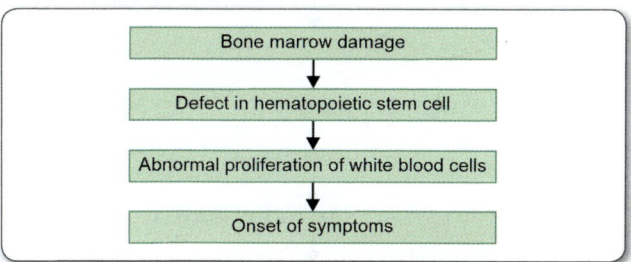

Chronic Myeloid Leukemia

- Mutation in the myeloid stem cell leads to chronic myeloid leukemia (CML).
- CML typically affects in the older ages.

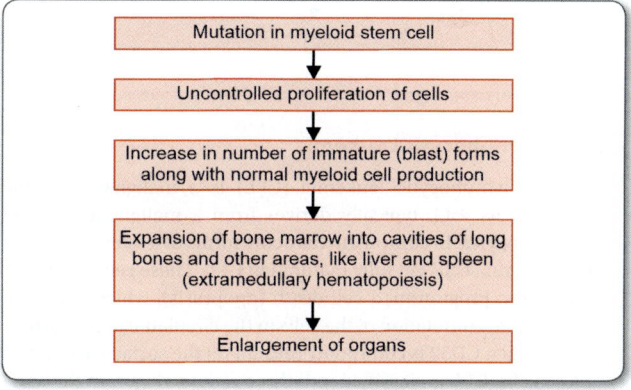

Acute Lymphocytic Leukemia

- An uncontrolled proliferation of immature cells, i.e. lymphoblasts, results into acute lymphocytic leukemia (ALL).
- ALL is most common in young children and the peak incidence is seen in four years of age. It affects boys more often than girls.

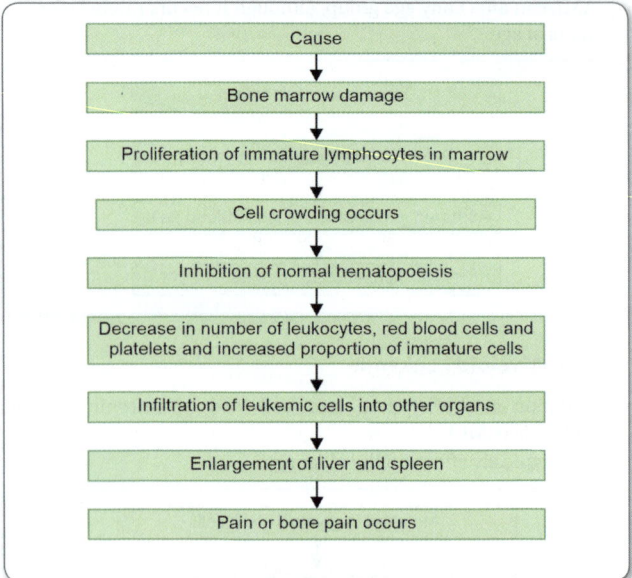

```
                    Cause
                      ↓
             Bone marrow damage
                      ↓
   Proliferation of immature lymphocytes in marrow
                      ↓
              Cell crowding occurs
                      ↓
         Inhibition of normal hematopoeisis
                      ↓
 Decrease in number of leukocytes, red blood cells and
 platelets and increased proportion of immature cells
                      ↓
      Infiltration of leukemic cells into other organs
                      ↓
         Enlargement of liver and spleen
                      ↓
            Pain or bone pain occurs
```

Chronic Lymphocytic Leukemia

- Chronic lymphocytic leukemia (CLL) is a malignancy of the older adults. CLL typically derives from a malignant clone of B lymphocytes. In contrary to the acute forms of leukemia, most of the leukemia cells get fully matured in CLL. These cells can break away from programmed cell death (apoptosis), which results in excessive accumulation of the cells in the circulation and marrow. The antigen CD52 is commonly present on the surface of many of these cells. CLL is classified into three or four stages. In the early stage, elevation of lymphocyte count occurs even above 100,000/mm³. Lymphocytes can travel through the small capillaries easily because of their small size, and the cerebral and pulmonary complications of leukocytosis are not usually found in CLL.

- The lymphocytes can be trapped within the lymph nodes resulting in lymphadenopathy. The nodes can sometimes be very large and painful. Hepatomegaly and splenomegaly can then develop.
- Thrombocytopenia and anemia may be developed in later stages. Treatment is typically started in the later stages.

MYELOMAS

- Myeloma is the malignant disease of the mature form of B lymphocytes. An increased amount of a specific immunoglobulin, which is nonfunctional, is produced by the malignant plasma cells in myeloma. Nonmalignant plasma cells still produce functional types of immunoglobulin, but in lower quantity than normal.
- Myeloma cells secrete specific immunoglobulin that is noticeable in the blood or urine, and is known as M protein or monoclonal protein. This protein helps to check the extent of disease and patient's response to treatment.
- Additionally, due to the M protein production, elevation of the patient's total protein level occurs. Certain substance secreted by the malignant plasma cells, stimulates the creation of new blood vessels and this process is known as angiogenesis.
- In rare cases, the plasma cells may infiltrate the other tissue and are called as plasmacytomas. Median survival time is 3–5 years. Infection may result in the death.

LYMPHOMAS

- Neoplasms of lymphoid cells are called lymphomas. These tumors usually initiate affecting lymph nodes but can affect lymphoid tissue in the liver, the gastrointestinal tract, the spleen, or the bone marrow.
- Lymphomas are classified into two types: Hodgkin's disease and non-Hodgkin's lymphoma (NHL).

Hodgkin's Disease

Hodgkin's disease begins in a single node, thus is unicentric in origin. The disease spreads along the lymphatic system by contiguous extension. The exact cause of Hodgkin's disease is not clear, but suspected to be caused by a viral etiology. In 40–50% of patients, fragments of the Epstein-Barr virus (EBV) have been found. It commonly affects the younger population. The malignant cell of Hodgkin's disease is the Reed-Sternberg cell.

Non-Hodgkin's Lymphomas (NHLs)

The neoplastic growth of lymphoid tissue is the origin of Non-Hodgkin's lymphomas. Morphologically, the cells may vary in NHL. In most of the NHLs, malignant B lymphocytes are involved, but only in 5% of the NHLs, T lymphocytes are involved. In contrary to Hodgkin's disease, malignant cells get largely penetrated in the involved lymphoid tissues. These malignant lymphoid cells spread unexpectedly. NHLs may affect the sites outside the lymphoid system (extranodal tissue).

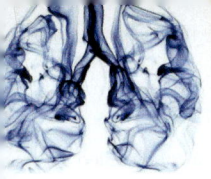

Pathophysiology of Respiratory Disorders

INTRODUCTION

The respiratory system is primarily involved in the gas exchange function. When exchange of gases occurs, oxygen is absorbed from the environment and carbon dioxide is excreted out from the blood. Oxygen is required for normal metabolism to take place and carbon dioxide is the waste product of this metabolism.

The respiratory system is divided into upper and lower respiratory tracts (Figs 1A and B).

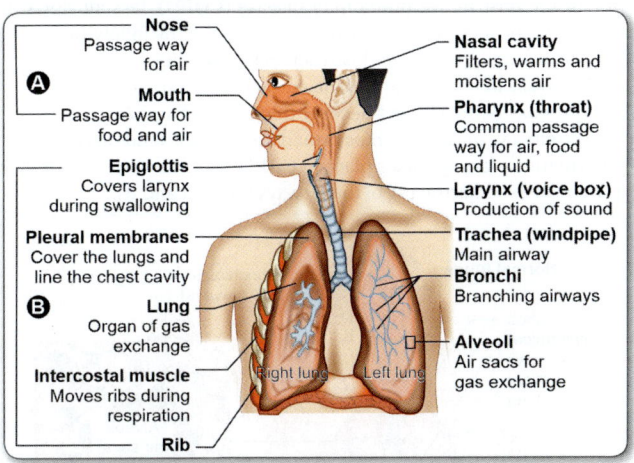

Nose
Passage way for air

A

Mouth
Passage way for food and air

Epiglottis
Covers larynx during swallowing

Pleural membranes
Cover the lungs and line the chest cavity

B

Lung
Organ of gas exchange

Intercostal muscle
Moves ribs during respiration

Rib

Nasal cavity
Filters, warms and moistens air

Pharynx (throat)
Common passage way for air, food and liquid

Larynx (voice box)
Production of sound

Trachea (windpipe)
Main airway

Bronchi
Branching airways

Alveoli
Air sacs for gas exchange

Right lung   Left lung

Figs 1A and B: A. Upper respiratory system; **B.** Lower respiratory system

The contraction of skeletal muscles occurs during an active process of breathing. The muscles responsible for respiration include the intercostal muscles and the diaphragm.

The walls of alveoli are coated with a thin film of water. Water molecules, including those on the alveolar walls, are more attracted

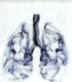
to each other than to air, and this attraction creates a force called surface tension. This surface tension increases as water molecules come closer, which happens during exhalation and the alveoli become smaller (like air leaving a balloon). Potentially, alveolar collapse may result because of this surface tension, which in turn would make re-expansion of alveoli difficult during inhalation. The collapse of the alveoli is prevented by substance produced by the lungs known as 'pulmonary surfactant'. The pulmonary surfactant is a mixture of lipids and proteins secreted by the epithelial type II cells into the alveolar space.

Role of Pulmonary Surfactant

Surfactant decreases surface tension, which:
- Increases pulmonary compliance (reducing the effort needed to expand the lungs)
- Reduces tendency for alveoli to collapse

In this chapter, the discussion regarding the pathophysiological changes that alter the normal respiratory functions are discussed one by one.

CHRONIC OBSTRUCTIVE PULMONARY DISEASE

In chronic obstructive pulmonary disease (COPD), less air flows in and out of the airways because of one or more of the following:
- The airways and air sacs lose their elastic quality.
- The walls between many of the air sacs are destroyed.
- The walls of the airways become thick and inflamed.
- The airways make more mucus than usual, which tends to clog them.

A permanent damage takes place in COPD. Chronic symptoms occur as there is fixed narrowing of the airways (Figs 2A and B).

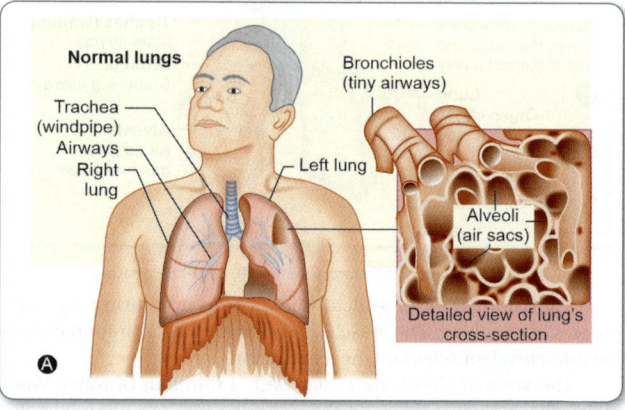

Fig. 2A:

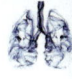

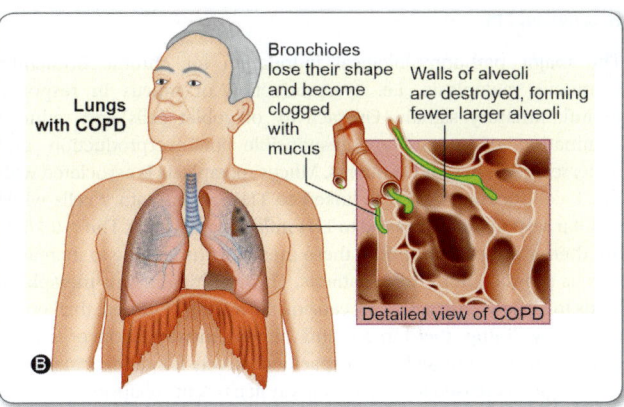

Bronchioles lose their shape and become clogged with mucus

Walls of alveoli are destroyed, forming fewer larger alveoli

Lungs with COPD

Detailed view of COPD

Ⓑ

Figs 2A and B: Comparison between normal lungs and lungs with chronic obstructive pulmonary disease

In case of asthma, airways get inflamed causing the constriction of respiratory muscles, further leading to narrowing of airways. The symptoms vary in severity and are periodical. Chronic cough with sputum is the main feature of COPD than asthma.

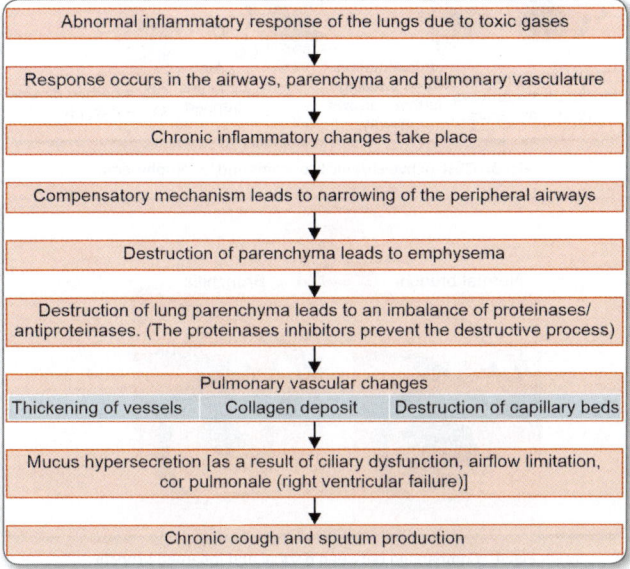

Abnormal inflammatory response of the lungs due to toxic gases

↓

Response occurs in the airways, parenchyma and pulmonary vasculature

↓

Chronic inflammatory changes take place

↓

Compensatory mechanism leads to narrowing of the peripheral airways

↓

Destruction of parenchyma leads to emphysema

↓

Destruction of lung parenchyma leads to an imbalance of proteinases/antiproteinases. (The proteinases inhibitors prevent the destructive process)

↓

Pulmonary vascular changes

| Thickening of vessels | Collagen deposit | Destruction of capillary beds |

↓

Mucus hypersecretion [as a result of ciliary dysfunction, airflow limitation, cor pulmonale (right ventricular failure)]

↓

Chronic cough and sputum production

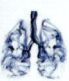

BRONCHITIS

The major pathophysiological foundation for chronic bronchitis is mucus metaplasia, i.e. overproduction of mucus in response to inflammatory signals. Overactivity of goblet cells and reduced elimination of mucus are responsible for overproduction and hypersecretion in COPD patients. Mucus metaplasia is associated with the T cell function and it is linked to TH1 inflammatory cells while cellular response is attributed to TH1 inflammatory cells. The cytokines are then produced by both of these mechanisms leading to increased mucus production in these patients. This resulting mucus metaplasia leads to airflow obstruction by causing narrowing of lumen, thickening of airway lining the lumen and altered airway surface tension (Figs 3 and 4). Ultimately, the capacity of airway for gas exchange and airflow get decreased leaving the airway at a risk of collapsing.

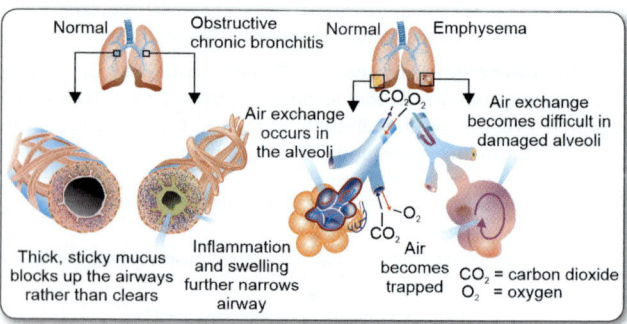

Fig. 3: Obstructive chronic bronchitis and/or emphysema

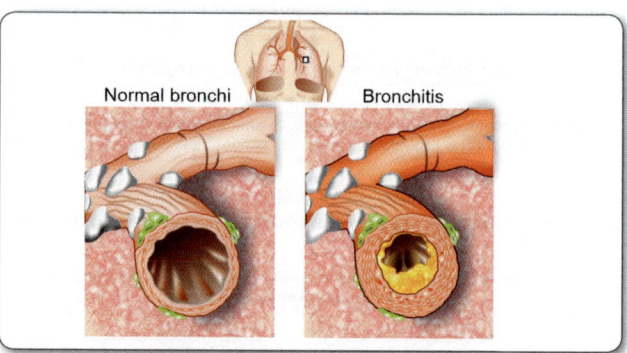

Fig. 4: Comparison between normal and inflamed bronchi

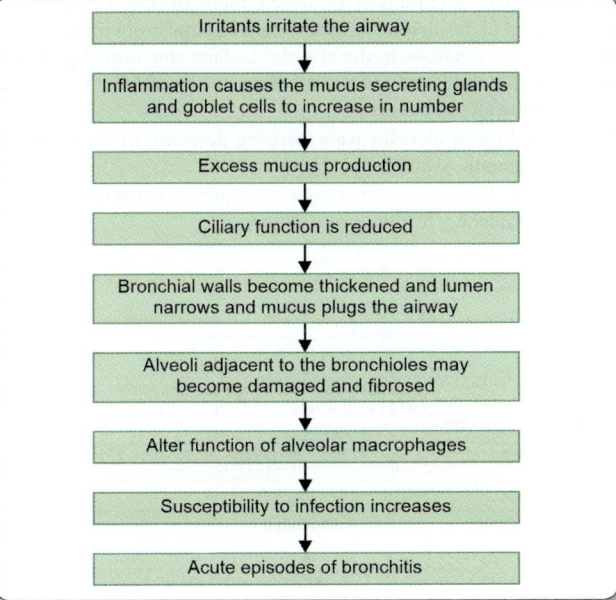

Irritants irritate the airway

↓

Inflammation causes the mucus secreting glands and goblet cells to increase in number

↓

Excess mucus production

↓

Ciliary function is reduced

↓

Bronchial walls become thickened and lumen narrows and mucus plugs the airway

↓

Alveoli adjacent to the bronchioles may become damaged and fibrosed

↓

Alter function of alveolar macrophages

↓

Susceptibility to infection increases

↓

Acute episodes of bronchitis

EMPHYSEMA

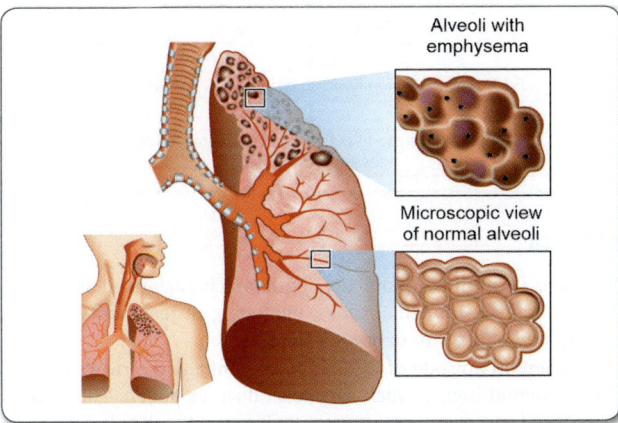

Alveoli with emphysema

Microscopic view of normal alveoli

Fig. 5: Alveoli with emphysema

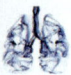
Emphysema is a condition in which there occurs a permanent enlargement of the airspaces distal to the terminal bronchioles. Then, there occurs a decrease in the alveolar surface area available for gas exchange (Fig. 5). There are two mechanisms by which limitation of airflow in the alveoli occurs:

1. First is loss of alveolar walls causing decrease in elastic recoil leading finally to airflow limitation.
2. Secondly, loss of alveolar supporting structure leads to narrowing of airway, which further limits airflow.

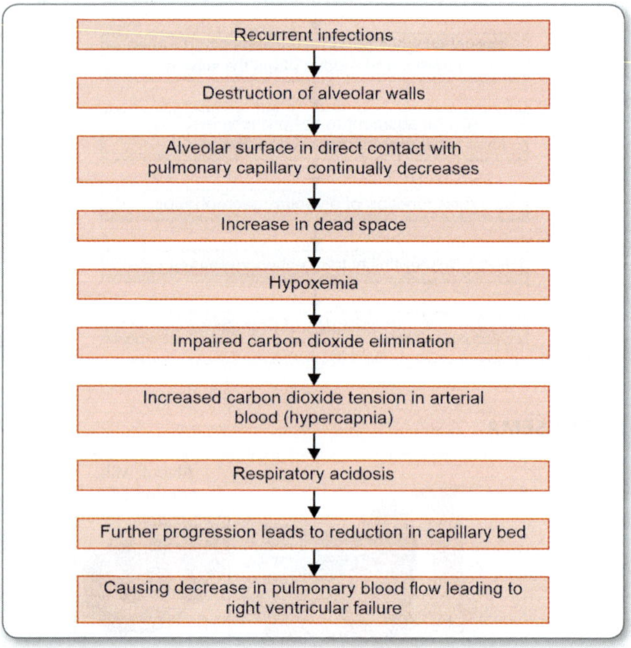

Recurrent infections
↓
Destruction of alveolar walls
↓
Alveolar surface in direct contact with pulmonary capillary continually decreases
↓
Increase in dead space
↓
Hypoxemia
↓
Impaired carbon dioxide elimination
↓
Increased carbon dioxide tension in arterial blood (hypercapnia)
↓
Respiratory acidosis
↓
Further progression leads to reduction in capillary bed
↓
Causing decrease in pulmonary blood flow leading to right ventricular failure

ASTHMA

Asthma is a common pulmonary condition characterized by chronic inflammation of bronchial tubes, tightening of respiratory smooth muscle, and paroxysms of bronchoconstriction.

When an episode of asthma occurs, inflamed airways react to environmental triggers such as smoke, dust, or pollen. The airways narrow and produce excess mucus, making it difficult to breathe. The immune response in the bronchial airways ultimately leads to asthma (Figs 6A to C).

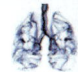

The airways of asthma patients are hypersensitive to certain triggers also known as stimuli. In response to exposure to these triggers, large airways contract into spasm (an asthma attack). Soon, there occurs an inflammation leading to further narrowing of the airways and excessive production of mucus, which leads to coughing and other breathing difficulties. Bronchospasm may resolve spontaneously in 1–2 hours, or in about 50% of patients, may become part of a 'late' response, further causing bronchoconstriction and inflammation about 3–12 hours later.

Regardless of the asthma trigger type, the response is characterized by inflammation, edema, bronchoconstriction, and build-up of mucus in the airways, leading to coughing, wheezing, chest tightness, and shortness of breath.

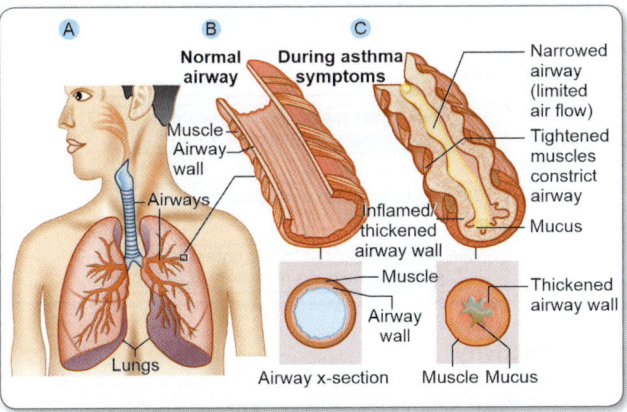

Figs 6A to C: **A.** Airways and lungs; **B.** Normal airway; **C.** During asthma symptoms

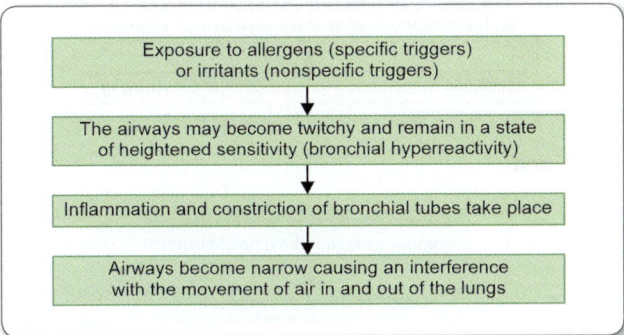

Inflammation

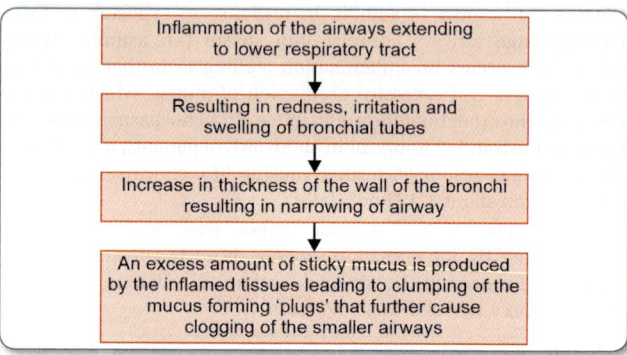

Inflammation of the airways extending to lower respiratory tract

↓

Resulting in redness, irritation and swelling of bronchial tubes

↓

Increase in thickness of the wall of the bronchi resulting in narrowing of airway

↓

An excess amount of sticky mucus is produced by the inflamed tissues leading to clumping of the mucus forming 'plugs' that further cause clogging of the smaller airways

Bronchospasm

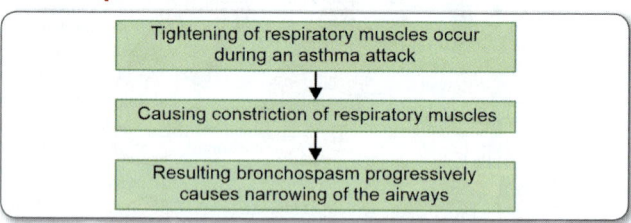

Tightening of respiratory muscles occur during an asthma attack

↓

Causing constriction of respiratory muscles

↓

Resulting bronchospasm progressively causes narrowing of the airways

Hyperreactivity

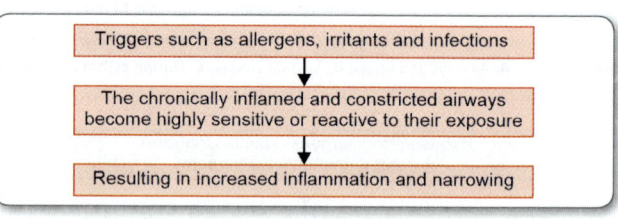

Triggers such as allergens, irritants and infections

↓

The chronically inflamed and constricted airways become highly sensitive or reactive to their exposure

↓

Resulting in increased inflammation and narrowing

Combined

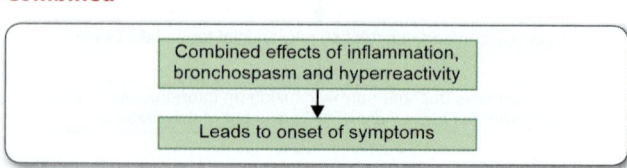

Combined effects of inflammation, bronchospasm and hyperreactivity

↓

Leads to onset of symptoms

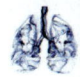

PLEURAL EFFUSION

About 10–20 mL of pleural fluid normally flows between visceral and parietal pleurae. The fluid enters the pleural space from systemic capillaries present in the parietal pleurae and leaves the space through parietal pleural openings. Accumulation of pleural fluid occurs when either too much fluid enters or too little is able to exit the pleural space.

A combination of an increase in hydrostatic pressure and decrease in plasma oncotic pressure leads to **transudative effusions**.

Exudative effusions are caused by an increased capillary permeability leading to exudation of fluid, protein, cells, and other constituents of serum. The most common causes include pneumonia, cancer, pulmonary embolism, viral infection, and tuberculosis.

Transudative Pleural Effusion

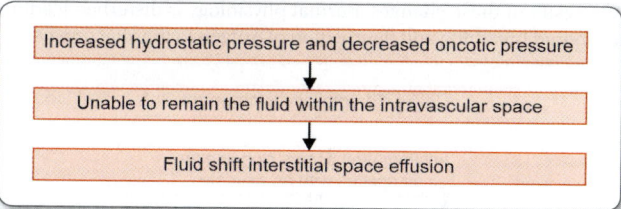

Exudative Effusion

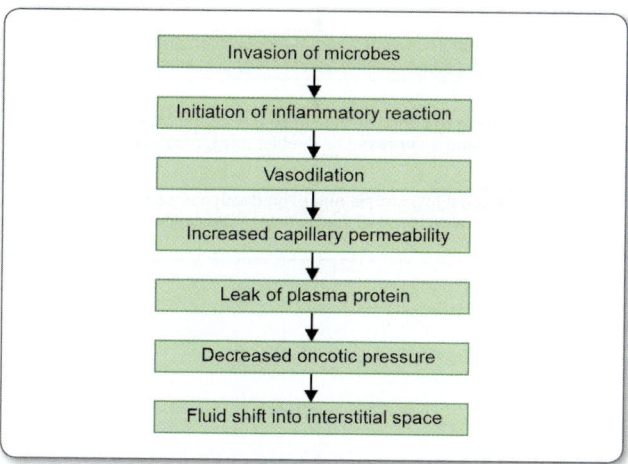

PNEUMONIA

Pneumonia is an infection that causes inflammation of air sacs in one or both the lungs. The alveoli may fill with fluid or pus, causing cough with phlegm, fever, chills, and difficulty in breathing. The organisms like bacteria, viruses and fungi, can cause pneumonia. Since the host's physical defense mechanism is invaded by the infectious organisms, they are thus highly virulent.

Consequently, the macrophages also become overwhelmed by these organisms, leading to the production of fibrin-rich exudate that fills the infected as well as adjacent alveoli. This makes the alveoli stick together acquiring an airless state. Proliferation of neutrophils also occur in response to the inflammation, which further leads to damage of lung tissues, causing fibrosis and pulmonary edema, thereby impairing expansion of the lungs. Pleural effusion also results from the inflammatory response causing reduction in gaseous exchange. As a result of these changes, normal physiology is disturbed leading to labored breathing and deprivation of oxygen to the vital organs.

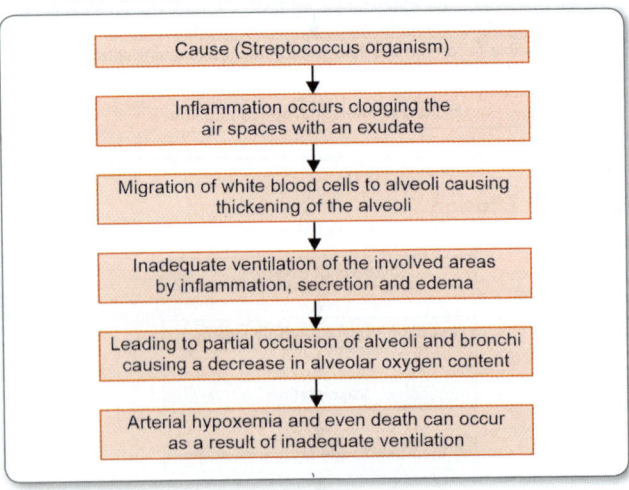

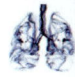

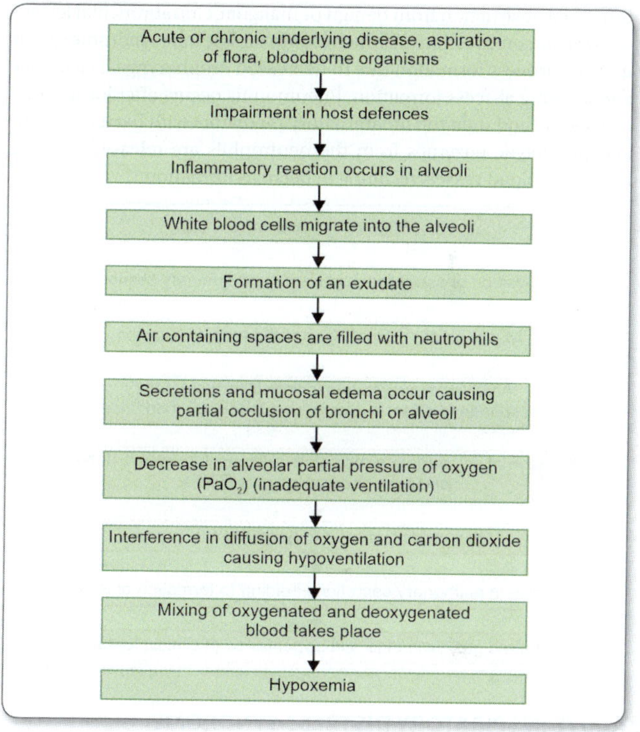

```
┌─────────────────────────────────────────────┐
│  Acute or chronic underlying disease, aspiration │
│         of flora, bloodborne organisms           │
└─────────────────────────────────────────────┘
                       ↓
┌─────────────────────────────────────────────┐
│           Impairment in host defences            │
└─────────────────────────────────────────────┘
                       ↓
┌─────────────────────────────────────────────┐
│      Inflammatory reaction occurs in alveoli     │
└─────────────────────────────────────────────┘
                       ↓
┌─────────────────────────────────────────────┐
│     White blood cells migrate into the alveoli   │
└─────────────────────────────────────────────┘
                       ↓
┌─────────────────────────────────────────────┐
│            Formation of an exudate               │
└─────────────────────────────────────────────┘
                       ↓
┌─────────────────────────────────────────────┐
│  Air containing spaces are filled with neutrophils │
└─────────────────────────────────────────────┘
                       ↓
┌─────────────────────────────────────────────┐
│  Secretions and mucosal edema occur causing      │
│     partial occlusion of bronchi or alveoli      │
└─────────────────────────────────────────────┘
                       ↓
┌─────────────────────────────────────────────┐
│  Decrease in alveolar partial pressure of oxygen │
│        (PaO₂) (inadequate ventilation)           │
└─────────────────────────────────────────────┘
                       ↓
┌─────────────────────────────────────────────┐
│ Interference in diffusion of oxygen and carbon dioxide │
│          causing hypoventilation                 │
└─────────────────────────────────────────────┘
                       ↓
┌─────────────────────────────────────────────┐
│     Mixing of oxygenated and deoxygenated        │
│             blood takes place                    │
└─────────────────────────────────────────────┘
                       ↓
┌─────────────────────────────────────────────┐
│                  Hypoxemia                       │
└─────────────────────────────────────────────┘
```

Decrease in alveolar partial pressure of oxygen (PaO_2) (inadequate ventilation)

LUNG ABSCESS

Lung abscess is defined as necrosis of the pulmonary tissue and formation of cavities containing necrotic debris or fluid caused by microbial infection. The formation of multiple small (<2 cm) abscesses is occasionally referred to as necrotizing pneumonia or lung gangrene. It is commonly caused by aspiration of anaerobic bacteria from oropharynx in patients who are unconscious, have an absence of gag reflex or have an inability to swallow. The defense mechanisms in the healthy individuals are able to cope with the small amounts of aspirates without any serious effects but patients with alcoholism, diabetes mellitus and immunocompromised status will have a decline in the activity of alveolar macrophages and leukocyte mobility.

In secondary lung abscess, abscess formation depends on the underlying lung disease and predisposing factors, for example,

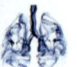

bronchial obstruction from benign or malignant intrabronchial lesions or extrinsic compression of bronchus as in middle lobe syndrome results in distal abscess formation due to decreased oropharyngeal clearance and favoring abscess formation. Pneumonitis occurs after localization of aspirate, and then the inflammatory mediators with bacterial toxins and proteolytic enzymes from the neutrophils are released, causing rupture of blood vessels resulting in necrosis formation.

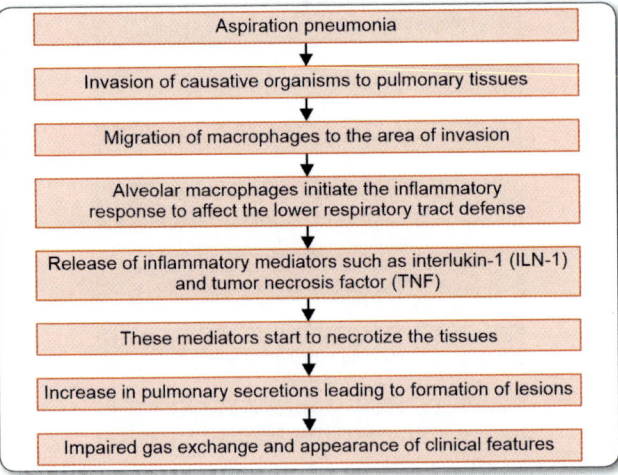

ACUTE RESPIRATORY DISTRESS SYNDROME

The ARDS (Fig. 7) occurs when fluid builds up in the alveoli of lungs. This causes reduction in air entry into the lungs and thus there is deficit in oxygenation of blood. The pathophysiology of ARDS is characterized by pulmonary edema, decreased lung compliance and arterial hypoxemia. The triggers of ARDS include endothelial cells and polymorphonuclear neutrophils. The interaction of these cells leads to binding of leukocytes, transendothelial migration and injury to the lungs.

This injury to the lungs leads to release of mediators including oxidants and proteases, elastase being the significant in case of pulmonary injury. The potential targets of these mediators are endothelial cell membrane, glycocalyx and basement membrane. Destruction of these elements appears to be responsible for increased pulmonary microvascular permeability and lung edema formation and may also facilitate neutrophil-transendothelial migration.

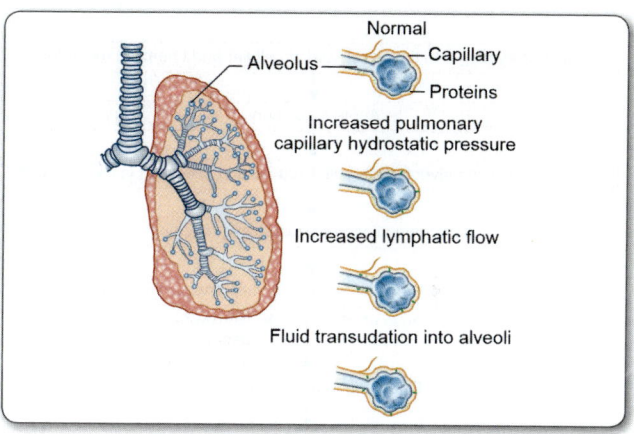

Fig. 7: Acute respiratory distress syndrome

Stages of Edema Formation in Acute Respiratory Distress Syndrome (ARDS)

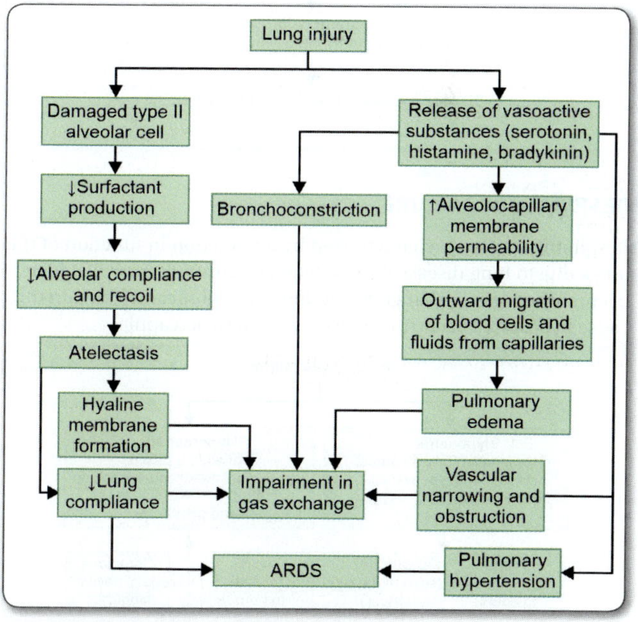

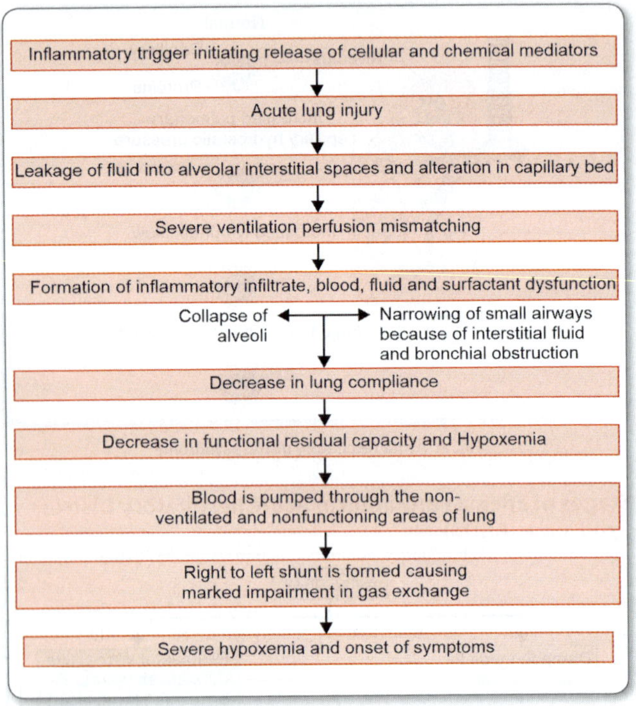

Inflammatory trigger initiating release of cellular and chemical mediators

↓

Acute lung injury

↓

Leakage of fluid into alveolar interstitial spaces and alteration in capillary bed

↓

Severe ventilation perfusion mismatching

↓

Formation of inflammatory infiltrate, blood, fluid and surfactant dysfunction

Collapse of ← → Narrowing of small airways
alveoli   because of interstitial fluid
                  and bronchial obstruction

Decrease in lung compliance

↓

Decrease in functional residual capacity and Hypoxemia

↓

Blood is pumped through the non-ventilated and nonfunctioning areas of lung

↓

Right to left shunt is formed causing marked impairment in gas exchange

↓

Severe hypoxemia and onset of symptoms

RESPIRATORY FAILURE

Respiratory failure is characterized by a reduction in function of the lungs due to lung disease or a skeletal or neuromuscular disorder. It occurs when gas exchange at the lungs is significantly impaired to cause hypoxemia occurring with or without hypercapnia.

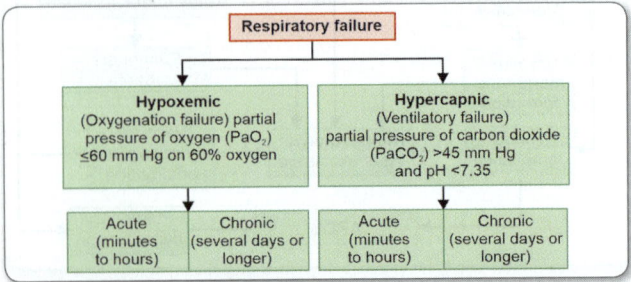

Respiratory failure

Hypoxemic
(Oxygenation failure) partial pressure of oxygen (PaO_2) ≤60 mm Hg on 60% oxygen

Hypercapnic
(Ventilatory failure) partial pressure of carbon dioxide ($PaCO_2$) >45 mm Hg and pH <7.35

Acute (minutes to hours) | Chronic (several days or longer)

Acute (minutes to hours) | Chronic (several days or longer)

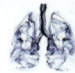

Hypoxemic Respiratory Failure

Causes

- **Ventilation-perfusion (V/Q) mismatch:**
  - COPD
  - Pneumonia
  - Asthma
  - Atelectasis
  - Pulmonary embolus
- **Range of V/Q relationships:**
  - Normal V/Q = 1 (1 mL air/1 mL of blood)
  - Ventilation = lungs
  - Perfusion or Q = perfusion
  - Pulmonary embolus (VQ scan)
- **Shunt:**
  - Anatomic—passes through an anatomic channel of the heart and does not pass through the lungs, e.g. ventricular septal defect
  - Intrapulmonary shunt—blood flows through pulmonary capillaries without participating in gas exchange, e.g. alveoli filled with fluid

    * Patients with shunts are more hypoxemic than those with VQ mismatch and they may require mechanical ventilators
- **Diffusion limitation:** Gas exchange is compromised by a process that thickens or destroys the membrane
  - Severe emphysema
  - Recurrent pulmonary emboli
  - Pulmonary fibrosis

    * A classic sign of diffusion limitation is hypoxemia during exercise but not at rest
- **Alveolar hypoventilation:** Mainly due to hypercapnic respiratory failure but can cause hypoxemia. The conditions are:
  - Restrictive lung disease
  - Central nervous system disease
  - Chest wall dysfunction
  - Neuromuscular disease
- **Interrelationship of mechanisms:**
  - Combination of two or more physiologic mechanisms

Hypercapnic Respiratory Failure

Causes

- Imbalance between ventilatory supply and demand
- **Airways and alveoli:** Air flow obstruction and air trapping
  - Asthma
  - Emphysema
  - Chronic bronchitis
  - Cystic fibrosis
- **Central nervous system:**
  - Drug overdose
  - Brainstem infarction
  - Spinal cord injuries
- **Chest wall:**
  - Flail chest
  - Fractures
  - Mechanical restriction
  - Muscle spasm
- **Neuromuscular conditions:**
  - Muscular dystrophy
  - Multiple sclerosis

Cause 1: Decreased respiratory drive

Severe brain injury, large lesions of brain stem, use of sedatives and metabolic disorders such as hypothyroidism

↓

Impair the normal response of chemoreceptors in brain to normal respiratory stimulation

↓

Impairment leads to decreased respiratory drive

Cause 2: Dysfunction of chest wall

Musculoskeletal disorders, neuromuscular junction disorders and spinal cord disorders

↓

Affect the pathway of impulses arising in respiratory center and traveling through the nerves extending from brain to spinal cord to receptors in muscles of respiration

↓

Hypoventilation and onset of symptoms

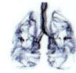

Cause 3: Dysfunction of lung parenchyma

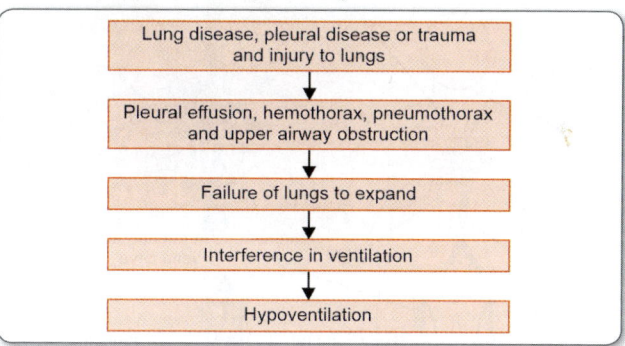

Cause 4: Other causes

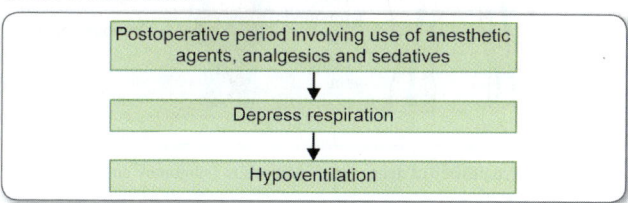

PULMONARY EMBOLISM

Once a thrombus separates from its site of origin, it travels through the circulation to the inferior vena cava. From the inferior vena cava, it then passes through the right ventricle, which pumps the thrombus into the pulmonary arteries where it finally lodges. Once a pulmonary embolism has lodged in an artery, a disruption of both pulmonary hemodynamics and gas exchange occurs (Fig. 8).

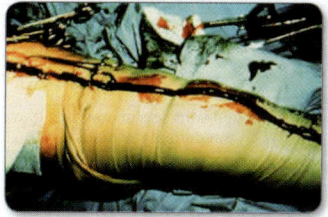

Fig. 8: Deep vein thrombosis

At least 90% of pulmonary emboli originate from major leg veins (Fig. 9).

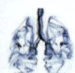

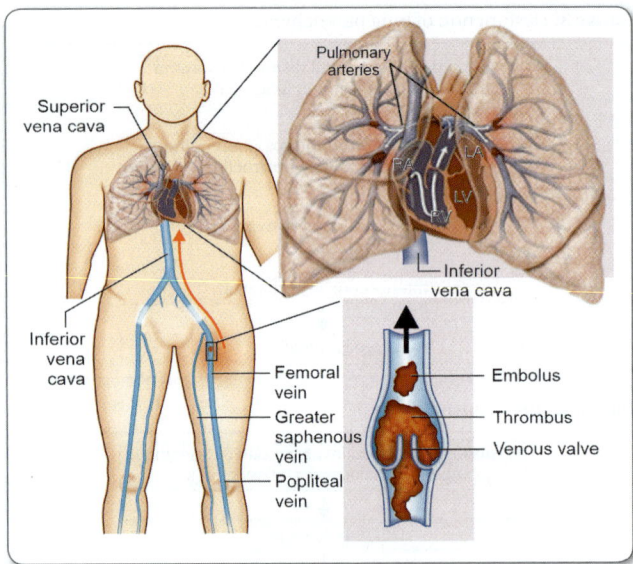

Fig. 9: Progression of deep vein thrombosis to pulmonary embolism

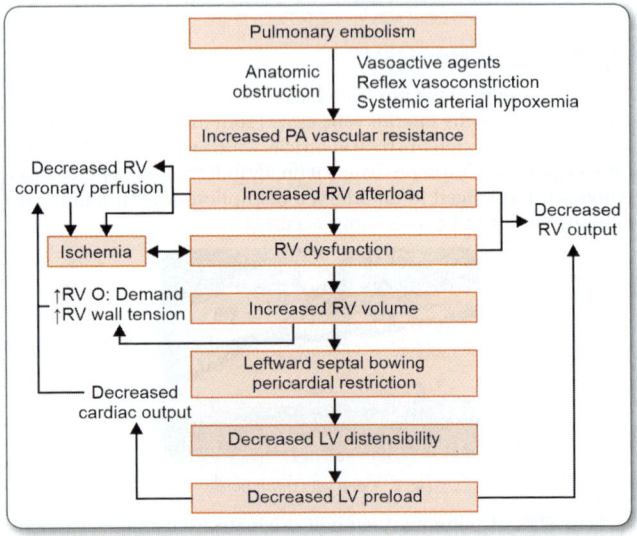

Abbreviations: LV, left ventricular; PA, pulmonary arterial; RV, right ventricular

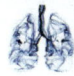

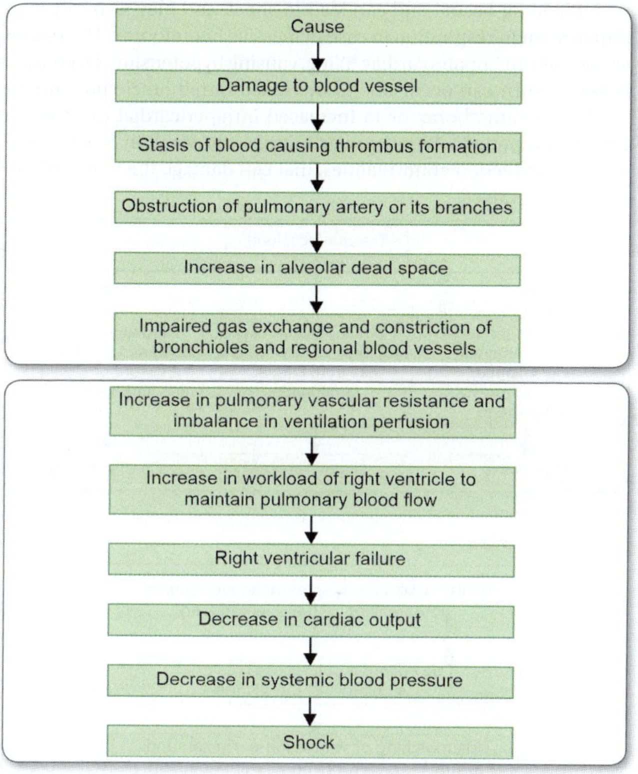

```
                    ┌─────────────────────────────┐
                    │            Cause            │
                    └─────────────────────────────┘
                                   ↓
                    ┌─────────────────────────────┐
                    │    Damage to blood vessel   │
                    └─────────────────────────────┘
                                   ↓
                 ┌────────────────────────────────────┐
                 │ Stasis of blood causing thrombus   │
                 │            formation               │
                 └────────────────────────────────────┘
                                   ↓
             ┌────────────────────────────────────────────┐
             │ Obstruction of pulmonary artery or its     │
             │                branches                    │
             └────────────────────────────────────────────┘
                                   ↓
                 ┌────────────────────────────────────┐
                 │  Increase in alveolar dead space   │
                 └────────────────────────────────────┘
                                   ↓
             ┌────────────────────────────────────────────┐
             │ Impaired gas exchange and constriction of  │
             │  bronchioles and regional blood vessels    │
             └────────────────────────────────────────────┘
```

```
           ┌────────────────────────────────────────────┐
           │ Increase in pulmonary vascular resistance  │
           │    and imbalance in ventilation perfusion  │
           └────────────────────────────────────────────┘
                                   ↓
           ┌────────────────────────────────────────────┐
           │  Increase in workload of right ventricle   │
           │     to maintain pulmonary blood flow       │
           └────────────────────────────────────────────┘
                                   ↓
                 ┌────────────────────────────────────┐
                 │     Right ventricular failure      │
                 └────────────────────────────────────┘
                                   ↓
                 ┌────────────────────────────────────┐
                 │     Decrease in cardiac output     │
                 └────────────────────────────────────┘
                                   ↓
             ┌────────────────────────────────────────────┐
             │  Decrease in systemic blood pressure       │
             └────────────────────────────────────────────┘
                                   ↓
                 ┌────────────────────────────────────┐
                 │                Shock               │
                 └────────────────────────────────────┘
```

CHEST INJURIES

Chest injuries have a high rate of morbidity and mortality as these primarily interfere with respiration, circulation or both.

The direct damage to the lungs or airways or alteration in breathing mechanism are mainly responsible for causing respiratory compromise.

Injuries that directly damage the lung or airways include pulmonary contusion and tracheobronchial disruption. Chest injuries that cause alteration in breathing include hemothorax, pneumothorax and flail chest. Both respiration and circulation are impaired in tension pneumothorax.

Circulation can be impaired by bleeding, decreased venous return and direct cardiac injury.

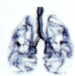

Bleeding occurs and can lead to shock and may also cause an impairment in respiration in case of massive hemothorax. Decreased venous return impairs cardiac filling, causing hypotension. Decreased venous return can occur due to increased intrathoracic pressure in tension pneumothorax or to increased intrapericardial pressure in cardiac tamponade. Blunt cardiac injuries can result in heart failure and/or conduction abnormalities, that can damage the myocardium or the heart valves.

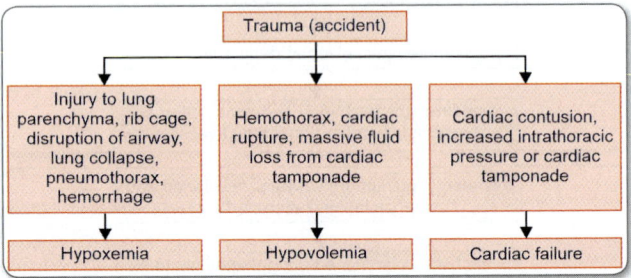

Pneumothorax

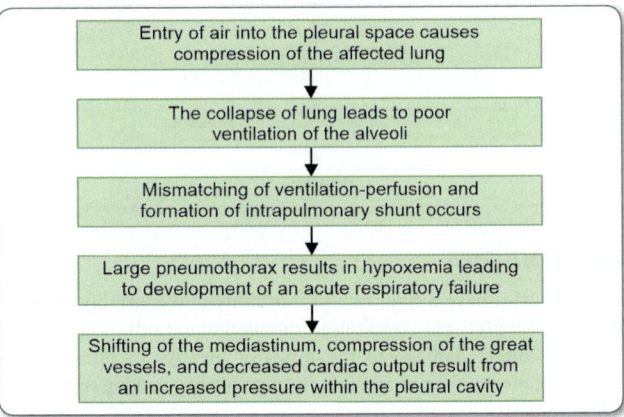

TUBERCULOSIS

The four possible outcomes that occur because of inhalation of *Mycobacterium tuberculosis* are:

- Immediate clearance of the organism
- Latent infection

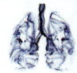

- The onset of active disease (primary disease)
- Active disease many years later (reactivation disease)

Primary Disease

The tubercle bacilli carried in the droplets reach the alveolar spaces and initiate infection. In case, there is a failure of the host defense mechanism, multiplication of bacilli occurs in the alveolar macrophages, eventually killing the cells. The cytokines are then produced by the infected macrophages that attract other phagocytic cells, leading to the formation of tubercle. An uncontrolled replication of bacteria causes an enlargement of tubercle and entry of bacilli in the lymph nodes. This leads to lymphadenopathy, a characteristic clinical manifestation of primary tuberculosis (TB). This expansion of the tubercle into the lung parenchyma and involvement of lymph nodes forms a lesion called as Ghon's complex.

Disseminated TB, also known as miliary TB, is produced by hematogenous spread of bacilli caused by an unrestricted growth of bacteria. Repeated episodes of healing by fibrotic changes around the lesions and breakdown of tissues are responsible for chronic disease.

Reactivation Disease

Reactivation TB results from multiplication of a formerly dormant bacterium fixed in the lungs at the time of the primary infection. A localized disease process occurs in reactivation TB with very less involvement of lymph nodes and formation of lesion (Fig. 10).

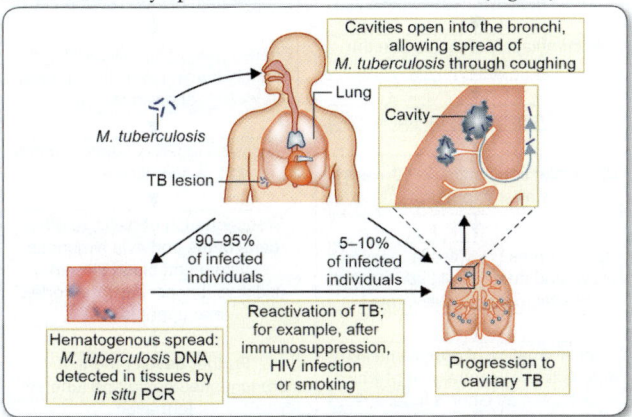

Fig. 10: Progression of tuberculosis

Abbreviations: DNA, deoxyribonucleic acid, HIV, human immunodeficiency virus; PCR, polymerase chain reaction; TB, tuberculosis

Susceptible
or
Mycobacterium tuberculosis
Latent infection
Recovery
Reactivation
Pulmonary tuberculosis
Active tuberculosis
Extrapulmonary tuberculosis
Miliary tuberculosis

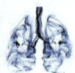

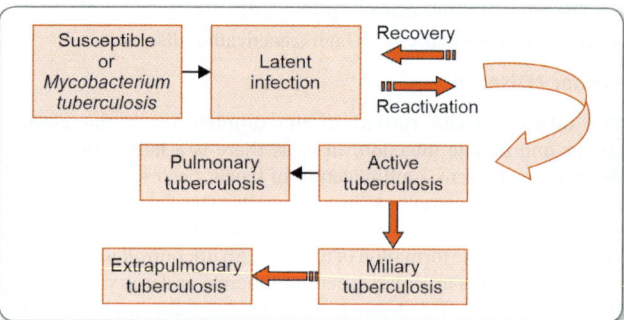

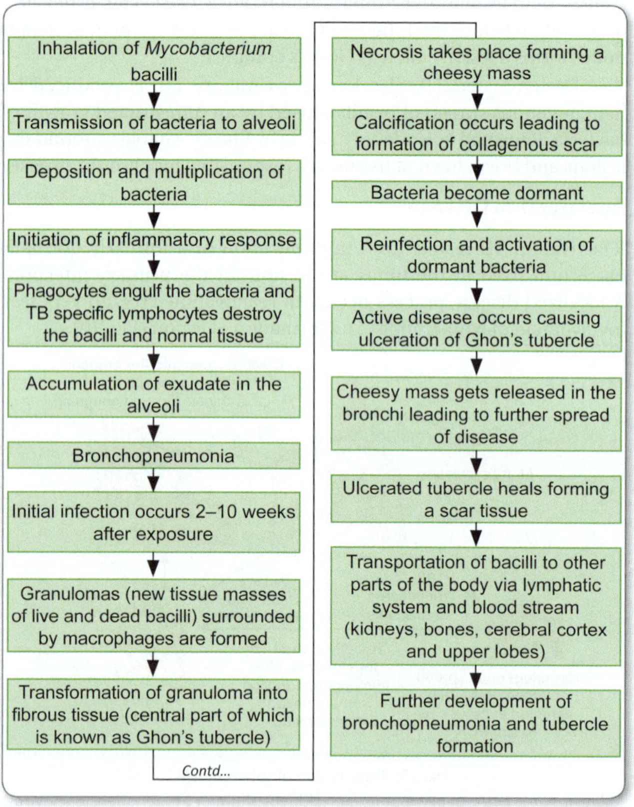

Inhalation of *Mycobacterium* bacilli
Transmission of bacteria to alveoli
Deposition and multiplication of bacteria
Initiation of inflammatory response
Phagocytes engulf the bacteria and TB specific lymphocytes destroy the bacilli and normal tissue
Accumulation of exudate in the alveoli
Bronchopneumonia
Initial infection occurs 2–10 weeks after exposure
Granulomas (new tissue masses of live and dead bacilli) surrounded by macrophages are formed
Transformation of granuloma into fibrous tissue (central part of which is known as Ghon's tubercle)
Contd...
Necrosis takes place forming a cheesy mass
Calcification occurs leading to formation of collagenous scar
Bacteria become dormant
Reinfection and activation of dormant bacteria
Active disease occurs causing ulceration of Ghon's tubercle
Cheesy mass gets released in the bronchi leading to further spread of disease
Ulcerated tubercle heals forming a scar tissue
Transportation of bacilli to other parts of the body via lymphatic system and blood stream (kidneys, bones, cerebral cortex and upper lobes)
Further development of bronchopneumonia and tubercle formation

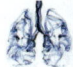

ATELECTASIS

Atelectasis describes the loss of lung volume due to the collapse of lung tissue. It can be classified according to the pathophysiologic mechanism, i.e., compressive atelectasis, the amount of lung involved, e.g., lobar, segmental, or subsegmental atelectasis, or the location, i.e., specific lobe or segment location.

Obstructive

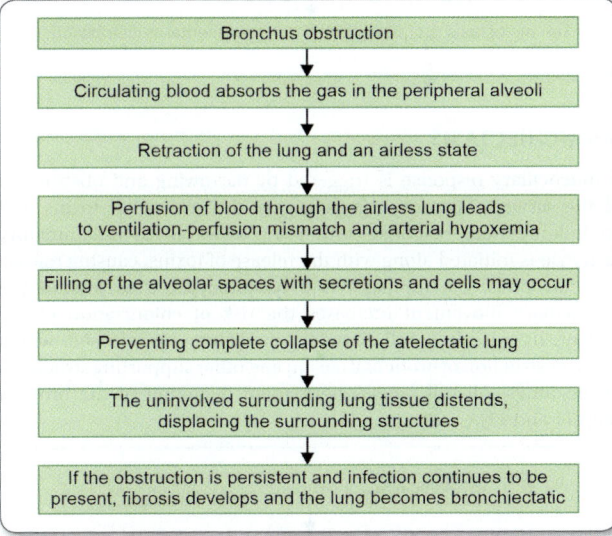

Bronchus obstruction

↓

Circulating blood absorbs the gas in the peripheral alveoli

↓

Retraction of the lung and an airless state

↓

Perfusion of blood through the airless lung leads to ventilation-perfusion mismatch and arterial hypoxemia

↓

Filling of the alveolar spaces with secretions and cells may occur

↓

Preventing complete collapse of the atelectatic lung

↓

The uninvolved surrounding lung tissue distends, displacing the surrounding structures

↓

If the obstruction is persistent and infection continues to be present, fibrosis develops and the lung becomes bronchiectatic

Nonobstructive

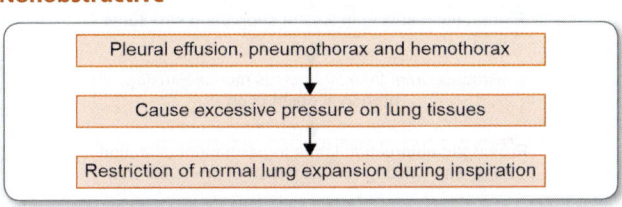

Pleural effusion, pneumothorax and hemothorax

↓

Cause excessive pressure on lung tissues

↓

Restriction of normal lung expansion during inspiration

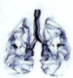

Postoperative Atelectasis

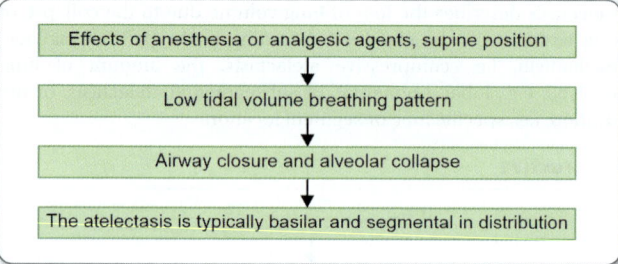

Effects of anesthesia or analgesic agents, supine position

Low tidal volume breathing pattern

Airway closure and alveolar collapse

The atelectasis is typically basilar and segmental in distribution

BRONCHIECTASIS

A mucociliary response is triggered by narrowing and obstruction of the airway. Microorganisms trigger the release of toxins and an inflammatory response within the airways. An inflammatory response is initiated along with the release of toxins, causing release of neutrophils, macrophages and lymphocytes. This loss in the mucociliary movement increases the risk of colonization of the airways by microbes. Inflammatory mediators are released, which cause destruction of bronchial elastin and other supporting structures of the lungs. All this causes permanent dilatation of the bronchi (Figs 11 and 12).

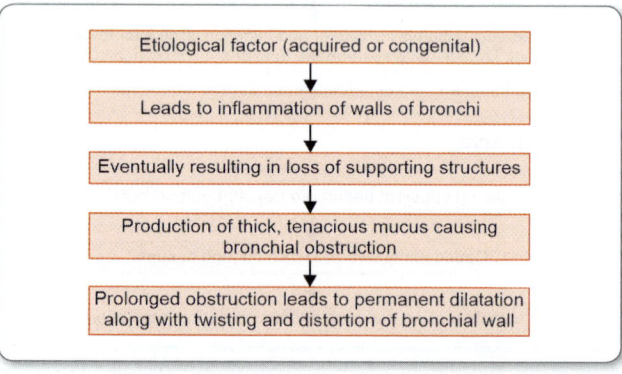

Etiological factor (acquired or congenital)

Leads to inflammation of walls of bronchi

Eventually resulting in loss of supporting structures

Production of thick, tenacious mucus causing bronchial obstruction

Prolonged obstruction leads to permanent dilatation along with twisting and distortion of bronchial wall

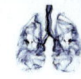

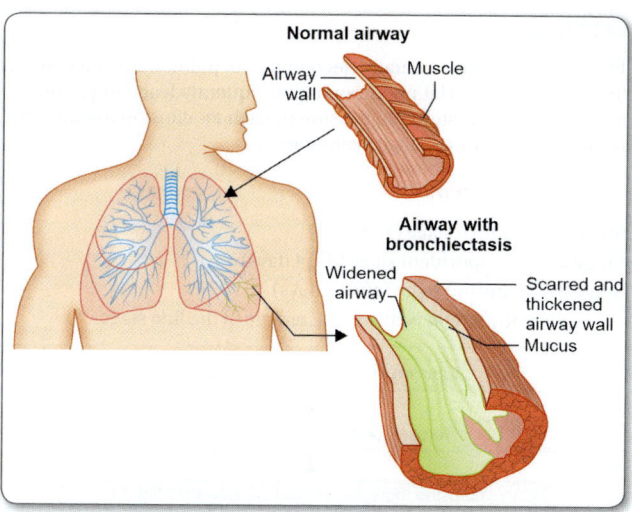

Fig. 11: Comparison between normal airway and airway with bronchiectasis

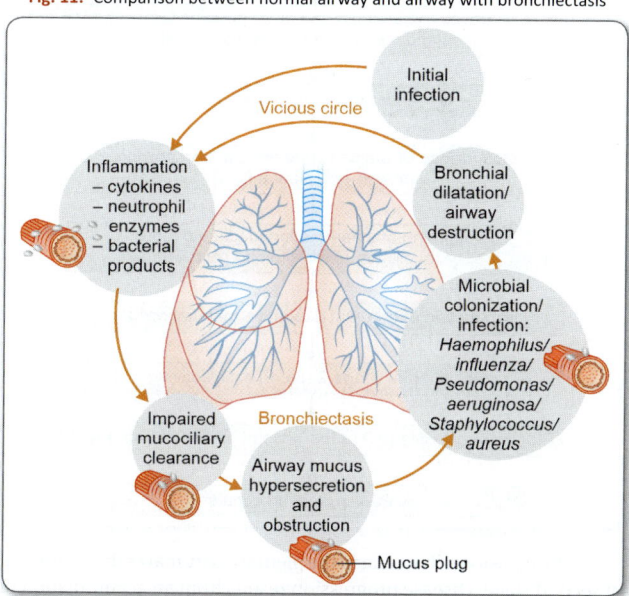

Fig. 12: Vicious circle of bronchiectasis

EMPYEMA

Pleural empyema is usually secondary to pulmonary infection at another site. Bacterial pneumonia consequently leads to parapneumonic pleural effusion. Progression of such an effusion to empyema is said to have a three-stage evolution.

Stages of Empyema

Stage 1: Exudative stage (1–3 days)
Stage 2: Fibrinopurulent stage (4–14 days)
Stage 3: Organizing stage (after 1 days)
An exudate formation is the characteristic of the first stage.

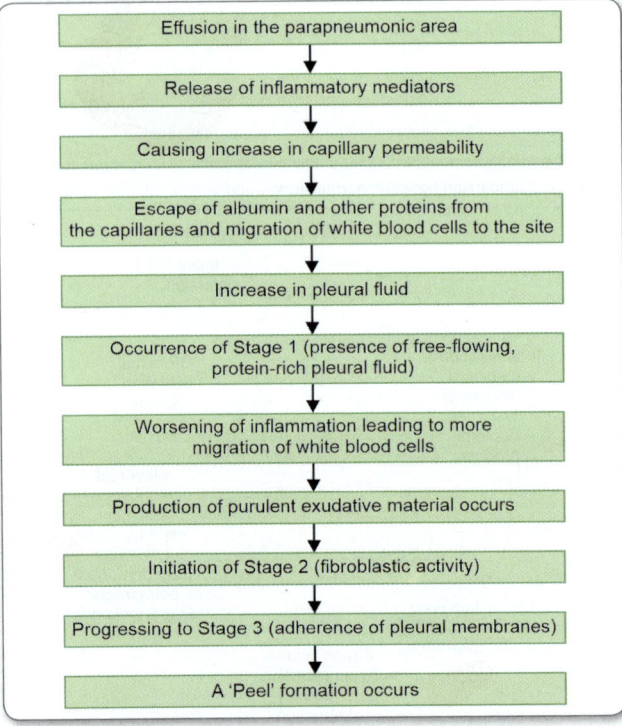

Effusion in the parapneumonic area

↓

Release of inflammatory mediators

↓

Causing increase in capillary permeability

↓

Escape of albumin and other proteins from the capillaries and migration of white blood cells to the site

↓

Increase in pleural fluid

↓

Occurrence of Stage 1 (presence of free-flowing, protein-rich pleural fluid)

↓

Worsening of inflammation leading to more migration of white blood cells

↓

Production of purulent exudative material occurs

↓

Initiation of Stage 2 (fibroblastic activity)

↓

Progressing to Stage 3 (adherence of pleural membranes)

↓

A 'Peel' formation occurs

The invasion of bacteria in the pleural cavity marks the beginning of second stage. Disease progression results from an accumulation of neutrophils along with the deposition of fibrin. The pH of pleural fluid

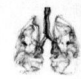

and concentration of glucose decrease, whereas there is an increase in the concentration of lactic acid dehydrogenase.

The third stage is characterized by organization. There is a growth of fibroblasts into the exudate within the pleural surfaces. A restriction in respiration occurs by the formation of the *pleural peel* that encases the lung. A pleurocutaneous or a bronchopleural fistula may be produced by a spontaneous drainage of the thick tenaceous exudate through the chest wall.

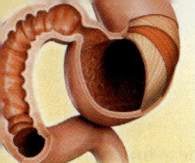

Pathophysiology of Gastrointestinal Disorders

INTRODUCTION

The digestive tract is a tube starting from the mouth to the anus along with the associated organs, which secrete fluids into the digestive tract. Technically gastrointestinal tract is the term that only refers to the stomach and intestine but is often used as the other name of digestive tract. The internal environment of the digestive tract is continuous with the external environment at the opening of the mouth and anus. Nutrients enter the circulation by crossing the wall of the digestive tract.

The digestive tract extends from the oral cavity, through the pharynx, esophagus, stomach, small intestine, large intestine, and ends in anus. There are accessory glands, which are associated with the digestive tract. The salivary glands open into the oral cavity, and the liver and pancreas are connected to the small intestine.

The primary function of the digestive tract is to break down food into nutrients, which can be absorbed by the body so as to provide energy. Firstly, food must be ingested by the mouth to get mechanically processed and moistened. Secondly, digestion occurs mainly in the stomach and small intestine where proteins, fats and carbohydrates are chemically broken down into their basic building blocks. Smaller molecules are then absorbed across the epithelium of the small intestine and subsequently enter the circulation. The large intestine plays a key role in reabsorbing excess water. Finally, undigested material and secreted waste products are excreted from the body via defecation (passing of feces).

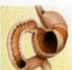

In case of gastrointestinal diseases or disorders, these functions of the gastrointestinal tract get altered (Fig. 1).

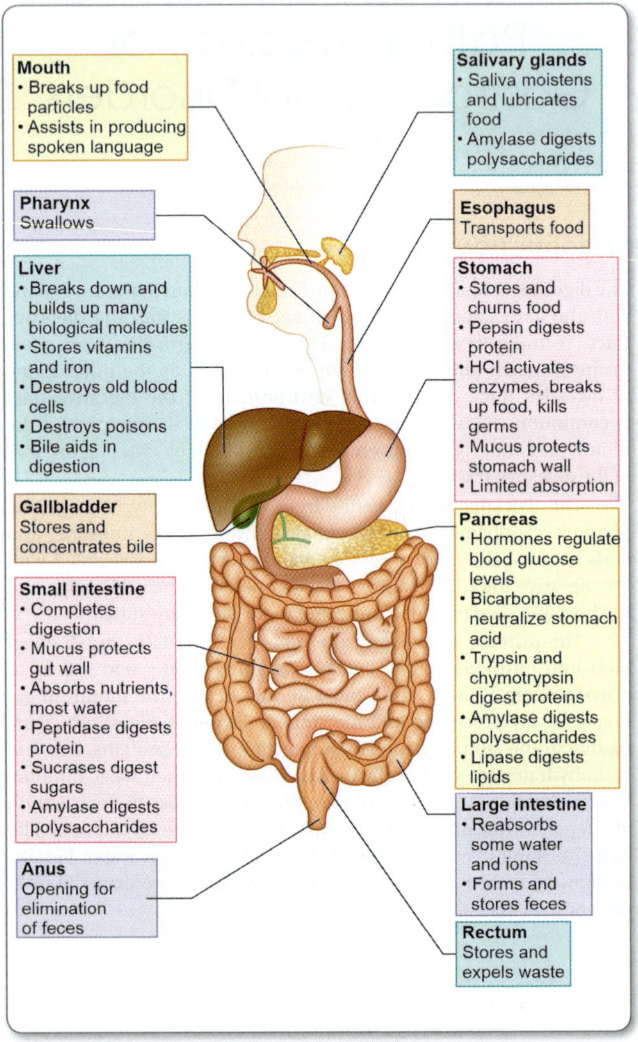

Mouth
• Breaks up food particles
• Assists in producing spoken language

Salivary glands
• Saliva moistens and lubricates food
• Amylase digests polysaccharides

Pharynx
Swallows

Esophagus
Transports food

Liver
• Breaks down and builds up many biological molecules
• Stores vitamins and iron
• Destroys old blood cells
• Destroys poisons
• Bile aids in digestion

Stomach
• Stores and churns food
• Pepsin digests protein
• HCl activates enzymes, breaks up food, kills germs
• Mucus protects stomach wall
• Limited absorption

Gallbladder
Stores and concentrates bile

Pancreas
• Hormones regulate blood glucose levels
• Bicarbonates neutralize stomach acid
• Trypsin and chymotrypsin digest proteins
• Amylase digests polysaccharides
• Lipase digests lipids

Small intestine
• Completes digestion
• Mucus protects gut wall
• Absorbs nutrients, most water
• Peptidase digests protein
• Sucrases digest sugars
• Amylase digests polysaccharides

Large intestine
• Reabsorbs some water and ions
• Forms and stores feces

Anus
Opening for elimination of feces

Rectum
Stores and expels waste

Fig. 1: Functions of gastrointestinal system

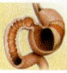
GASTRITIS

Gastritis involves inflammation of mucosal lining of stomach. It produces inflammation via the production of a number of toxins and enzymes. The intense inflammation can result in the loss of gastric glands. Consequently, gastric acid production drops.

The stomach has a protective lining of mucus called the mucosa. It protects the stomach from the strong stomach acid that digests food. When something damages or weakens this protective lining, the mucosa becomes inflamed, causing gastritis. A type of bacteria called *Helicobacter pylori (H. pylori)* is the most common bacterial cause of gastritis.

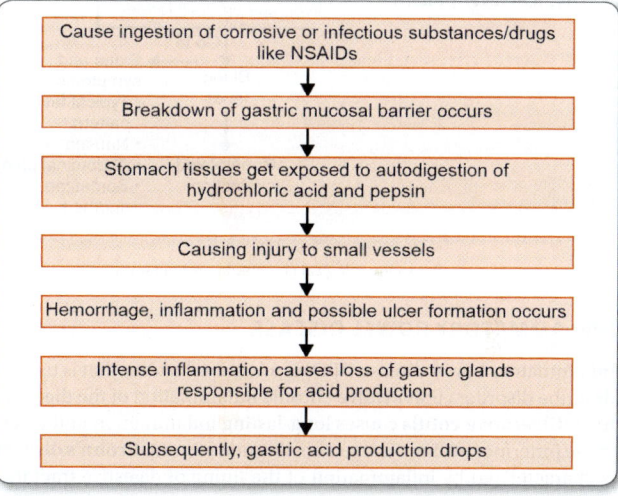

Abbreviation: NSAIDs, nonsteroidal anti-inflammatory drugs

TYPHOID FEVER

Typhoid fever also termed as Enteric fever is caused by *Salmonella typhi* leading to multisystem illness. Salmonellosis is a foodborne disease that spreads by the ingestion of contaminated food. The epithelial layer of small bowel is penetrated by salmonella after ingestion, which then enters the lymphoid tissue and later gets disseminated through the lymphatic or the hematogenous route. The proximal part of the colon is mainly affected by this infection leading to ulceration and bleeding (Fig. 2).

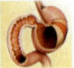

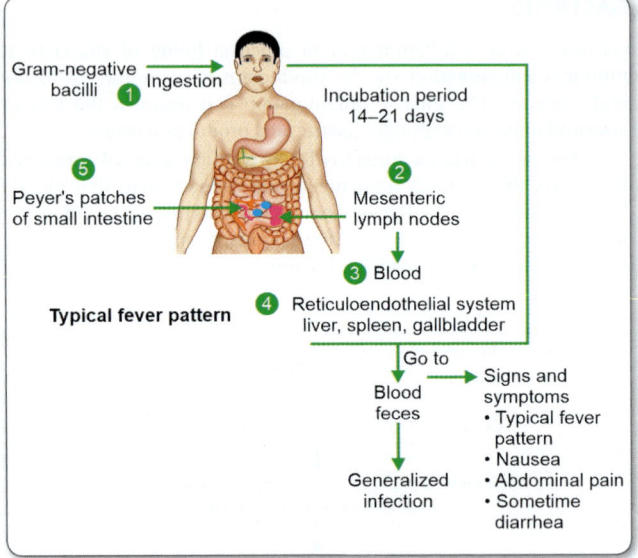

Fig. 2: Pathophysiological changes in typhoid fever

INFLAMMATORY BOWEL DISEASE

Inflammatory bowel disease (IBD) is an umbrella term that is used to describe disorders that involve chronic inflammation of the digestive tract. **Ulcerative colitis** causes long-lasting inflammation and ulcers in the innermost lining of large intestine and rectum. **Crohn's disease** is characterized by inflammation of the lining of digestive tract that spreads deep into affected tissues.

Subacute and chronic inflammation, which affects all layers of the bowel wall from the intestinal mucosa is called regional enteritis (Fig. 3). In the beginning of the disease process, edema and thickening of the mucosa occurs and ulcers appear on the inflamed mucosa later. These lesions appear as skip lesions. As the inflammation spreads into the peritoneum, fistulas, fissures, and abscesses are formed. In the advance stage, the bowel wall thickens and becomes fibrotic, and the intestinal lumen narrows. Affected bowel loops sometimes stick to other loops surrounding them.

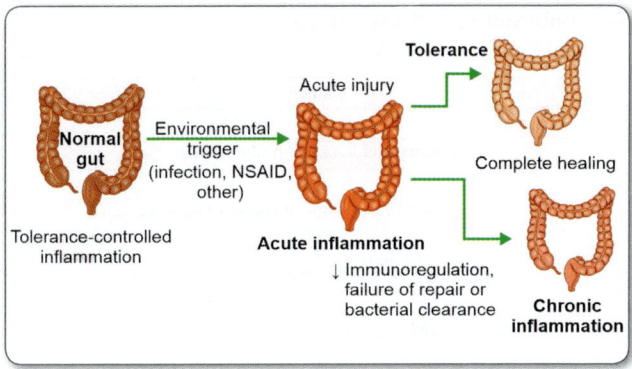

Fig. 3: Normal gut, acute inflammation and chronic inflammation

Pathophysiology: Crohn's Disease

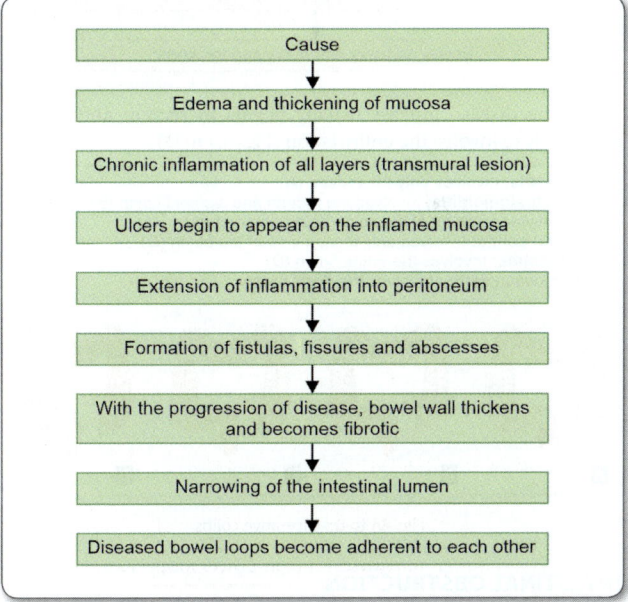

Pathophysiology: Ulcerative Colitis

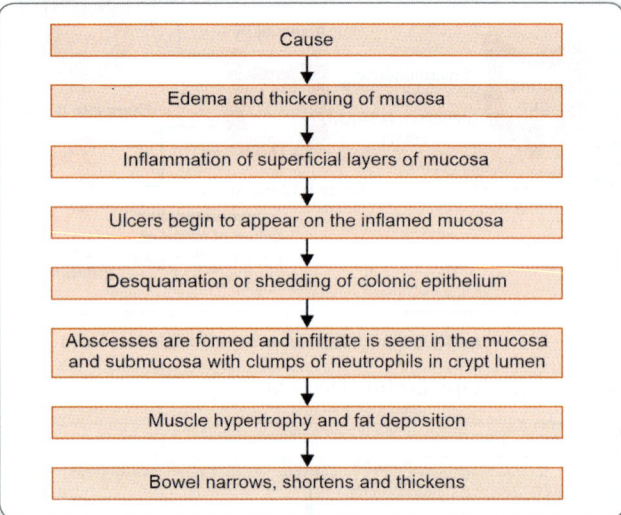

Note: The disease process usually begins in rectum and spreads proximally to involve the entire colon (Figs 4A to D).

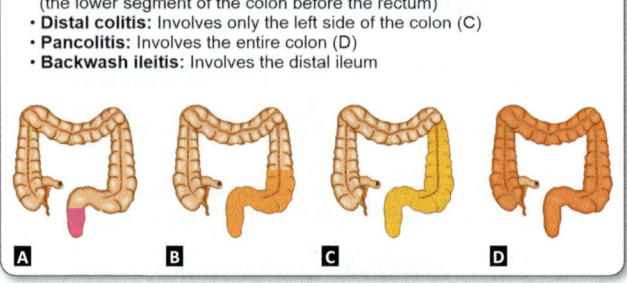

Figs 4A to D: Ulcerative colitis

INTESTINAL OBSTRUCTION

It is a significant mechanical impairment or a complete arrest of the passage of contents through the intestine due to blockage of the bowel.

Small Intestinal Obstruction

Intestinal contents, fluid and gas accumulate above the intestinal obstruction. Gastric secretion is stimulated more by the reduction of the absorption of fluid caused due to abdominal distention and retention of fluid. Pressure within the intestinal lumen is increased with the increasing distention, leading to a decrease in venous and arteriolar capillary pressure. This may cause edema, congestion, necrosis, and eventual rupture or perforation of the intestinal wall, which may result in resultant peritonitis.

Vomiting, caused because of abdominal distention, results in a loss of hydrogen ions and potassium from the stomach. This loss causes a reduction of chlorides and potassium in the blood and leads to metabolic alkalosis. Loss of water and sodium causes dehydration and acidosis. Hypovolemic shock may occur because of acute fluid losses.

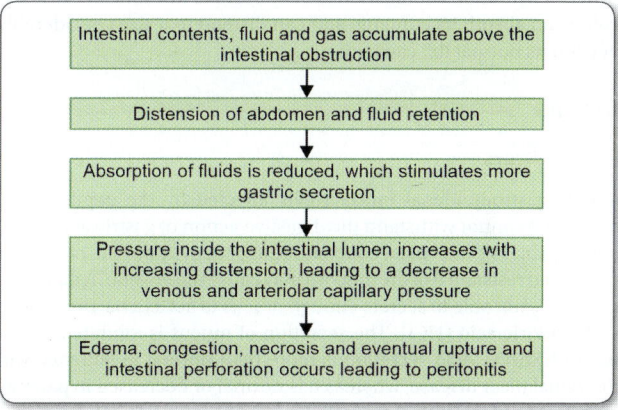

Large Intestinal Obstruction

Large bowel (intestinal) obstruction occurs when there is a blockage in the colon or rectum that prevents food or gas from passing through. The normal secretory and absorptive functions of the mucosa are depressed, and the bowel wall becomes edematous and congested. If the blockage and swelling are severe, the bowel can rupture, or the blood supply to the bowel can be cut off leading to bowel death.

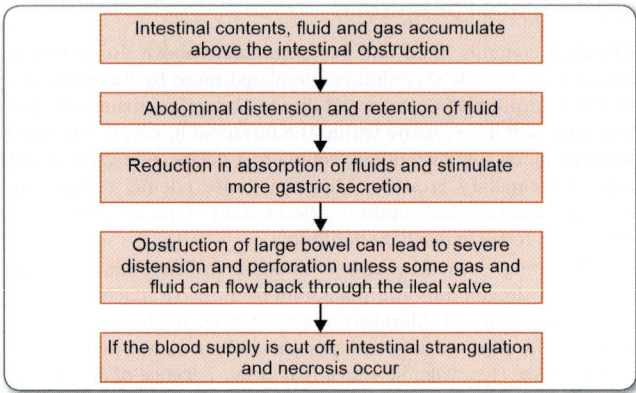

Note: Dehydration occurs more slowly in small intestine because the colon can absorb its contents and can distend to a size considerably beyond its normal full capacity.

ULCERS

Peptic Ulcers

Mainly gastroduodenal mucosa gets affected by the peptic ulcers because it cannot withstand the digestive action of gastric acid (HCl) and pepsin. The increased concentration or activity of acid–pepsin, or decreased resistance of the mucosa may cause the erosion. A damaged mucosa is not able to secrete enough mucus to act as a barrier against hydrochloric acid (HCl). The secretion of mucus is inhibited by the use of NSAIDs. Acid secretion is more than normal in patients with duodenal ulcer disease, whereas it is normal or decreased in patients with gastric ulcer (Fig. 5).

Acute mucosal ulceration of the duodenal or gastric area is called Stress ulcer that occurs after stressful events, such as burns, shock, severe sepsis and multiple organ traumas (Fig. 6).

These stress ulcers should be distinguished from Cushing's ulcers and Curling's ulcers. Cushing's ulcers are common in patients with trauma to the brain. These ulcers affect esophagus, stomach, or duodenum. These are usually deeper and more penetrating than stress ulcers. Curling's ulcer is frequently observed about 72 hours after extensive burns. It involves the antrum of the stomach or the duodenum.

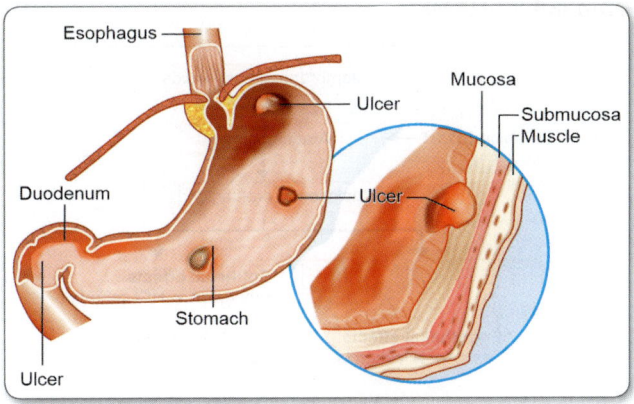

Fig. 5: Peptic ulcer disease

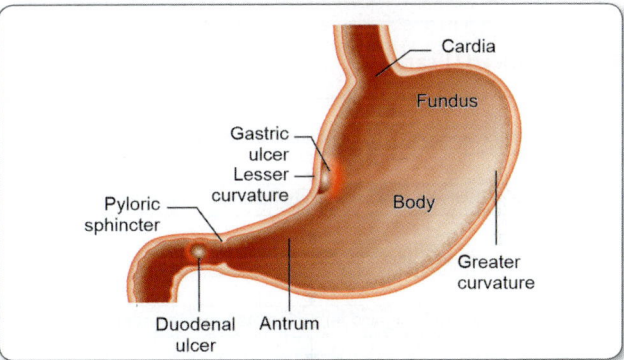

Fig. 6: Gastric and duodenal ulcers

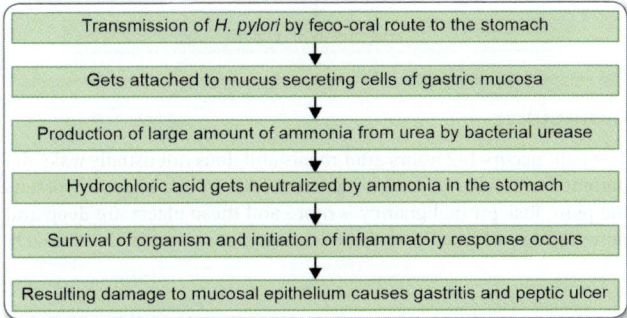

Drug-induced Ulcer

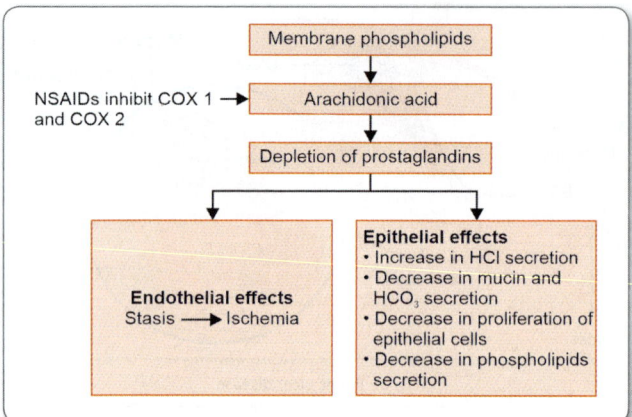

Stress-induced Ulcer

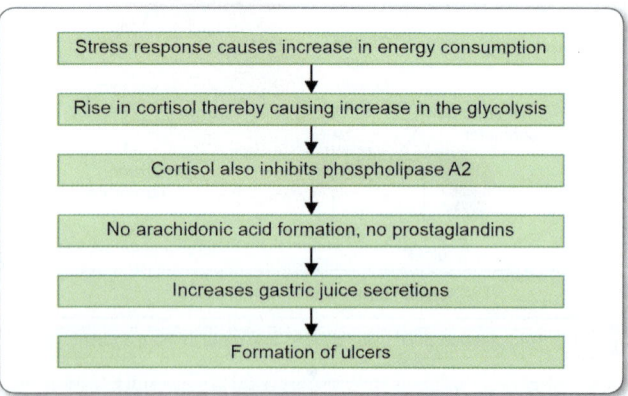

Gastric Ulcer

The pain occurs 1–2 hours after meals and does not usually wake the patient from sleep in case of gastric ulcer. Intake of food worsens the pain. Risk for malignancy is more and these ulcers are deep and penetrating and usually occur on the lesser curvature of the stomach.

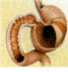

Duodenal Ulcer

First portion of the duodenum is usually affected. Pain occurs 2–4 hours after meals and this pain wakes up the patient. Administration of food relives the pain and there is very little risk for malignancy.

MALABSORPTION

Malabsorption refers to the impaired absorption of nutrients. It includes defects that occur during the digestion and absorption of food nutrients by infections of the gastrointestinal tract. The digestion or absorption of a single nutrient component may be impaired (e.g., lactose intolerance due to lactase deficiency). When a diffuse disorder, such as celiac disease or Crohn's disease, affects the intestine, the absorption of almost all nutrients is impaired.

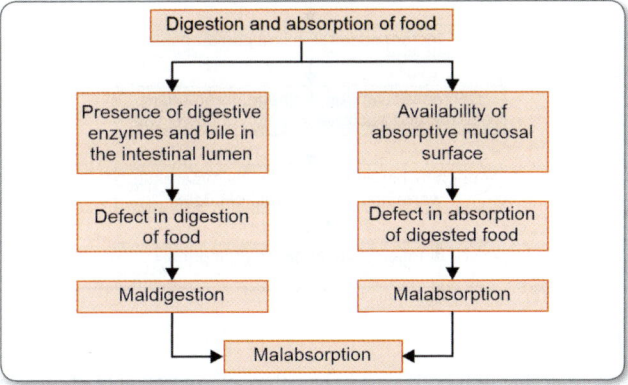

APPENDICITIS

The appendix becomes inflamed and edematous as a result of either becoming kinked or occluded by a fecalith (i.e., hardened mass of stool), tumor, or foreign body (Figs 7A and B). As it gets obstructed, there is **reduced blood flow to the tissue** and thus favors multiplication of **bacteria**. Lumen obstruction increases the pressure in the appendix and this obstructs the venous drainage leading to ischemia. Necrosis and gangrene may occur, if ischemia is not treated. **Risk of perforation** of the appendix increases at this stage. **Perforation may occur at around 72 hours, if the appendix gets obstructed**. Bacteria and inflammatory cells get released into the surrounding structures, once the perforation occurs. This leads to peritonitis.

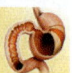

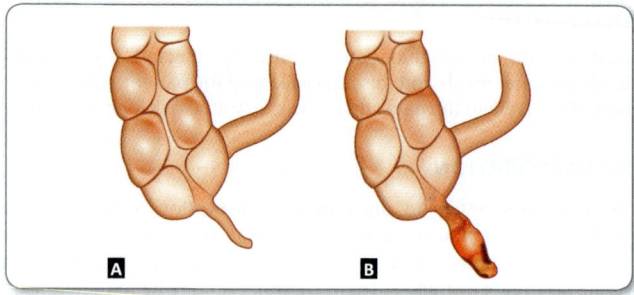

Figs 7A and B: **A.** Normal appendix; **B.** Inflamed appendix

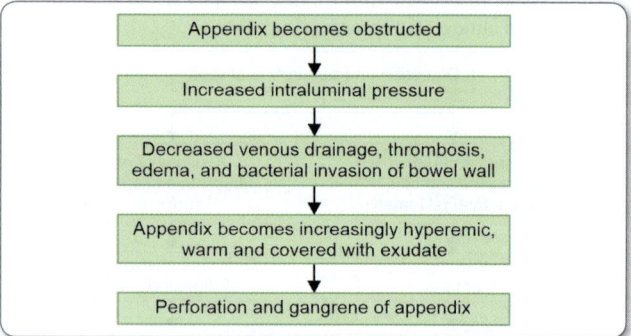

HERNIAS

When an internal body part bulges through a weak area of muscle or the surrounding tissue wall, it is called a hernia. Hernias are often asymptomatic, but a swelling may occur in the abdomen or groin.

Inguinal Hernia

When a loop of intestine bulges into the inguinal canal through a hole in the abdominal wall, it is called inguinal hernia. Formation of the testes occurs in the abdomen, while a male fetus is in the womb and they move down into the scrotum via the inguinal canal before birth.

A hernia, which occurs as a congenital lesion is known as **indirect inguinal hernia**. It occurs when the deep inguinal ring fails to close during embryogenesis after a testicle has moved through it. Once bowel or other abdominal tissue moves into the empty space, a visible bulge is formed and the hernia is clinically evident (Figs 8A and B).

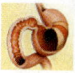

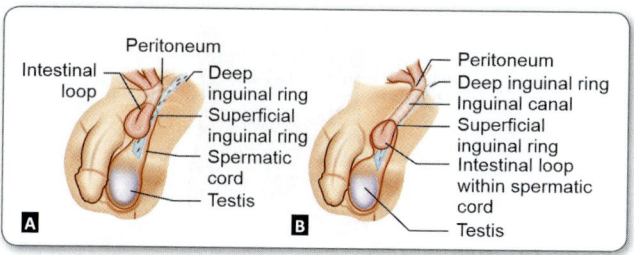

Figs 8A and B: A. Direct inguinal hernia; **B.** Indirect inguinal hernia

Direct hernias occur in people who are aged 25 or above and are not congenital, but acquired. The cause of direct hernias is the degeneration and fatty changes in the inguinal area or posterior wall in an area called the Hesselbach triangle.

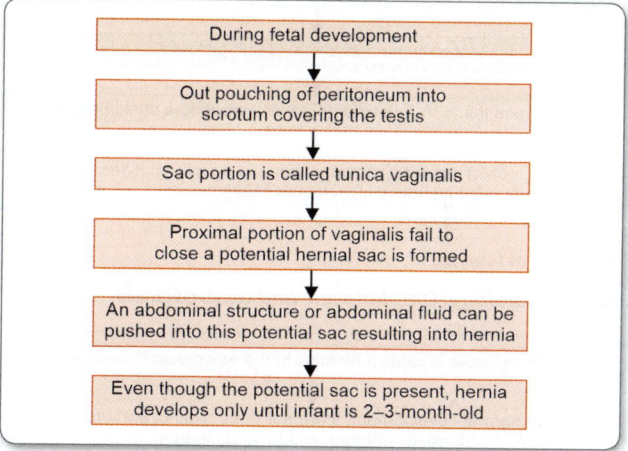

Umbilical Hernia

An umbilical hernia forms when part of the intestine or fatty tissue protrudes through an opening in the abdominal muscles near to the navel, causing swelling of the belly button. This type of hernia may develop in babies if the opening that the umbilical cord passes through does not close properly after birth. In adults, umbilical hernia occurs, possibly due to repeated abdominal strain (Fig. 9).

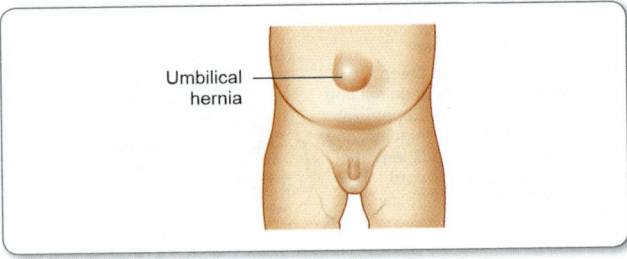

Fig. 9: Umbilical hernia

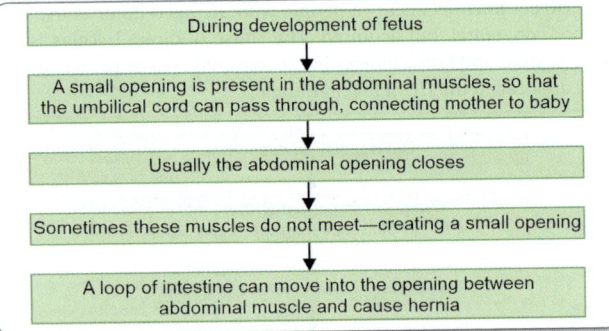

During development of fetus
↓
A small opening is present in the abdominal muscles, so that the umbilical cord can pass through, connecting mother to baby
↓
Usually the abdominal opening closes
↓
Sometimes these muscles do not meet—creating a small opening
↓
A loop of intestine can move into the opening between abdominal muscle and cause hernia

Congenital Hernia

Pathophysiology: Omphalocele and Gastroschisis

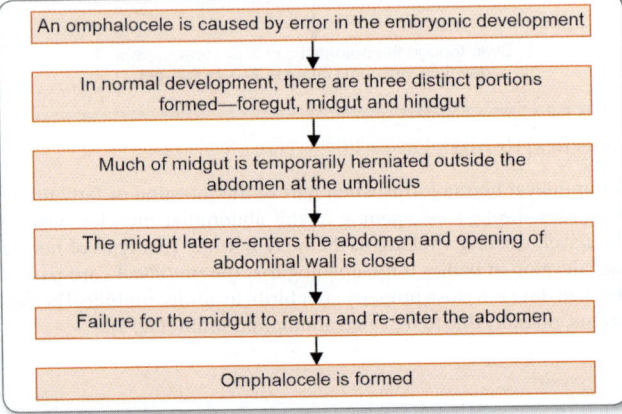

An omphalocele is caused by error in the embryonic development
↓
In normal development, there are three distinct portions formed—foregut, midgut and hindgut
↓
Much of midgut is temporarily herniated outside the abdomen at the umbilicus
↓
The midgut later re-enters the abdomen and opening of abdominal wall is closed
↓
Failure for the midgut to return and re-enter the abdomen
↓
Omphalocele is formed

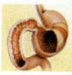

Pathophysiology: Congenital Diaphragmatic Hernia

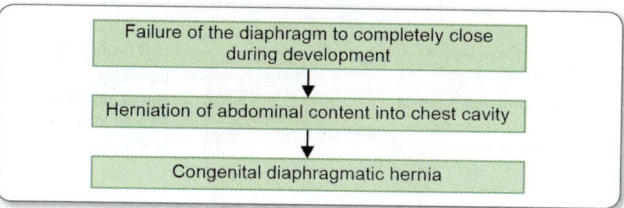

Types

- **Hiatus hernia:** Hiatus hernia refers to when a part of the stomach protrudes into the chest via an opening in the diaphragm. The diaphragm has a small opening (hiatus) that the esophagus passes through to connect to the stomach. Hiatus hernia results from the pushing up of stomach through this opening (Fig. 10).

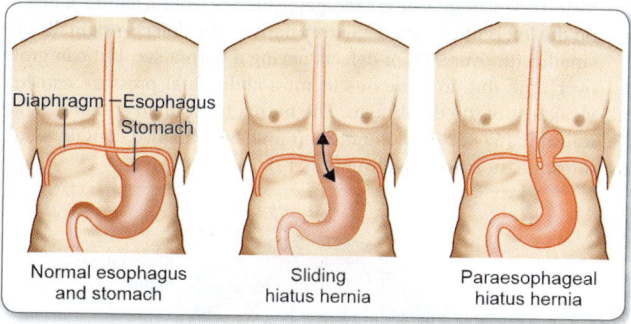

Fig. 10: Types of hernia

- **Bochdalek hernia:** A Bochdalek hernia is a type of congenital hernia due to a developmental defect in the formation of the diaphragm. The diaphragm starts to form at around 4 weeks of gestation. The central tendon is formed anteriorly from the septum transversum. Posterolateral infoldings form the pleuroperitoneal membranes. The pleuroperitoneal canal, in turn, communicates between the pleural and peritoneal cavities via the foramen of Bochdalek at the posterior aspect of the developing diaphragm. This communication normally closes around 8th week of gestation. Bochdalek hernias result from failure of closure of this communication. Since the right canal closes before the left canal, most Bochdalek hernias (85%) are left-sided (Fig. 11).

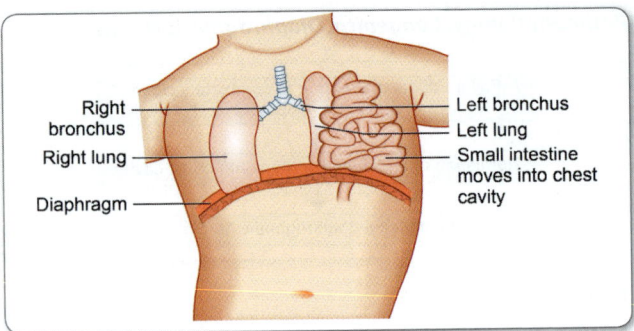

Fig. 11: Bochdalek in hernia (congenital diaphragmatic hernia)

- **Morgagni hernia:** A Morgagni hernia is located posterolaterally to the sternum and is caused by the failure of the pars tendinatis part of the costochondral arches to fuse with the pars sternalis. Failure of fusion on the right side is a Morgagni hernia, while a failure of fusion on the left is often called a Larrey hernia. The defects originally are small, with over 90% of defects having a hernia sac, but can grow over time due to increases in intra-abdominal pressure causing weakness of the diaphragm. The hernia most often contains large intestine (54–72%) or omentum (65%), but can also contain small intestine, stomach, and liver (Fig. 12).

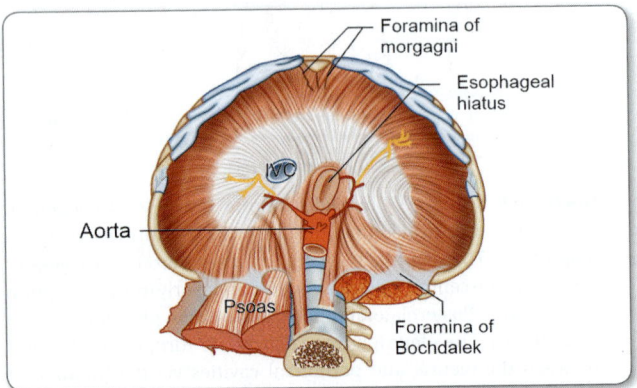

Fig. 12: Morgagni hernia

- **Diaphragm eventration:**
  - In **diaphragmatic eventration**, because of lack of muscle or nerve function, the diaphragm is present in an abnormally

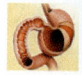

high position. The muscle, if not contracts, compresses against the lung and it may cause difficulty in breathing.

■ It can be **congenital**. It occurs because of the damage of the nerve, which controls the movement of the diaphragm muscle. It is said to be acquired when it results from the injury to phrenic nerve from birth trauma or chest surgery.

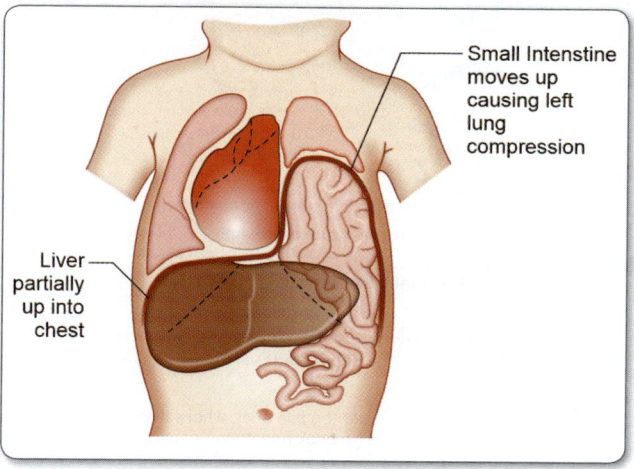

Fig. 13: Diaphragmatic hernia

ACUTE PANCREATITIS

The pathophysiology of acute pancreatitis is characterized by a loss of intracellular and extracellular compartmentation, by an obstruction of pancreatic secretory transport and by an activation of pancreatic enzymes. Proteolytic enzymes, primarily trypsin causes self-digestion of the pancreas, which leads to acute pancreatitis. Gallstones lodge at the ampulla of Vater that obstruct the flow of pancreatic juice or cause a reflux of bile from the common bile duct into the pancreatic duct, thus activates the powerful enzymes within the pancreas. Activation of the enzymes can cause vasodilation, increased vascular permeability, necrosis, and hemorrhage (Fig. 14).

● **Trypsinogen—(a proteolytic enzyme)**
  ■ Normally released into the small intestine, where it is activated to trypsin
  ■ Activated trypsin in the pancreas causes autodigestion of pancreas

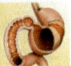

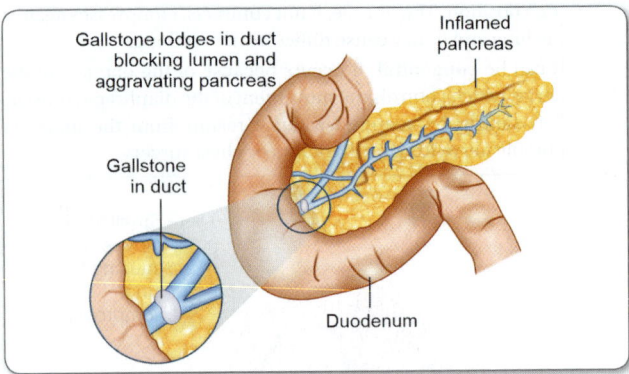

Gallstone lodges in duct blocking lumen and aggravating pancreas

Inflamed pancreas

Gallstone in duct

Duodenum

Fig. 14: Acute pancreatitis

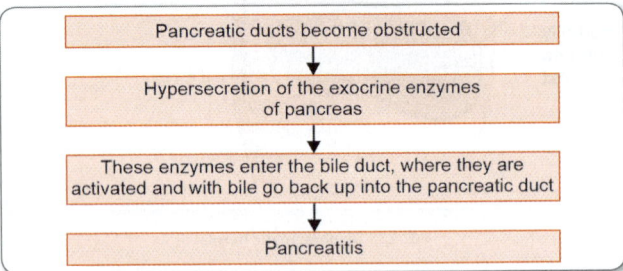

Pancreatic ducts become obstructed

Hypersecretion of the exocrine enzymes of pancreas

These enzymes enter the bile duct, where they are activated and with bile go back up into the pancreatic duct

Pancreatitis

Progression of Disease

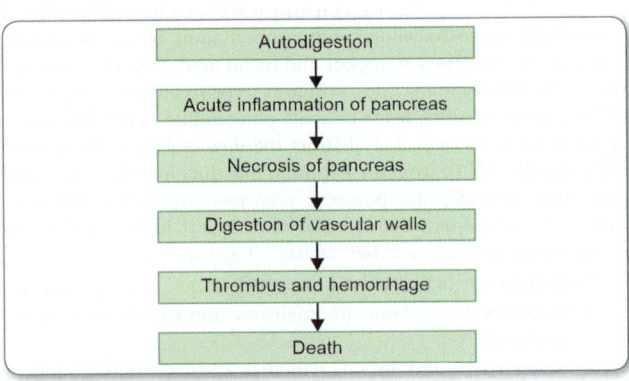

Autodigestion

Acute inflammation of pancreas

Necrosis of pancreas

Digestion of vascular walls

Thrombus and hemorrhage

Death

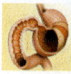

CHRONIC PANCREATITIS

Chronic pancreatitis (CP) is the inflammation of the pancreas, which has the characteristic feature of progressive fibrotic destruction of the pancreatic secretory parenchyma. This causes irreversible morphological and structural changes, which result in impairment of both exocrine as well as endocrine functions.

Common changes in chronic pancreatitis are shown below:

- Cells are replaced by fibrous tissues with repeated episodes of pancreatitis, pressure within the pancreas increases, this results in obstruction of common bile ducts and the duodenum.
- Additionally, there is atrophy of epithelium of the ducts.
- Inflammation and destruction of the secreting cells of the pancreas.

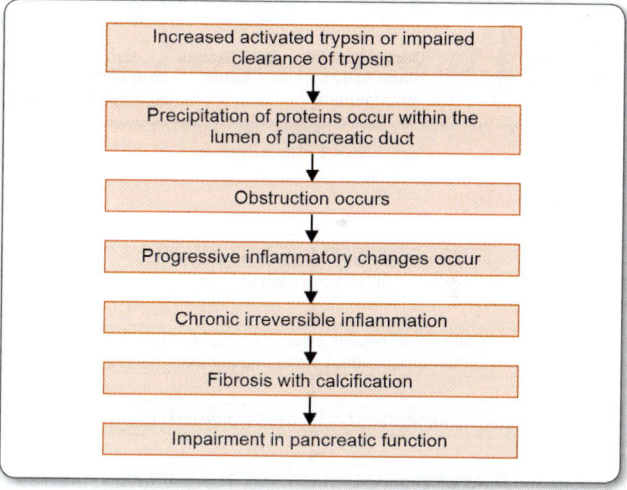

LIVER CIRRHOSIS

Cirrhosis is characterized by regenerative nodules surrounded by dense fibrotic tissue.

In response to injury and loss, growth regulators (cytokines and hepatic growth factors) induce hepatocellular hyperplasia (producing regenerating nodules) and angiogenesis. The development of the nodules is determined by insulin, glucagon, and patterns of intrahepatic blood flow.

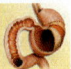
New vessels are produced within the fibrous sheath of the nodules by angiogenesis. These vessels restore the intrahepatic circulatory pathways by connecting the hepatic artery and portal vein to hepatic venules. These vessels allow relatively low-volume, high-pressure venous drainage than normal resulting in increased portal vein pressure. This obstruction in blood flow leads to portal hypertension, which is increased due to the compression of the hepatic venules by the regenerating nodules (Fig. 15).

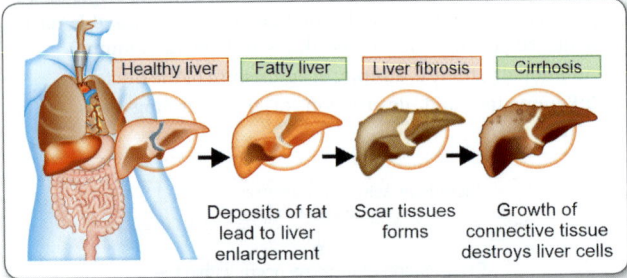

Fig. 15: Stages of liver damage

Pathophysiology

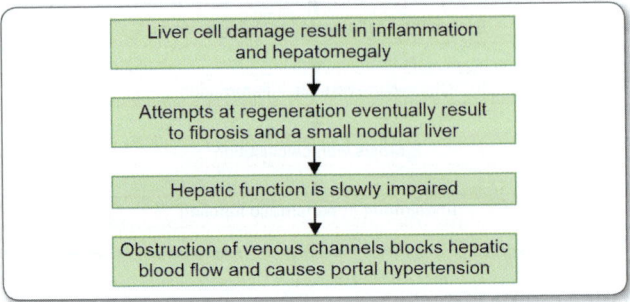

CHOLELITHIASIS

There are two major types of gallstones: those composed predominantly of pigment and those composed primarily of cholesterol. Pigment stones probably form when unconjugated pigments in the bile precipitate to from stones. Pigment stones cannot be dissolved and must be removed surgically.

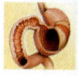

Cholesterol, a normal constituent of bile, is insoluble in water. Its solubility depends on bile acids and lecithin (phospholipids) in bile. In gallstone-prone patients, there is decreased bile acid synthesis and increased cholesterol, which precipitates out of the bile to form stones. The cholesterol-saturated bile predisposes to the formation of gallstones, which act as irritant, producing inflammatory changes in the gallbladder.

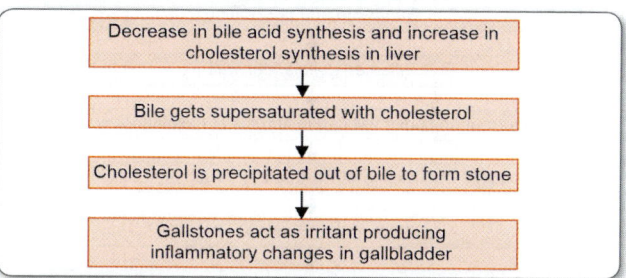

CHOLECYSTITIS

The pathophysiological changes in cholecystitis most commonly involve the gallstone impaction in the bladder neck, Hartmann's pouch, or the cystic duct. As the pressure on the gallbladder increases, it gets enlarged, the walls get thicken, the blood supply decreases, and there may be a formation of an exudate as well.

Cholecystitis can be either acute or chronic, with repeated episodes of acute inflammation potentially leading to chronic cholecystitis (Fig. 16). The gallbladder can become infected by various microorganisms, including those that are gas forming. An inflamed gallbladder can undergo necrosis and gangrene and, if left untreated, may progress to symptomatic sepsis. Failure of adequate treatment of cholecystitis may result in perforation of the gallbladder.

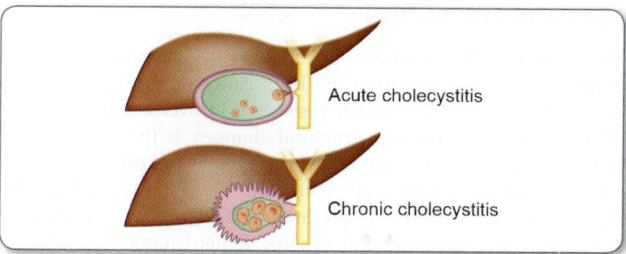

Fig. 16: Acute and chronic cholecystitis

Growth of bacteria
↓
Localized cellular irritation, infiltration or both
↓
Development of areas of ischemia
↓
Gangrene and perforation
↓
Inflamed gallbladder wall
↓
Recurrent episodes will cause fibrosis of gallbladder wall
↓
Stone causes obstruction at Hartmann's pouch or in cystic duct
↓
Obstruction causes stasis
↓
It leads to edema of the wall
↓
Bacterial infection occurs
↓
Leads to acute cholecystitis
↓
Impacted stone—mucosal erosion
↓
Thereby bile salts will act on submucosal tissue
↓
Bile is toxic to tissues
↓
Leads to necrosis, infection and perforation

PORTAL HYPERTENSION

The pathological conditions, which raise the vascular resistance to the portal blood flow into the liver, cause portal hypertension. Increased intrahepatic vascular resistance in liver cirrhosis, which occurs because of massive structural changes, is the prime cause of portal hypertension. Formation of collateral vessels and arterial vasodilatation is progressed with the development of portal hypertension, which leads to the increase in the portal circulation. Ultimately the development of the hyperdynamic circulatory syndrome occurs that leads to esophageal varices or ascites.

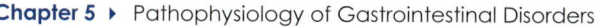

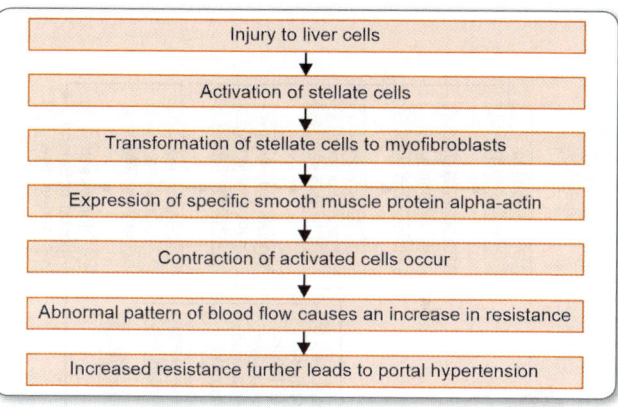

```
┌─────────────────────────────────────────────┐
│          Injury to liver cells              │
└─────────────────────────────────────────────┘
                      ↓
┌─────────────────────────────────────────────┐
│        Activation of stellate cells         │
└─────────────────────────────────────────────┘
                      ↓
┌─────────────────────────────────────────────┐
│  Transformation of stellate cells to myofibroblasts │
└─────────────────────────────────────────────┘
                      ↓
┌─────────────────────────────────────────────┐
│ Expression of specific smooth muscle protein alpha-actin │
└─────────────────────────────────────────────┘
                      ↓
┌─────────────────────────────────────────────┐
│      Contraction of activated cells occur    │
└─────────────────────────────────────────────┘
                      ↓
┌─────────────────────────────────────────────┐
│ Abnormal pattern of blood flow causes an increase in resistance │
└─────────────────────────────────────────────┘
                      ↓
┌─────────────────────────────────────────────┐
│ Increased resistance further leads to portal hypertension │
└─────────────────────────────────────────────┘
```

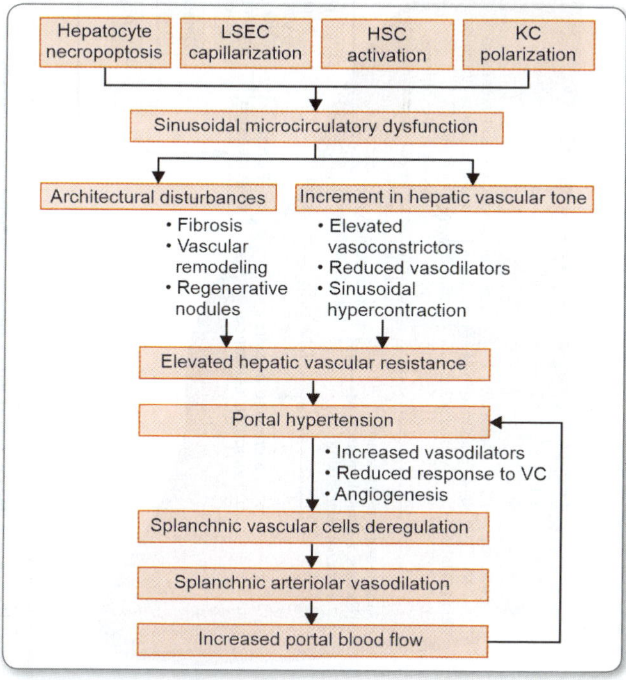

```
┌──────────────┬──────────────┬──────────────┬──────────────┐
│  Hepatocyte  │     LSEC     │     HSC      │      KC      │
│ necropoptosis│capillarization│  activation  │ polarization │
└──────────────┴──────────────┴──────────────┴──────────────┘
                      ↓
        ┌─────────────────────────────────────┐
        │ Sinusoidal microcirculatory dysfunction │
        └─────────────────────────────────────┘
              ↓                        ↓
┌──────────────────────────┐  ┌────────────────────────────┐
│ Architectural disturbances│  │ Increment in hepatic vascular tone │
└──────────────────────────┘  └────────────────────────────┘
   • Fibrosis                    • Elevated
   • Vascular                      vasoconstrictors
     remodeling                  • Reduced vasodilators
   • Regenerative                • Sinusoidal
     nodules                       hypercontraction
              ↓                        ↓
        ┌─────────────────────────────────────┐
        │  Elevated hepatic vascular resistance │
        └─────────────────────────────────────┘
                      ↓
        ┌─────────────────────────────────────┐◄──┐
        │         Portal hypertension         │   │
        └─────────────────────────────────────┘   │
                • Increased vasodilators           │
                • Reduced response to VC            │
                • Angiogenesis                      │
                      ↓                             │
        ┌─────────────────────────────────────┐    │
        │ Splanchnic vascular cells deregulation │  │
        └─────────────────────────────────────┘    │
                      ↓                             │
        ┌─────────────────────────────────────┐    │
        │  Splanchnic arteriolar vasodilation  │    │
        └─────────────────────────────────────┘    │
                      ↓                             │
        ┌─────────────────────────────────────┐    │
        │     Increased portal blood flow     │────┘
        └─────────────────────────────────────┘
```

Abbreviations: HSC, hepatic stellate cell; KC, Kupffer cells; LSEC, liver sinusoidal endothelial cells; VC, vascular cells

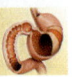

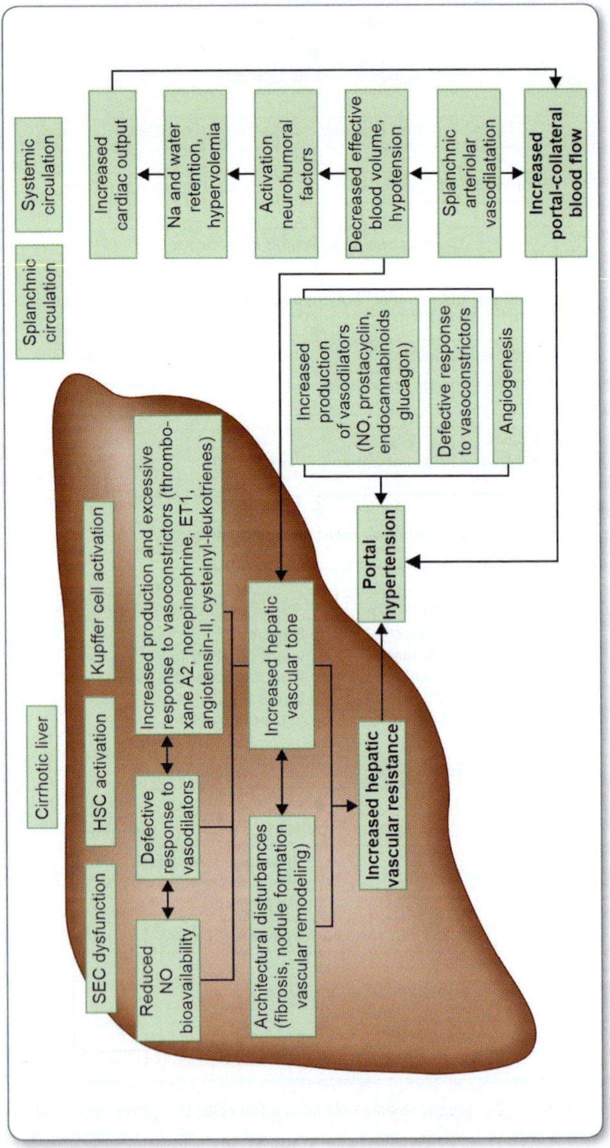

Cirrhotic liver

- SEC dysfunction
- HSC activation
- Kupffer cell activation

Reduced NO bioavailability

Defective response to vasodilators

Increased production and excessive response to vasoconstrictors (thromboxane A2, norepinephrine, ET1, angiotensin-II, cysteinyl-leukotrienes)

Architectural disturbances (fibrosis, nodule formation vascular remodeling)

Increased hepatic vascular tone

Increased hepatic vascular resistance

Portal hypertension

Splanchnic circulation

Increased production of vasodilators (NO, prostacyclin, endocannabinoids glucagon)

Defective response to vasoconstrictors

Angiogenesis

Increased portal-collateral blood flow

Systemic circulation

Increased cardiac output

Na and water retention, hypervolemia

Activation neurohumoral factors

Decreased effective blood volume, hypotension

Splanchnic arteriolar vasodilatation

Abbreviations: HSC, hepatic stellate cell; NO, nitric oxide; SEC, sinusoidal endothelial cells

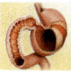

LIVER ABSCESS

Liver abscesses can be amebic or bacterial (pyogenic) in origin. *Entamoeba histolytica* is the causative agent in amebic abscess. It is contacted by ingestion of food or water contaminated by the cyst stage of the parasite. Amebiasis generally only involves the intestine but can invade the mesenteric venules resulting in liver abscesses. Its only host is the human. The usual pathophysiology for pyogenic liver abscesses is bowel content leakage and peritonitis. Bacteria travel to the liver via the portal vein and reside there. Infection can also originate in the biliary system (Fig. 17).

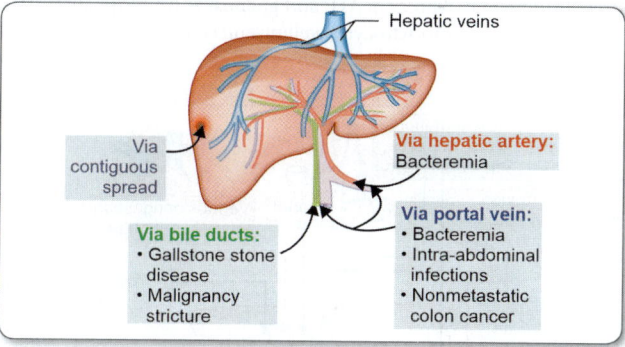

Fig. 17: Liver abscess

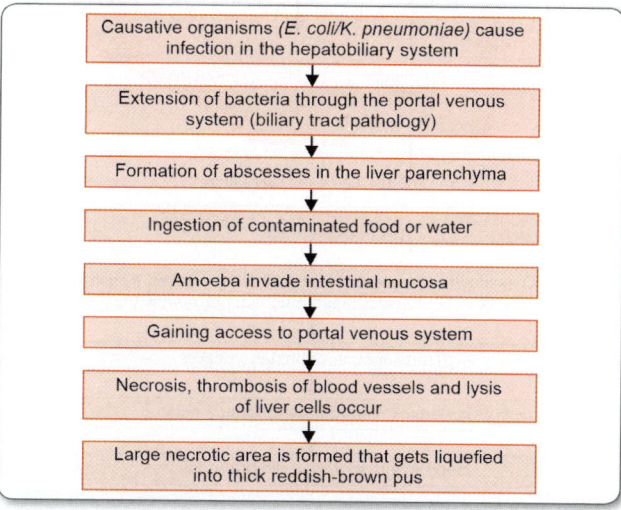

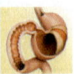

HEPATIC FAILURE

Most cases of acute liver failure (ALF) (except acute fatty liver of pregnancy and Reye syndrome) will have massive hepatocyte necrosis and/or apoptosis leading to liver failure. Hepatocyte necrosis occurs due to adenosine triphosphate (ATP) depletion causing cellular swelling and cell membrane disruption. ALF has a multifactorial pathophysiology of cerebral edema and hepatic encephalopathy and includes altered blood-brain barrier (BBB) secondary to inflammatory mediators leading to microglial activation, accumulation of glutamine secondary to ammonia crossing the BBB and subsequent oxidative stress leading to depletion of ATP and guanosine triphosphate (GTP). This ultimately leads to astrocyte swelling and cerebral edema (Fig. 18).

Causes of Liver Failure

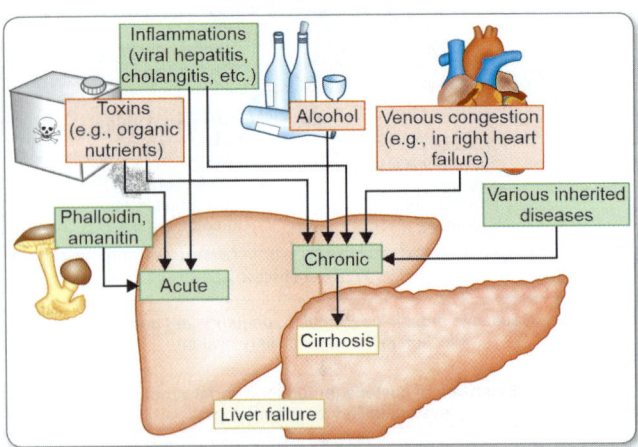

Fig. 18: Causes of liver failure

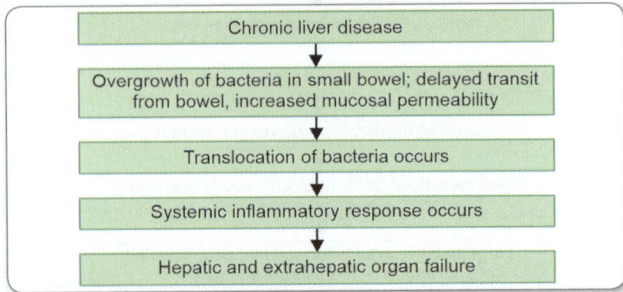

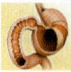

HEPATITIS

Hepatitis is an inflammation of the liver, resulting from various causes, both infectious (i.e., viral, bacterial, fungal, and parasitic organisms) and noninfectious (e.g., alcohol, drugs, autoimmune diseases, and metabolic diseases).

There are different types of hepatitis such as hepatitis A, B, C, D and E. viruses, which enter into liver through the blood stream, infect the hepatocytes and multiply. Self-mediated immune response of the body attempts to damage the hepatocytes.

Stages of Viral Hepatitis

There are three stages of viral hepatitis: prodromal, icteric and convalescent. The symptoms of the patient vary on the basis of the phase in which the patient is. In the prodromal stage, the virus releases chemicals in the blood, which cause symptoms such as fever, headache, fatigue, nausea, vomiting, skin rashes and joint pain. Due to the damage of hepatocytes and bile ducts, conjugated bilirubin and transaminases spill into the blood in the icteric stage. The patient appears yellow because of the conjugated and unconjugated bilirubin and the color of the patient's urine becomes dark. Hepatomegaly may also occur in this stage. In the convalescent stage, the patient starts returning to normal.

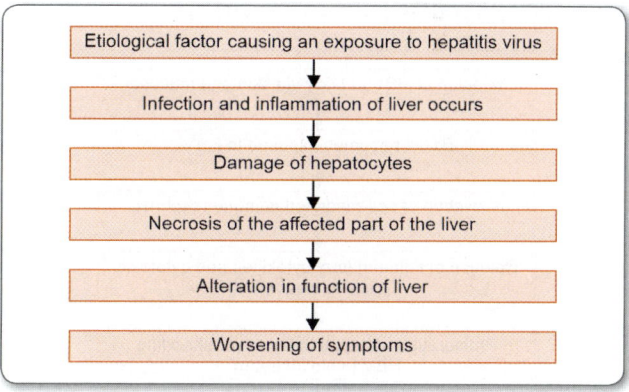

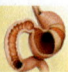

Pathophysiology of Hepatitis A Virus (HAV)

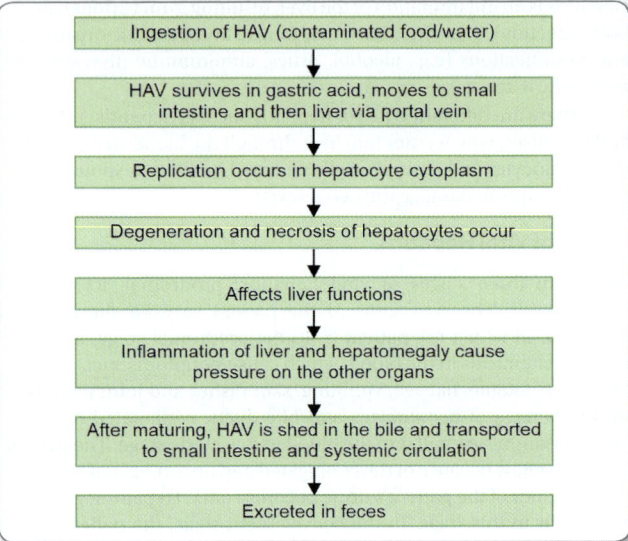

Ingestion of HAV (contaminated food/water)

↓

HAV survives in gastric acid, moves to small intestine and then liver via portal vein

↓

Replication occurs in hepatocyte cytoplasm

↓

Degeneration and necrosis of hepatocytes occur

↓

Affects liver functions

↓

Inflammation of liver and hepatomegaly cause pressure on the other organs

↓

After maturing, HAV is shed in the bile and transported to small intestine and systemic circulation

↓

Excreted in feces

Pathophysiology of Hepatitis B Virus (HBV)

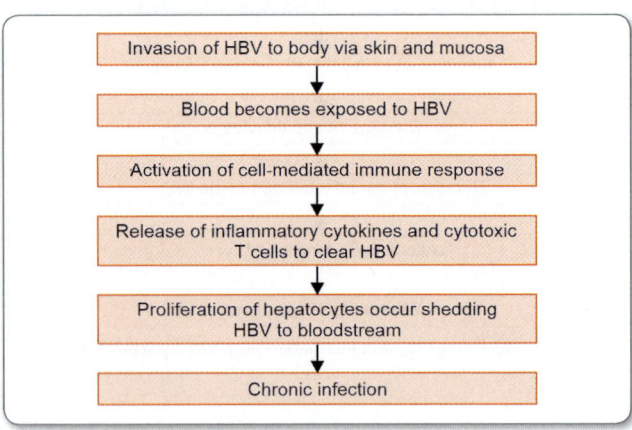

Invasion of HBV to body via skin and mucosa

↓

Blood becomes exposed to HBV

↓

Activation of cell-mediated immune response

↓

Release of inflammatory cytokines and cytotoxic T cells to clear HBV

↓

Proliferation of hepatocytes occur shedding HBV to bloodstream

↓

Chronic infection

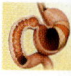

Pathophysiology of Hepatitis C Virus (HCV)

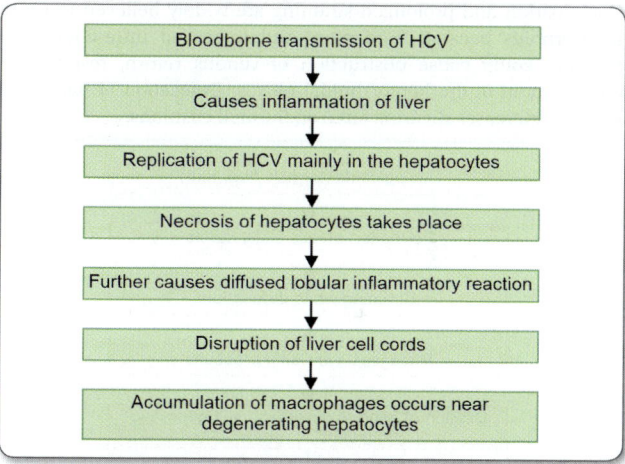

Pathophysiology of Hepatitis D Virus (HDV)

Transmission of HDV is similar to the HBV. HDV is transmitted sexually through contact with infected blood or blood products or percutaneously. Vertical transmission is also possible but it is rare. A person, who is already chronically infected with HBV, can also be infected. This superinfection of HDV on chronic hepatitis B leads to progression to a more severe disease, like cirrhosis, in all ages.

Pathophysiology of Hepatitis E Virus (HEV)

The virus is shed in the stools of infected persons and enters the human body through the intestine. It is transmitted mainly through contaminated drinking water. Usually the infection is self-limiting and resolves within 2–6 weeks. Other routes of transmission have been identified but appear to account for a much smaller number of clinical cases. These routes of transmission include:

- Ingestion of undercooked meat or meat products derived from infected animals (e.g., pork's liver)
- Transfusion of infected blood products
- Vertical transmission from a pregnant woman to her baby.

HEMORRHOIDS

Constipation and prolonged straining are widely believed to cause hemorrhoids because hard stool and increased intra-abdominal pressure could cause obstruction of venous return, resulting in engorgement of the hemorrhoidal plexus. Defecation of hard fecal material increases shearing force on the anal cushions.

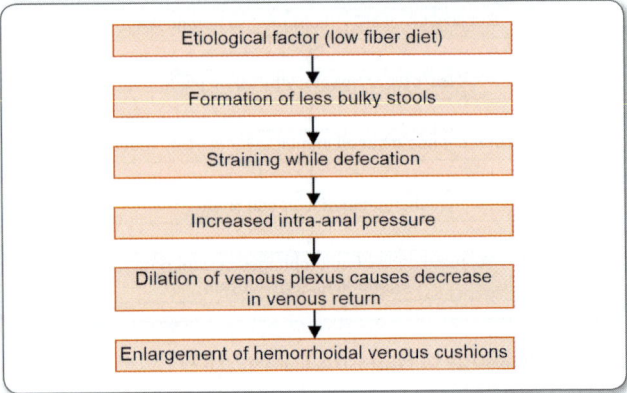

Classification of Hemorrhoids

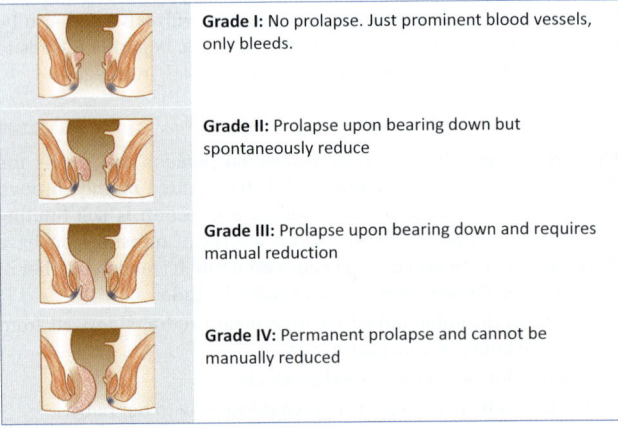

Grade I: No prolapse. Just prominent blood vessels, only bleeds.

Grade II: Prolapse upon bearing down but spontaneously reduce

Grade III: Prolapse upon bearing down and requires manual reduction

Grade IV: Permanent prolapse and cannot be manually reduced

Fig. 19: Classification of hemorrhoids

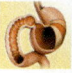

ANAL FISSURES

An anal fissure is a superficial linear tear in the anoderm that is distal to the dentate line. Anal fissures are often associated with local trauma such as the passage of hard stools or anal trauma, but can also be due to secondary causes such as inflammatory bowel disease.

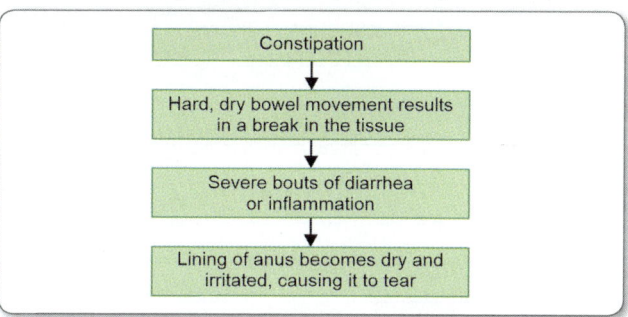

ANAL FISTULA

Most anal fistulas originate in anal crypts, which become infected with ensuing abscess formation. When the abscess is opened or when it ruptures, a fistula is formed.

A fistula is a tiny channel or tract that develops in the presence of inflammation and infection. It may or may not be associated with an abscess, but like abscesses, certain illnesses such as Crohn's disease can cause fistulas to develop. The fistulas being infected channels, drainage occurs from them. Often a draining fistula is not painful, but it can irritate the skin around it. An abscess and fistula often occur together.

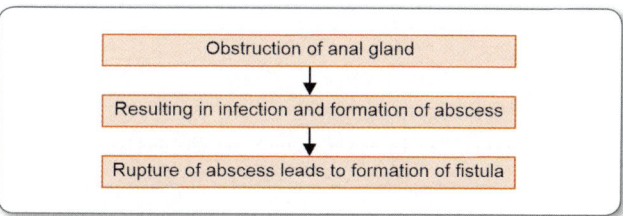

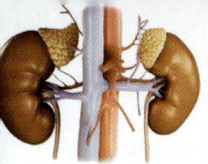

Pathophysiology of Renal System

INTRODUCTION

The renal or genitourinary system functions to remove the excess amount of fluid and toxic waste products from the bloodstream. The main functions of the renal system are to excrete out the wastes from the body, thereby, regulating the volume and pressure of blood. This system also maintains the electrolyte concentration and regulation of blood pH level (Fig. 1).

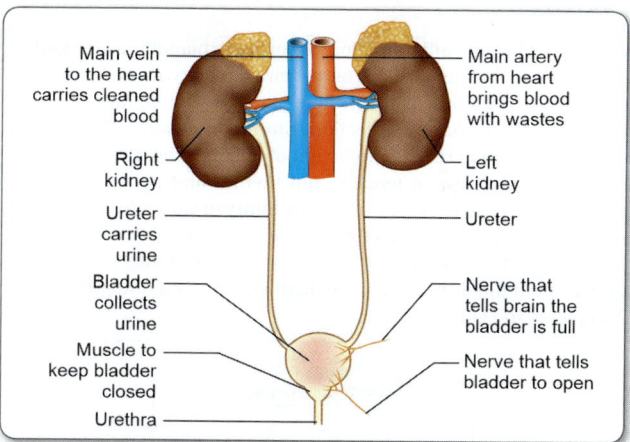

Fig. 1: Parts of renal system

Let us discuss about the pathophysiological changes occurring in various disorders related to renal system.

URINARY TRACT INFECTIONS

Infections mostly occur when bacteria gain access to the bladder, get attached and colonized in the epithelium of the urinary tract so that

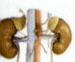

they don't get washed off with voiding, and are able to evade host defense mechanisms, and initiate inflammation.

A large number of bacteria can be cleared off from the bladder by increasing the slow shedding of epithelial cells lining the bladder.

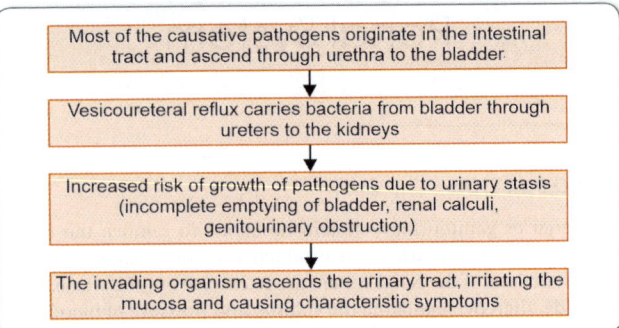

CYSTITIS

Acute or chronic inflammation of urinary bladder is termed as Cystitis. The bladder serves as a storage/reservoir for urine and also is lined with mucus membrane having a protein layer above it, that makes it resistant to infection. But the infection of the bladder occasionally is the result of infection of neighboring areas as vagina, urethra and kidneys in females and urethra and prostate gland in males. Obstruction, tumors, traumatic injury or stones in bladder also make it susceptible to infection. Acute cystitis mostly occurs in the course of urinary tract infection whereas chronic cystitis is a recurrent or persistent inflammation of the bladder. Pathophysiology of cystitis is depicted in Figure 2.

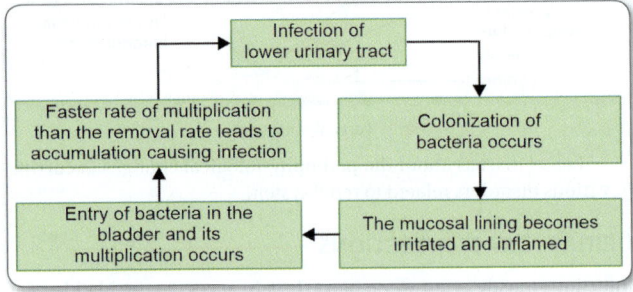

Fig. 2: Pathophysiology of cystitis

GLOMERULONEPHRITIS

An immune-mediated injury acts as a triggering factor for the occurrence of glomerulonephritis. With an onset of immune response, lymphocytes and macrophages infiltrate the glomeruli. The formation of immune deposit occurs in the glomerulus membrane. The circulating antibodies also become trapped in the glomerulus and get deposited there.

Acute Glomerulonephritis

Acute glomerulonephritis is mainly characterized by severe inflammation, renal insufficiency, swelling, increased blood pressure, and severe back pain. Kidneys get damaged because of infection and may progress on to subacute and chronic stages. Swelling of the kidneys occurs in the acute form of disease, the surface becomes smooth and grey and the capsule covering the kidneys is stretched.

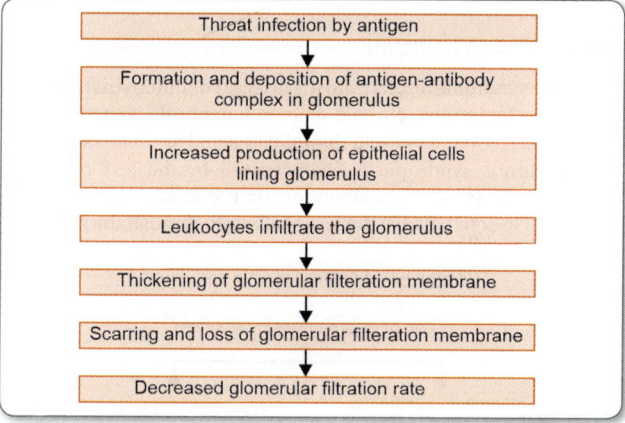

Chronic Glomerulonephritis

The repeated episodes of acute glomerulonephritis lead to occurrence of chronic glomerulonephritis, hypertensive nephrosclerosis, hyperlipidemia, chronic tubulointerstitial injury, or hemodynamically medicated glomerular sclerosis. The kidneys are reduced to as little as one-fifth their normal size (consisting primarily the fibrous tissue). The cortex shrinks, making the surface of the kidney rough and irregular. Numerous glomeruli and their tubules become scarred, and the branches of the renal artery are thickened.

The result is severe glomerular damage that results in end-stage renal disease (ESRD). Failure of kidneys to filter the waste products from the blood and accumulation of abnormal quantities of nitrogenous waste products is known as uremia.

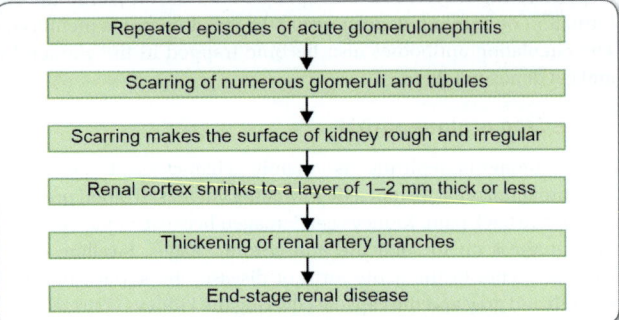

NEPHROTIC SYNDROME

Nephrotic syndrome results from the disease conditions that primarily affect the glomerulus, chronic glomerulonephritis, systemic lupus erythematosus and renal vein thrombosis being the main conditions.

Nephrotic syndrome is characterized by the loss of plasma protein in the urine. Hypoalbuminemia eventually results with an inability of liver to balance the loss of albumin through the kidneys.

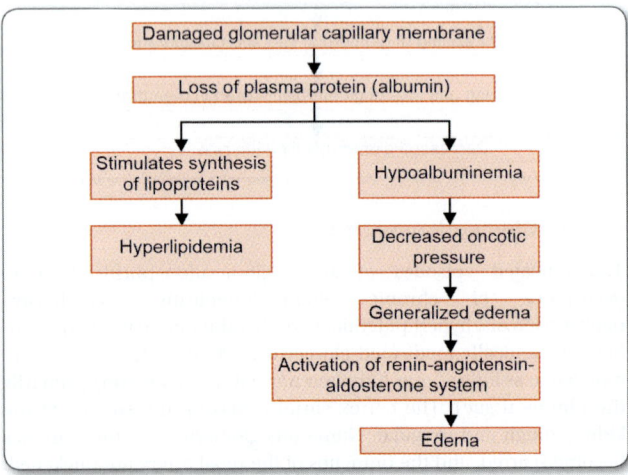

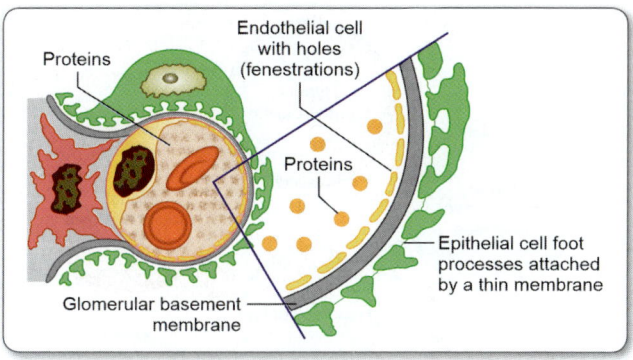

Fig. 3: Barriers that keep protein and blood cells out of the urine

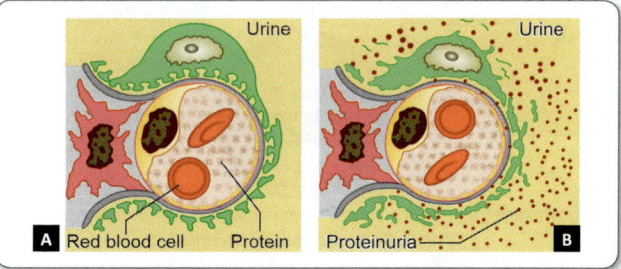

Figs 4A and B: **A.** Normal glomerular capillary; **B.** Capillary with proteinuria

RENAL CALCULI

The stones may be formed anywhere in the upper or lower urinary tract. Increased concentration of calcium oxalate, calcium phosphate, and uric acid whereas decrease in concentration of citrate, magnesium, nephrocalcin, and uropontin favors the formation of calculi.

Other factors contributing to the formation of stones include dehydration, infection, urinary stasis and episodes of immobility (Fig. 5).

Hyper-
parathyroidism
Myelo-
proliferative
diseases
Renal
tubular acidosis
Hypercalcemia
Granulomatous
diseases
Cancer
Excessive intake
of vitamin D,
milk and alkali

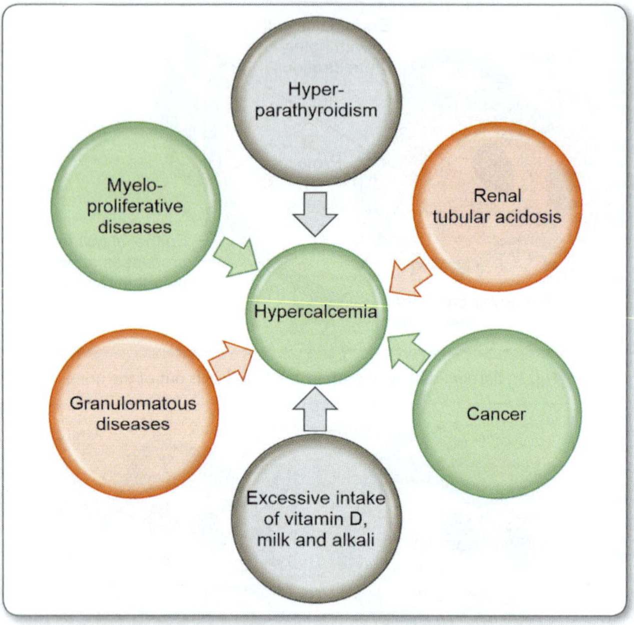

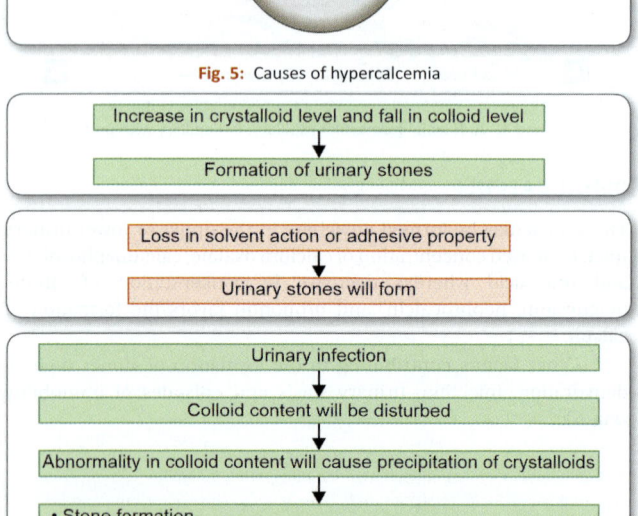

Fig. 5: Causes of hypercalcemia

Increase in crystalloid level and fall in colloid level
Formation of urinary stones

Loss in solvent action or adhesive property
Urinary stones will form

Urinary infection
Colloid content will be disturbed
Abnormality in colloid content will cause precipitation of crystalloids
• Stone formation
• Infection also changes urinary pH and also causes increase in concentration of crystalloids

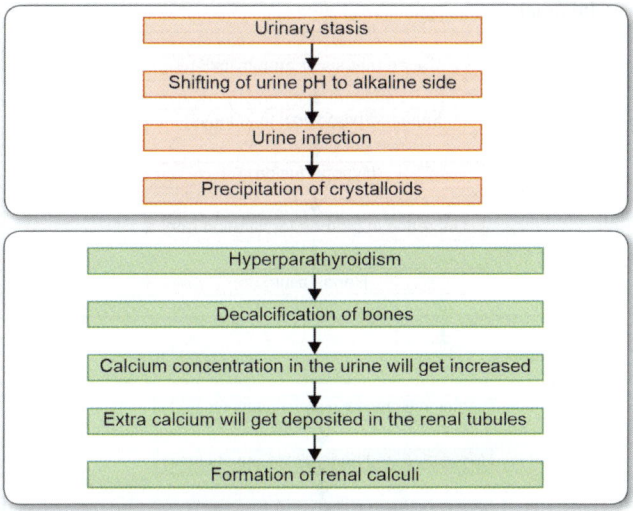

ACUTE RENAL FAILURE

Acute renal failure (ARF) is a sudden and nearly complete damage of kidney function. Oliguria (<400 mL/day of urine) is the most common manifestation seen in ARF; whereas anuria (<50 mL/day of urine) and normal urine output occur rarely. Even if the patient excretes normal urine output that normally doesn't occur, there will be an increase in the level of blood urea nitrogen (BUN) and serum creatinine including retention of other metabolic waste products.

The kidneys require an adequate blood supply, properly functioning glomeruli and renal capillaries and a normal elimination of urine from the body. Any interruption of these processes will lead to the occurrence of acute renal failure.

The classification of causes is in accordance with the disorders leading to disruption of these processes. Functional and structural causes that prevent a smooth supply of blood to kidneys are classified as prerenal. These include extracellular fluid (ECF) volume contraction, congestive heart failure (functional) and renal artery stenosis (structural). Diseases causing actual damage to the kidneys or any associated structure, are categorized as intrarenal causes like acute glomerulonephritis, acute tubular necrosis etc. The conditions causing an interference with normal drainage and excretion of urine are classified as postrenal, i.e., benign prostate hypertrophy or tumor of the prostate.

- **Prerenal**

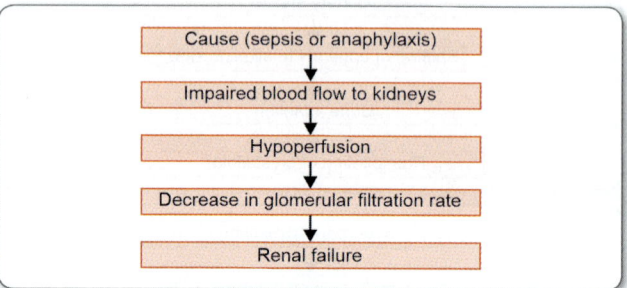

| Cause (sepsis or anaphylaxis) |
| ↓ |
| Impaired blood flow to kidneys |
| ↓ |
| Hypoperfusion |
| ↓ |
| Decrease in glomerular filtration rate |
| ↓ |
| Renal failure |

- **Intrinsic**

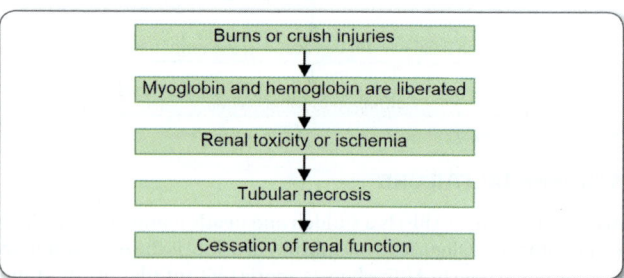

| Burns or crush injuries |
| ↓ |
| Myoglobin and hemoglobin are liberated |
| ↓ |
| Renal toxicity or ischemia |
| ↓ |
| Tubular necrosis |
| ↓ |
| Cessation of renal function |

- **Transfusion reaction**

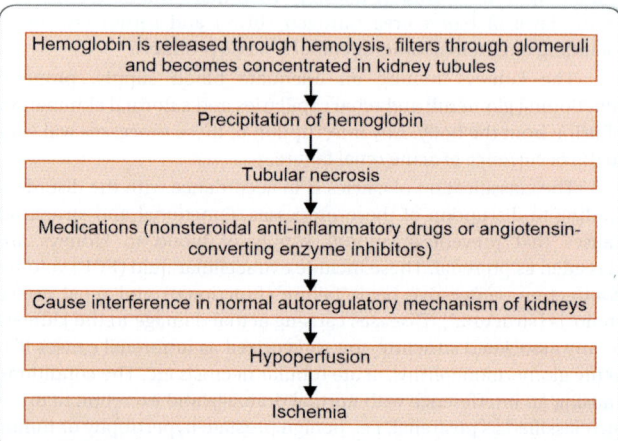

| Hemoglobin is released through hemolysis, filters through glomeruli and becomes concentrated in kidney tubules |
| ↓ |
| Precipitation of hemoglobin |
| ↓ |
| Tubular necrosis |
| ↓ |
| Medications (nonsteroidal anti-inflammatory drugs or angiotensin-converting enzyme inhibitors) |
| ↓ |
| Cause interference in normal autoregulatory mechanism of kidneys |
| ↓ |
| Hypoperfusion |
| ↓ |
| Ischemia |

- Postrenal

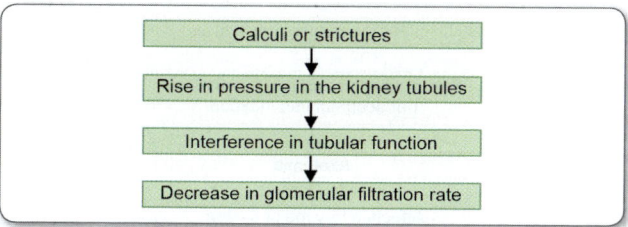

Phases of ARF

- **Initiation:** Begins with the injury of kidneys and ends with oliguria development.
- **Oliguria:** This period is accompanied by a rise in serum concentration of substances normally excreted by kidneys (urea, creatinine, uric acid, organic acids, intracellular cations). Hyperkalemia may also develop.
- **Diuresis:** Patient experiences gradually increasing urine output signaling that glomerular filtration has started to recover. Lab values start decreasing. Renal function may still be abnormal. Observe for dehydration during this period.
- **Recovery period:** It signals the improvement of renal function and may take 3–12 months.

CHRONIC RENAL FAILURE

Chronic renal failure also known as end-stage renal failure or ESRD is a progressive, irreversible deterioration in renal function in which the body's ability to maintain metabolic and fluid and electrolyte balance fails, resulting in uremia.

With the decline in renal function, the metabolic waste products start accumulating in the blood. Increase in blood urea nitrogen levels (uremia) results from this accumulation affecting every major system of the body. The severity of symptoms depends upon the extent of build-up of such waste products. The chronic renal disease is categorized in three stages as reduced renal reserve, renal insufficiency, and ESRD.

Any underlying disease condition, presence of hypertension, loss of protein in urine, all exacerbate the progression of chronic renal failure and increased decline in renal function.

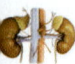

Pathophysiological Changes

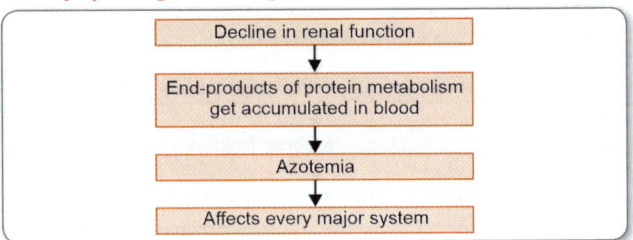

Decline in renal function

↓

End-products of protein metabolism get accumulated in blood

↓

Azotemia

↓

Affects every major system

Stages of ESRD

- **Reduced renal reserve:** 40–75% loss of nephron function. Patient usually does not have any symptom because remaining nephrons are able to carry out the normal functions of the kidney.
- **Renal insufficiency:** 75–90% of nephron function is lost. At this point, BUN and serum creatinine rise, kidney loses its ability to concentrate urine and anemia develops. Patient may report polyuria and nocturia.
- **ESRD:** It occurs when there is less than 10% nephron function remaining. Evidenced by elevated creatinine and BUN levels as well as electrolyte imbalances.

URETHRAL STRICTURE

A stricture refers to the narrowing of the lumen, which may be congenital or acquired. Urethral strictures arise from various causes and can result in a range of manifestations, from an asymptomatic presentation to severe discomfort secondary to urinary retention.

- Narrowing of the urethra can result from chronic infection that leads to inflammation of mucus membrane.
- The inflammation causes hyperplasia of the lining resulting in the development of stricture.
- Urethral anastomosis can also cause stricture.
- Pressure from a tumor against the exterior of urethra can result in the stricture of the lumen.
- A congenital stricture results from inadequate fusion of the anterior and posterior urethra, is short in length, and is not associated with an inflammatory process.

Urethral Stricture in Males

- **Posterior urethral stricture:** Posterior urethral strictures occur due to an injury related to pelvic fracture and is located in the first two inches of the urethra. There is a disruption of the urethra that may either be separated or completely cut due to which urine is not able to pass through.

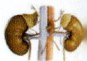

- **Anterior urethral stricture:** Main causes of anterior urethral stricture that is present in the last two inches of the urethra include direct traumatic injury to penis or catheterization.

BENIGN PROSTATE HYPERPLASIA/HYPERTROPHY

Benign prostatic hyperplasia (BPH) is a proliferative process of cellular elements of prostate, enlarged prostate or a voiding dysfunction that results from enlargement of prostate and bladder obstruction. The dominant role of the androgen system and the androgen receptor is well defined in the pathogenesis of BPH. Androgen receptors are expressed in BPH tissues in which they are activated by the potent androgen dihydrotestosterone. Synthesis of dihydrotestosterone is under control of the 5α-reductase enzyme, activity of which is antagonized by finasteride and dutasteride.

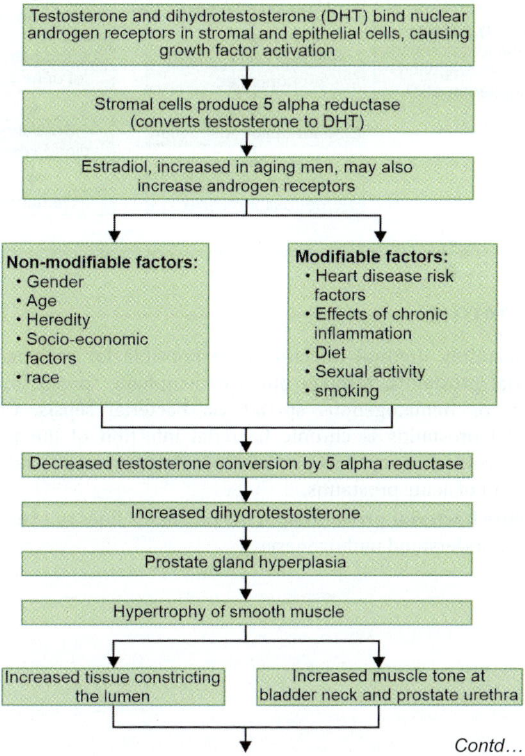

```
┌─────────────────────────────────────────────────────────┐
│  Testosterone and dihydrotestosterone (DHT) bind nuclear │
│  androgen receptors in stromal and epithelial cells,     │
│  causing growth factor activation                        │
│                         ↓                                │
│       Stromal cells produce 5 alpha reductase            │
│          (converts testosterone to DHT)                  │
│                                                          │
│       Estradiol, increased in aging men, may also        │
│              increase androgen receptors                 │
│                    ↓              ↓                       │
│  Non-modifiable factors:   Modifiable factors:           │
│   • Gender                  • Heart disease risk         │
│   • Age                       factors                    │
│   • Heredity                • Effects of chronic         │
│   • Socio-economic            inflammation               │
│     factors                 • Diet                       │
│   • race                    • Sexual activity            │
│                             • smoking                    │
│                                                          │
│     Decreased testosterone conversion by 5 alpha reductase│
│                         ↓                                │
│          Increased dihydrotestosterone                   │
│                         ↓                                │
│            Prostate gland hyperplasia                    │
│                         ↓                                │
│          Hypertrophy of smooth muscle                    │
│                    ↓              ↓                       │
│  Increased tissue constricting   Increased muscle tone at│
│        the lumen              bladder neck and prostate  │
│                                         urethra          │
│                         ↓                                │
│                                        Contd...          │
└─────────────────────────────────────────────────────────┘
```

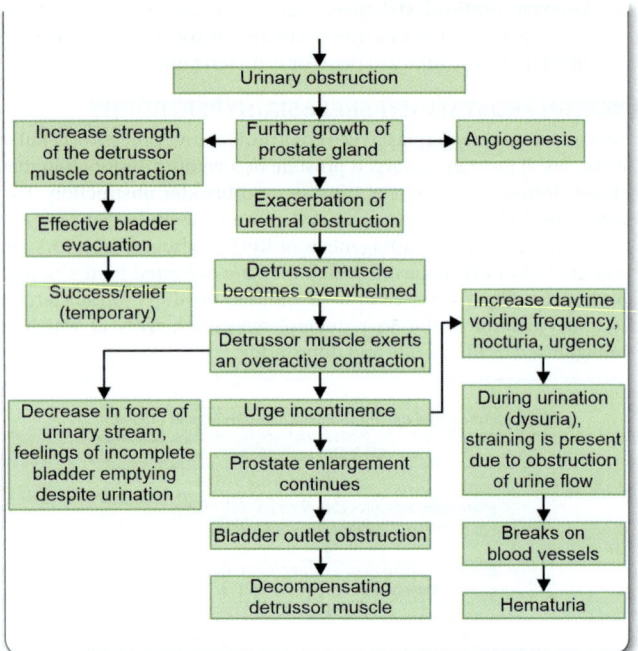

PROSTATITIS

An ascending urethral infection is responsible for causing acute bacterial prostatitis, through direct or lymphatic spread from the rectum or hematogenous spread via bacterial sepsis. Chronic bacterial prostatitis is chronic bacterial infection of the prostate with or without symptoms and also occurs because of inadequate treatment of acute prostatitis.

- **Acute bacterial prostatitis:** Acute prostatitis does not yet have a fully understood pathogenesis.

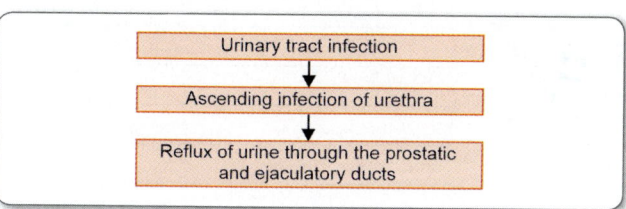

- **Chronic bacterial prostatitis:** Ascending infection from the distal part of urethra to the prostate is the possible cause of chronic prostatitis. Sometimes, any anatomical abnormality in the intra-prostatic ducts may also be responsible for the retrograde spread of infection.

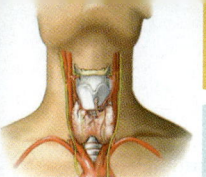

Pathophysiology of Endocrine Disorders

INTRODUCTION

The endocrine system consists of cells, tissues, and organs that secrete hormones. The primary function of these ductless glands is to secrete their hormones directly into the surrounding fluid. The interstitial fluid and the blood vessels then transport the hormones throughout the body.

The endocrine system consists of a collection of endocrine glands: the pituitary (anterior and posterior lobes), thyroid, parathyroid, adrenal (cortex and medulla), pancreas and gonads.

- **Pituitary gland:** The pituitary gland (hypophysis) is found in the inferior part of the brain, attached to the bottom of the hypothalamus by the infundibulum. The pituitary gland consists of two major regions, the anterior pituitary gland (adenohypophysis) and the posterior pituitary gland (neurohypophysis). The glandular secretion of the pituitary gland is controlled by the hypothalamus.

- **Posterior pituitary gland:** The neurosecretory cells are responsible for the communication between the hypothalamus and the posterior pituitary. Hormones produced by the cell bodies of the neurosecretory cells are packaged in vesicles and transported through the axon and stored in the axon terminals that lie in the posterior pituitary. The stimulation of neurosecretory cells triggers the release of stored hormones from those axon terminals to a network of capillaries within the posterior pituitary. The hormones released by the posterior pituitary are antidiuretic hormone (ADH) and oxytocin.

- **Anterior pituitary gland:** The anterior pituitary is involved in sending hormones that control all other hormones of the body. The releasing and inhibiting hormones that are produced by the hypothalamus and delivered to the anterior pituitary via a portal network of capillaries are responsible for the communication between the hypothalamus and the anterior pituitary.

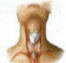

- **Thyroid gland:** This is one of the largest endocrine glands in the body. It is positioned on the neck just below the larynx and has two lobes, one on either side of the trachea. It is involved in the production of the hormones T_3 (triiodothyronine) and T_4 (thyroxine). The metabolic activity of body's cells is increased by these hormones. Calcitonin (thyrocalcitonin), which contributes to the regulation of blood calcium levels, is also produced and released by thyroid gland. Thyrocalcitonin is responsible for causing a decrease in calcium level in the blood and then it gets stored in the bones.

- **Parathyroid gland:** There are four parathyroid glands located on the sides of thyroid gland. Regulation of calcium and phosphorus levels is done by parathyroid gland. Parathyroid hormone (PTH) is also secreted from these glands that causes the release of calcium from the bones into the extracellular fluid. PTH is directly released into the bloodstream and reaches the target cells. Calcium-producing effects of PTH are counteracted by calcitonin.

- **Adrenal glands:** These are a pair of ductless glands that are situated atop both the kidneys. They are responsible for releasing hormones in response to stress through the synthesis of corticosteroids (cortisol) and catecholamines (epinephrine and norepinephrine) (Fig. 1).

- **Pancreas:** The pancreas plays an important role in maintaining the blood sugar level. It also forms insulin, glucagon, and other hormones that are released into the bloodstream to regulate blood sugar levels.

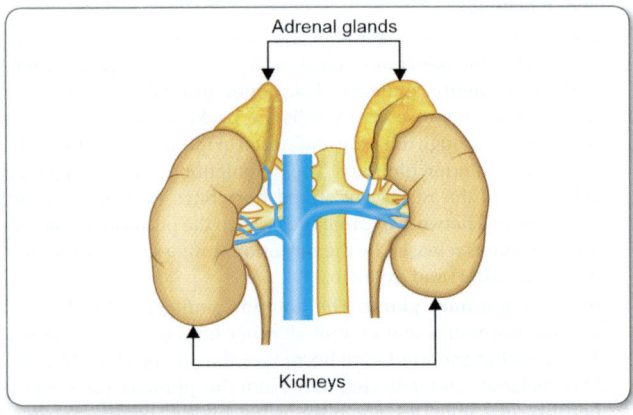

Fig. 1: Adrenal glands

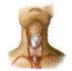

PITUITARY DISORDERS

Abnormalities of pituitary function are caused by over secretion or under secretion of any of the hormones produced or released by the gland. Hypersecretion most commonly involves adrenocorticotropic hormone (ACTH) or growth hormone and results in **Cushing's syndrome or acromegaly**. An excess of growth hormone in adults results in bone and soft tissue deformities. In children, over secretion of growth hormone results in **gigantism**, whereas an insufficient secretion results in **dwarfism**.

All anterior pituitary hormones are involved in hyposecretion. In this condition, there is an atrophy of the thyroid gland, the adrenal cortex, and the gonads as a result of loss of the trophic-stimulating hormones.

Diabetes insipidus is the most common disorder related to posterior lobe dysfunction in which less production of vasopressin leads to excretion of abnormally large volumes of dilute urine.

Hypopituitarism

Normally, a decreased concentration of the secondary hormones stimulates the pituitary gland to produce more hormones. However, in patients with hypopituitarism, the pituitary gland is unable to respond adequately to a reduction in the hormone levels of the target organ. As a result, there is a consistent decrease in the action of the target glands. This eventually leads to a deficiency in the hormones. The end result of this reduction is a failure of physiologic functions of body.

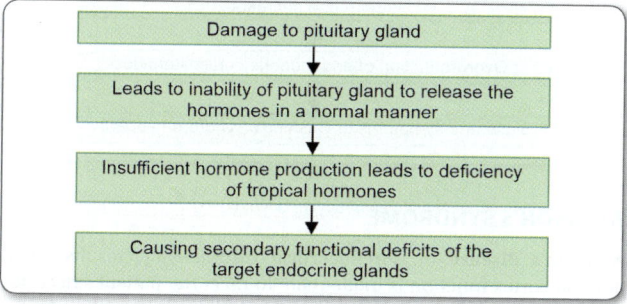

Hyperpituitarism

When the pituitary gland is overactive, it secretes excessive amounts of some hormones, usually due to the presence of a benign (noncancerous) tumor.

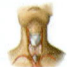

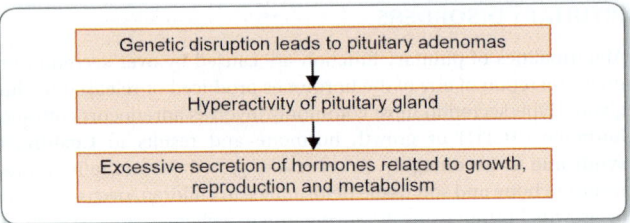

Genetic disruption leads to pituitary adenomas

↓

Hyperactivity of pituitary gland

↓

Excessive secretion of hormones related to growth, reproduction and metabolism

CUSHING'S SYNDROME

The most common cause of Cushing's syndrome is an excessive use of corticosteroid medications and less frequently due to excessive production of corticosteroid by the adrenal cortex. Other reasons include a tumor of the pituitary gland that produces ACTH and stimulates the adrenal cortex to cause an unnecessary increase of its hormone secretion. Regardless of the causes, the feedback mechanisms that control the adrenal cortex functions, start to become ineffective, leading to loss of the actual day-time pattern of cortisol.

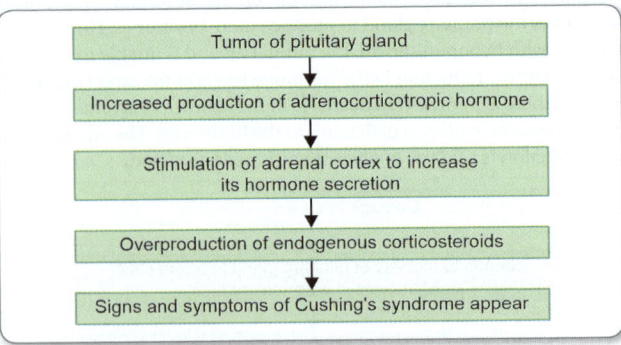

Tumor of pituitary gland

↓

Increased production of adrenocorticotropic hormone

↓

Stimulation of adrenal cortex to increase its hormone secretion

↓

Overproduction of endogenous corticosteroids

↓

Signs and symptoms of Cushing's syndrome appear

ADDISON'S SYNDROME

Addison's disease or adrenocortical insufficiency, results when adrenal cortex function is inadequate to meet the patient's need for cortical hormones. Autoimmune or idiopathic atrophy of the adrenal glands is responsible for 80% of cases. Other causes include surgical removal of both adrenal glands or infection of the adrenal glands. Inadequate secretion of ACTH from the pituitary gland also results in adrenal insufficiency because of decreased stimulation of the adrenal cortex.

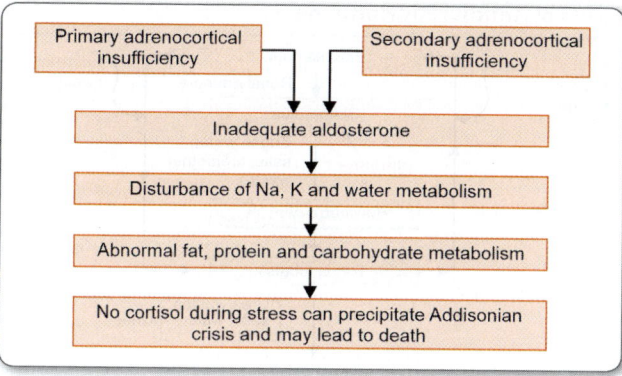

Diabetes Insipidus

The abnormality in the functioning of levels of ADH is mainly responsible for causing diabetes insipidus, which is characterized by increased amounts of dilute urine and excessive thirst.

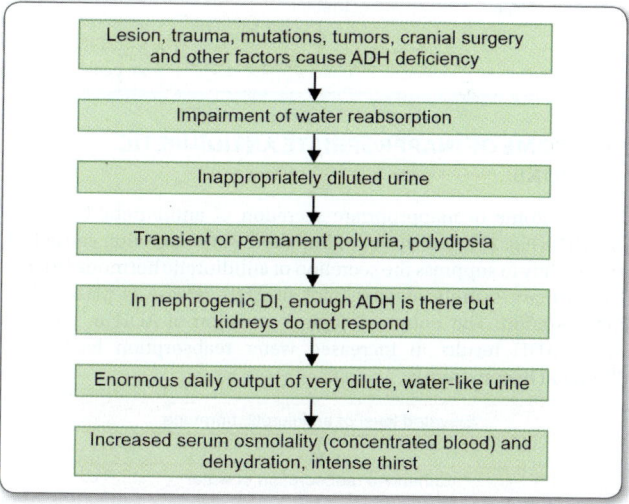

Abbreviations: ADH, antidiuretic hormone; DI, diabetes insipidus

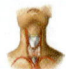

Action of Antidiuretic Hormone

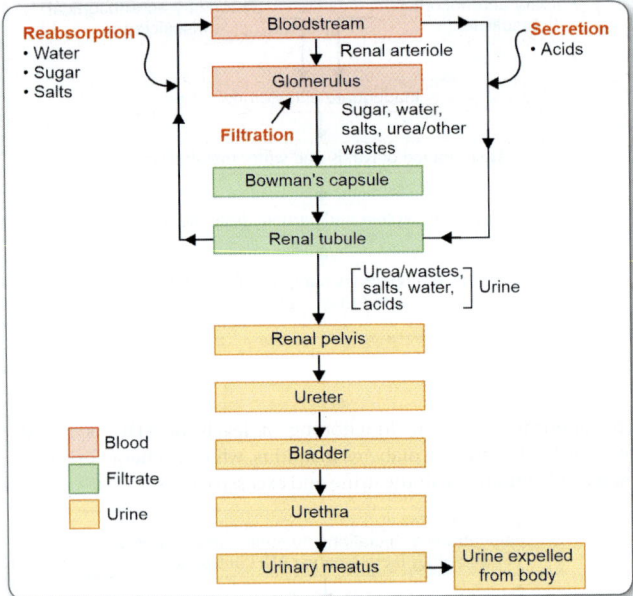

SYNDROME OF INAPPROPRIATE ANTIDIURETIC HORMONE

The syndrome of inappropriate secretion of antidiuretic hormone (SIADH) (Fig. 2) is a disorder of impaired water excretion caused by the inability to suppress the secretion of antidiuretic hormone (ADH). The primary osmotic determinant of ADH release is plasma Na^+ concentration. The nonphysiological secretion of ADH in patients with SIADH results in increased water reabsorption leading to dilutional hyponatremia.

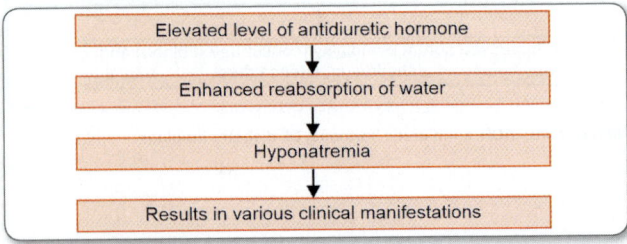

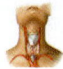

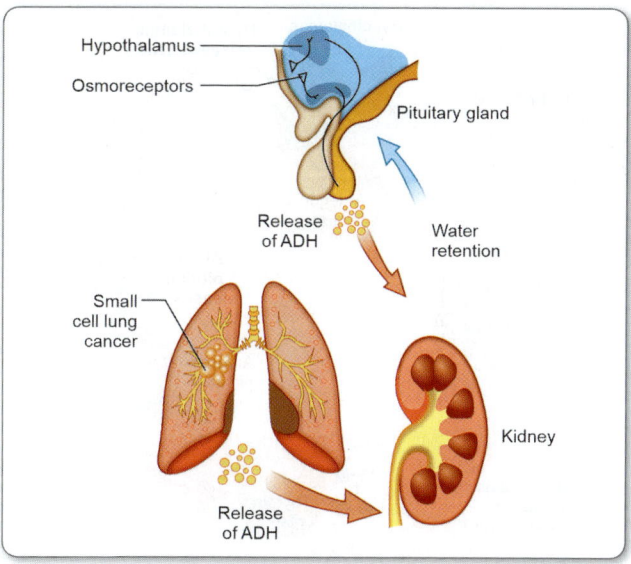

Fig. 2: Syndrome of inappropriate antidiuretic hormone
Abbreviation: ADH, antidiuretic hormone

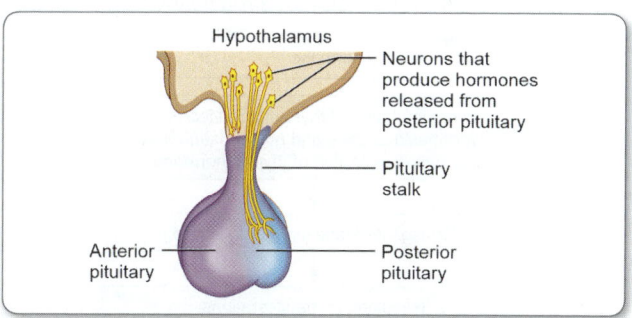

Fig. 3: Hypothalamic control of posterior pituitary

HYPERTHYROIDISM

Hyperthyroidism may result from increased synthesis and secretion of thyroid hormones (thyroxine [T_4] and triiodothyronine [T_3]) from the thyroid, caused by thyroid stimulators in the blood or by autonomous thyroid hyperfunction.

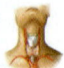
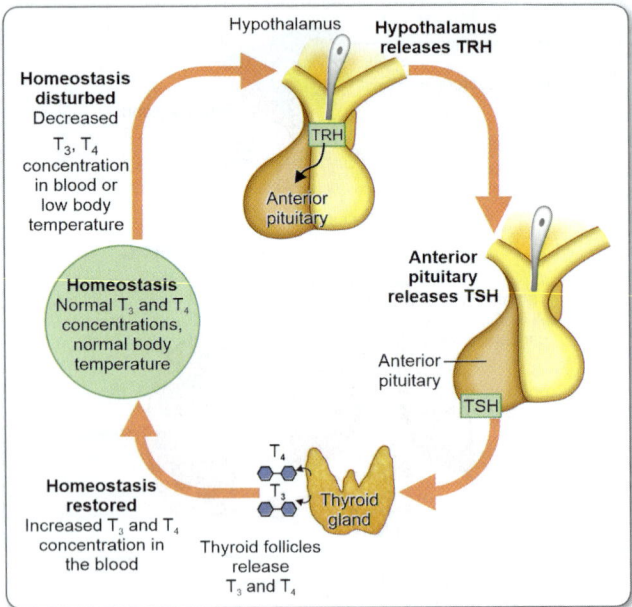

Fig. 4: Maintenance of homeostasis by thyroid gland

Abbreviations: T_3, triiodothyronine; T_4, thyroxine; TRH, thyrotropin releasing hormone; TSH, thyroid stimulating hormone

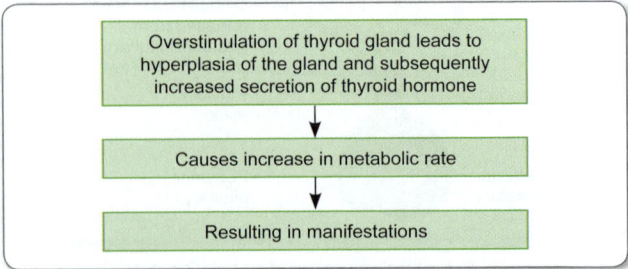

The manifestations are:

- Weight loss and muscular weakness due to accelerated metabolism of carbohydrates, fats and proteins.
- Increased cardiac output in conjunction with hormonal effects on the sympathetic nerves causing palpitation and tachycardia.
- Excessive absorption of glucose, which leads to hyperglycemia.

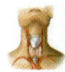

- The increased metabolic rate coupled with increased oxygen consumption lead to changes in perception and coordination.
- The skin becomes thinned and the hair is fine, soft and straight.
- The superficial capillaries dilate leading to increased peripheral blood flow and also an increase in cardiac output as the body tries to eliminate excess heat from the system. This accounts for warm, moist skin and perspiration.

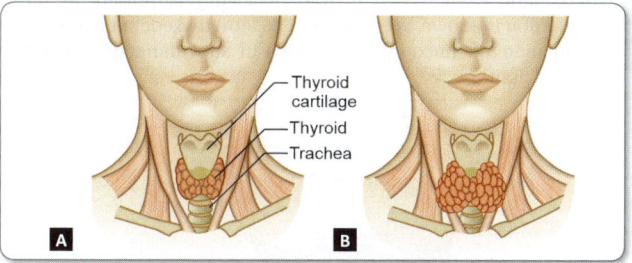

Figs 5A and B: **A.** Normal thyroid; **B.** Goiter

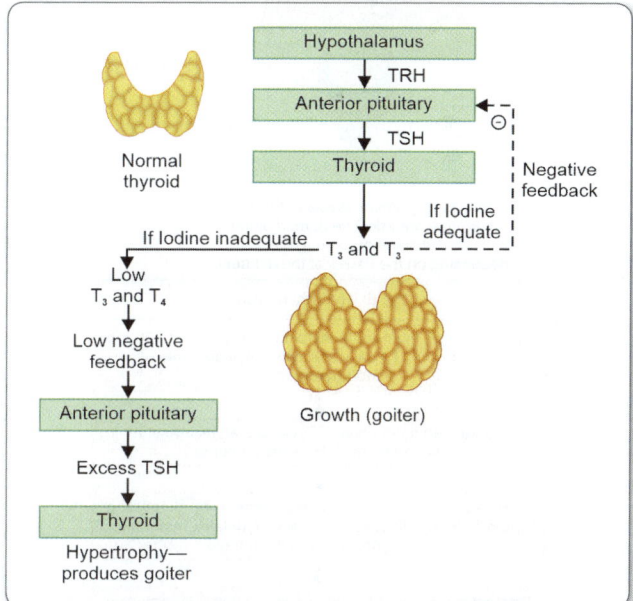

Abbreviations: TRH, thyrotropin releasing hormone; TSH, thyroid stimulating hormone

HYPOTHYROIDISM

In hypothyroidism, the thyroid gland is underactive, resulting in deficiency of the thyroid hormones triiodothyronine (T_3) and thyroxine (T_4). Rarely in some cases, there may be a sufficient production of hormones but the peripheral effects of these hormones may be insufficient (Fig. 6).

More than 95% of patients with hypothyroidism have primary or thyroidal hypothyroidism, which refers to dysfunction of the thyroid gland itself. When thyroid deficiency is present at birth, the condition is known as cretinism. The term myxedema refers to the accumulation of mucopolysaccharides in subcutaneous and other interstitial tissues.

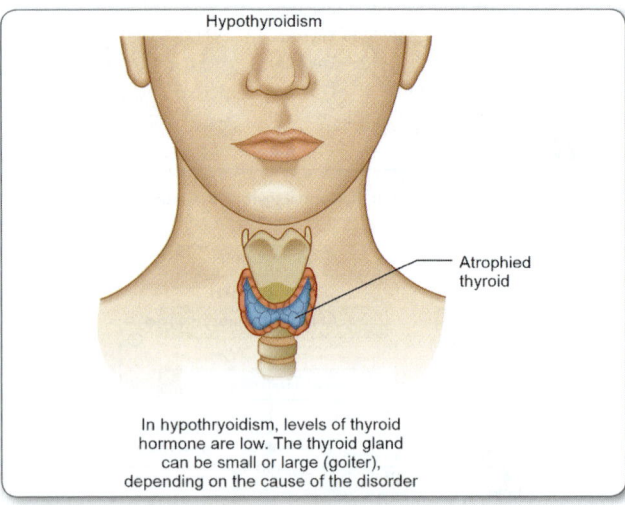

Hypothyroidism

Atrophied thyroid

In hypothryoidism, levels of thyroid hormone are low. The thyroid gland can be small or large (goiter), depending on the cause of the disorder

Fig. 6: Hypothyroidism

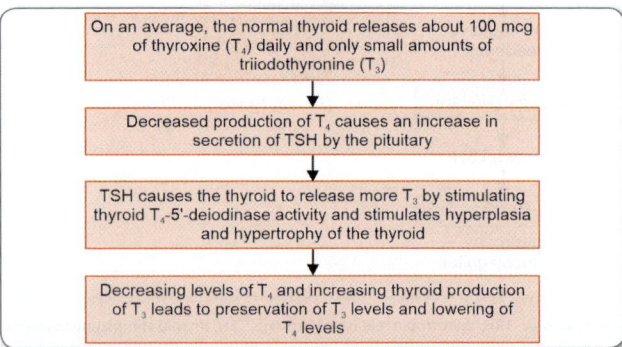

On an average, the normal thyroid releases about 100 mcg of thyroxine (T_4) daily and only small amounts of triiodothyronine (T_3)

↓

Decreased production of T_4 causes an increase in secretion of TSH by the pituitary

↓

TSH causes the thyroid to release more T_3 by stimulating thyroid T_4-5'-deiodinase activity and stimulates hyperplasia and hypertrophy of the thyroid

↓

Decreasing levels of T_4 and increasing thyroid production of T_3 leads to preservation of T_3 levels and lowering of T_4 levels

Abbreviations: T_3, triiodothyronine; T_4, thyroxine; TSH, thyroid stimulating hormone

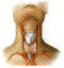

HYPERPARATHYROIDISM

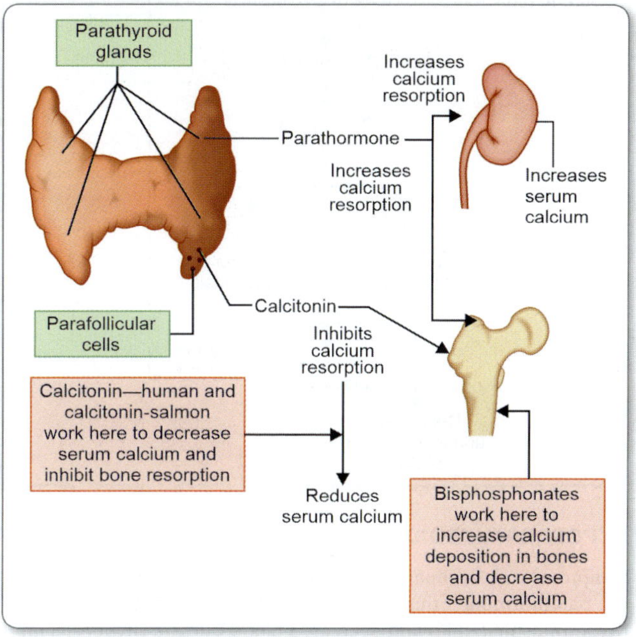

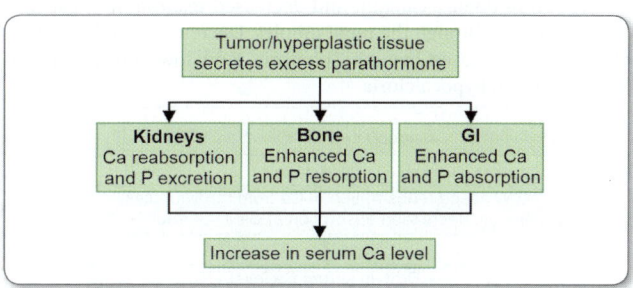

Fig. 7: Maintenance of calcium level by parathyroid gland

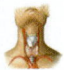

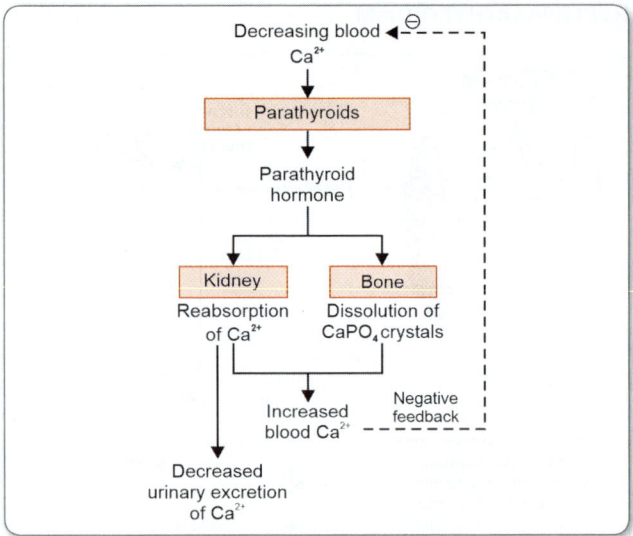

HYPOPARATHYROIDISM

Symptoms of hypoparathyroidism are caused by a deficiency of parathormone that results in elevated blood phosphate (hyperphosphatemia) and decreased blood calcium (hypocalcemia) levels. In the absence of parathormone, there is decreased intestinal absorption of dietary calcium and decreased resorption of calcium from bone and through the renal tubules. Decreased renal excretion of phosphate causes hypophosphaturia, and low serum calcium levels results in hypocalciuria.

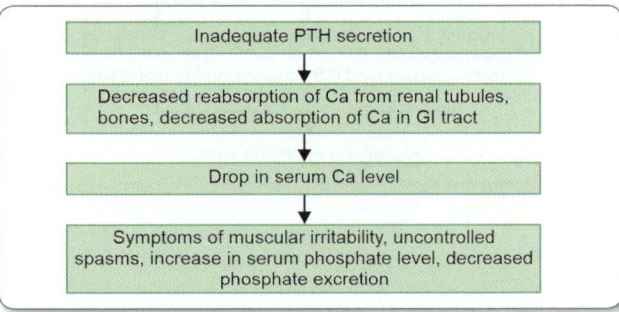

Abbreviations: GI, gastrointestinal; PTH, parathyroid hormone

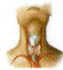

DIABETES MELLITUS

Insulin is a storage hormone that is secreted by beta cells in the islets of Langerhans in the pancreas. After eating food, secretion of insulin increases moving glucose from the blood to the muscle, liver and fat cells (Fig. 8).

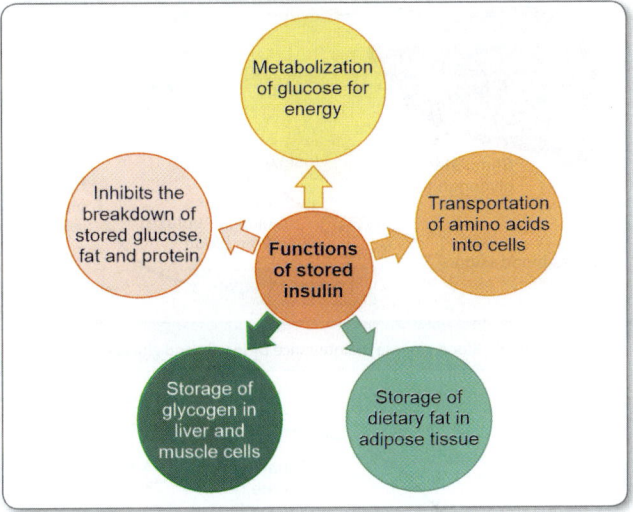

Fig. 8: Functions of stored insulin

Pancreas continues to release smaller amounts of insulin during fasting periods. Glucagon secreted by alpha cells is released when there is a decrease in blood glucose levels stimulating the liver to release the stored glucose. A constant level of glucose in the blood is maintained by insulin and glucagon together.

Initially, breakdown of glycogen occurs in liver, producing glucose. About 8–12 hours of not taking food, glucose is formed by the liver from the breakdown of noncarbohydrate substances, including amino acids (gluconeogenesis).

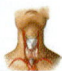

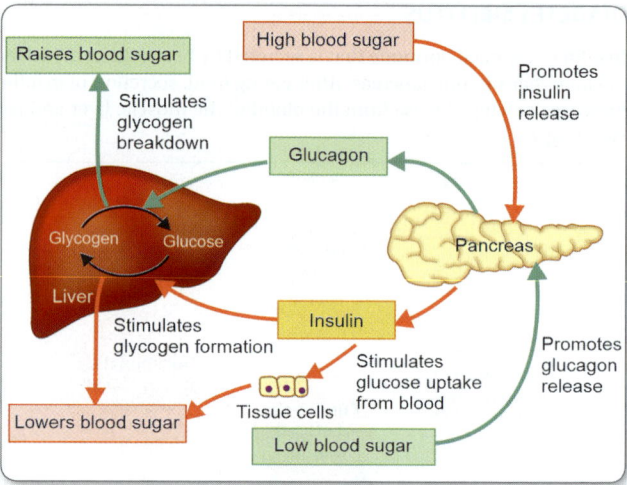

Fig. 9: Blood glucose maintenance by insulin and glucagon

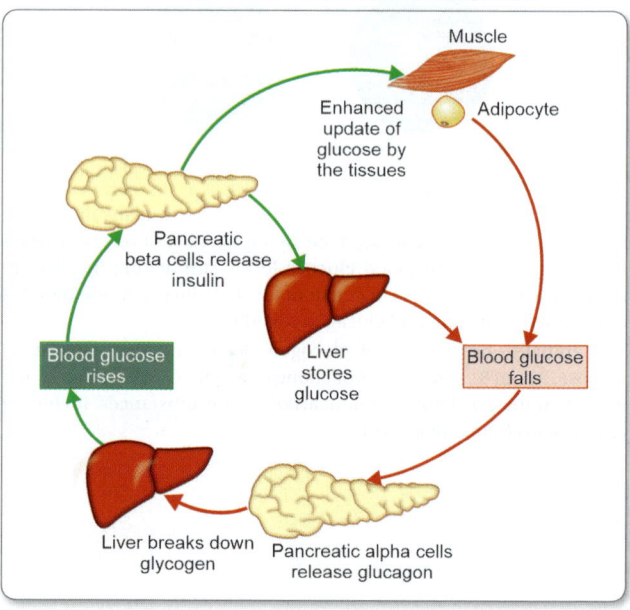

Fig. 10: Diabetes—insulin physiology

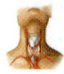

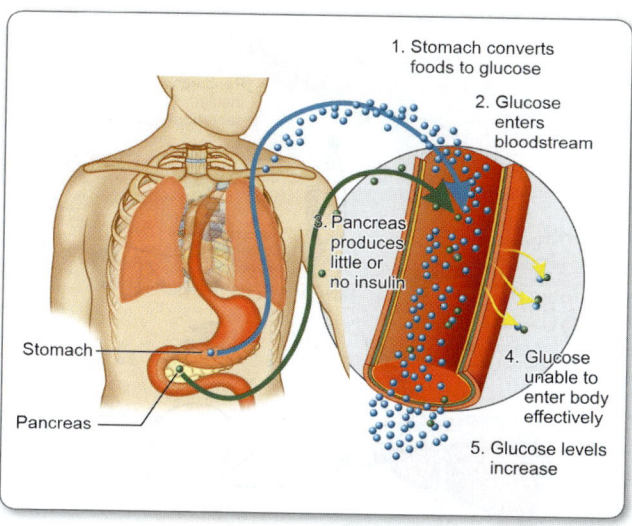

Fig. 11: Type I diabetes

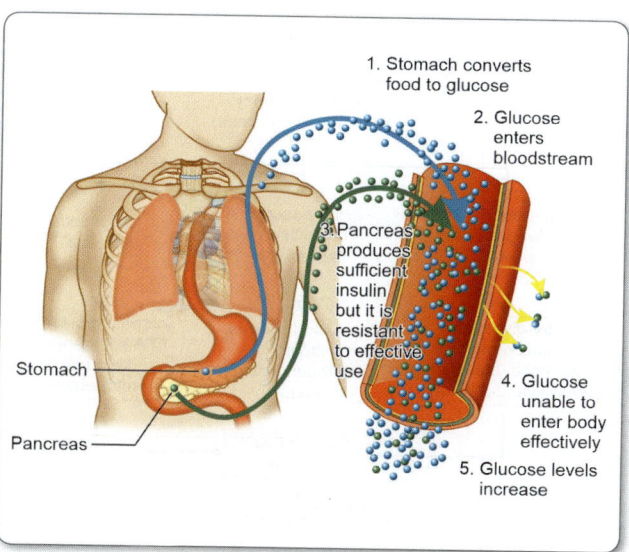

Fig. 12: Type II diabetes

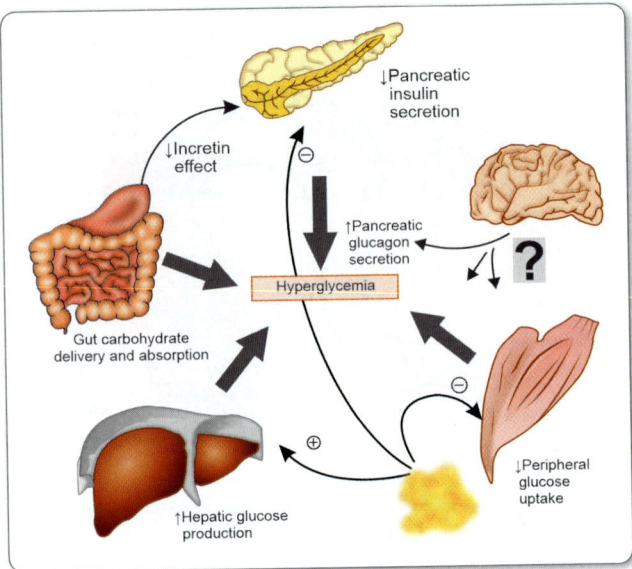

Fig. 13: Hyperglycemia

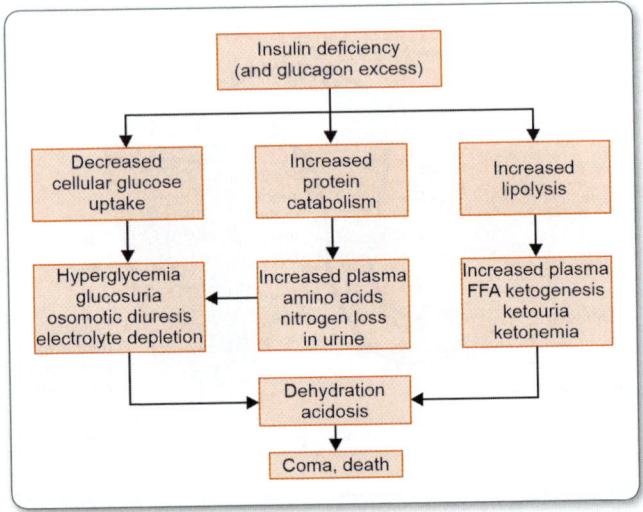

Abbreviation: FFA, free fatty acid

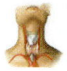

Pathophysiology of Diabetes Mellitus

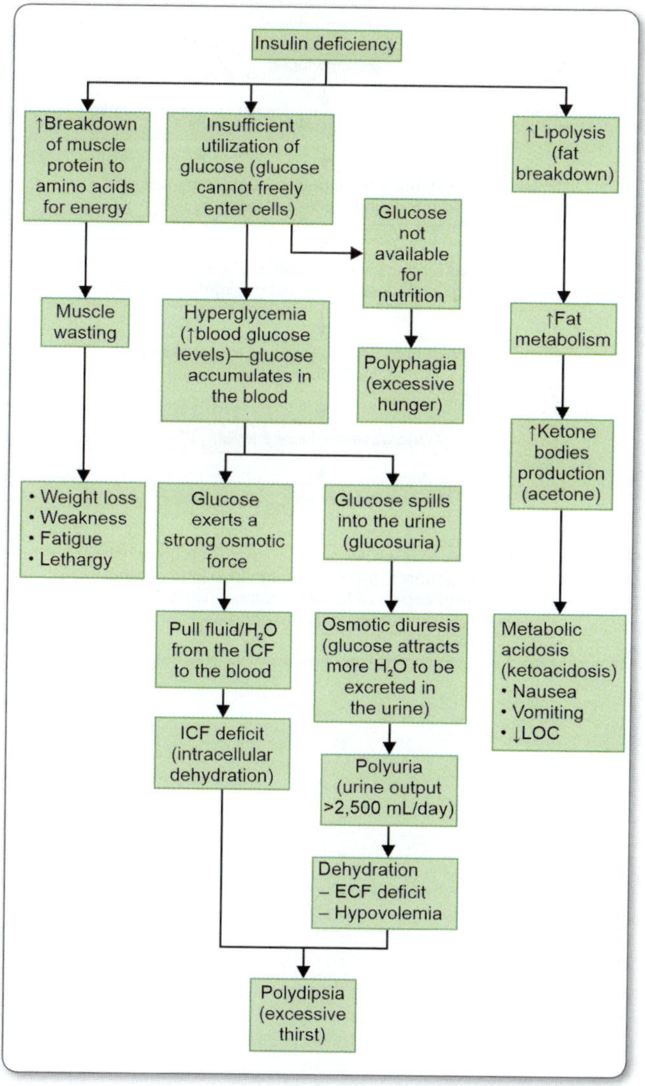

Insulin deficiency

↑Breakdown of muscle protein to amino acids for energy

Insufficient utilization of glucose (glucose cannot freely enter cells)

↑Lipolysis (fat breakdown)

Glucose not available for nutrition

Muscle wasting

Hyperglycemia (↑blood glucose levels)—glucose accumulates in the blood

↑Fat metabolism

Polyphagia (excessive hunger)

↑Ketone bodies production (acetone)

• Weight loss
• Weakness
• Fatigue
• Lethargy

Glucose exerts a strong osmotic force

Glucose spills into the urine (glucosuria)

Pull fluid/H_2O from the ICF to the blood

Osmotic diuresis (glucose attracts more H_2O to be excreted in the urine)

Metabolic acidosis (ketoacidosis)
• Nausea
• Vomiting
• ↓LOC

ICF deficit (intracellular dehydration)

Polyuria (urine output >2,500 mL/day)

Dehydration
− ECF deficit
− Hypovolemia

Polydipsia (excessive thirst)

Abbreviations: ECF, extracellular fluid; ICF, intracellular fluid; LOC, level of consciousness

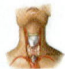

Pathophysiology (Type 2)

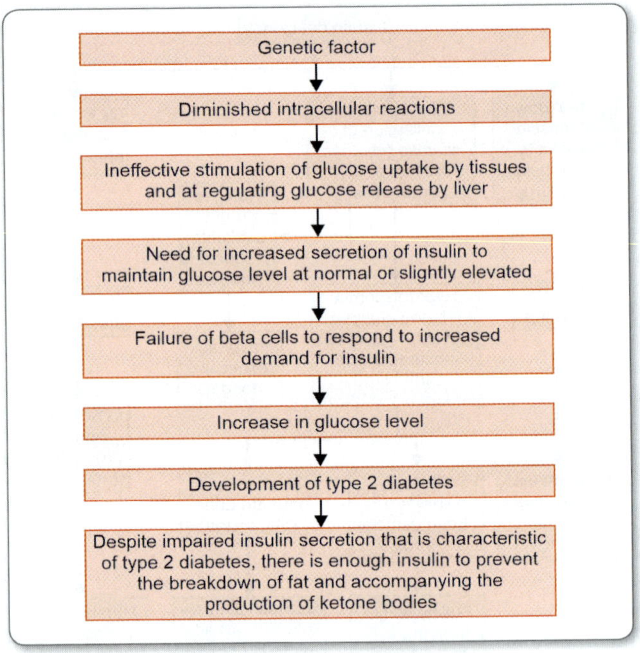

Genetic factor

↓

Diminished intracellular reactions

↓

Ineffective stimulation of glucose uptake by tissues and at regulating glucose release by liver

↓

Need for increased secretion of insulin to maintain glucose level at normal or slightly elevated

↓

Failure of beta cells to respond to increased demand for insulin

↓

Increase in glucose level

↓

Development of type 2 diabetes

↓

Despite impaired insulin secretion that is characteristic of type 2 diabetes, there is enough insulin to prevent the breakdown of fat and accompanying the production of ketone bodies

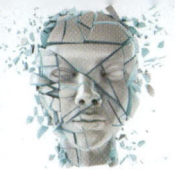

Pathophysiology of Nervous System Disorders

INTRODUCTION

The two main components of the nervous system are the central nervous system (CNS) and the peripheral nervous system (PNS). The brain and spinal cord make up the CNS, while PNS is composed of nerves exiting from the spinal cord and the autonomic nervous system that controls the nonvoluntary functions of the body (Fig. 1).

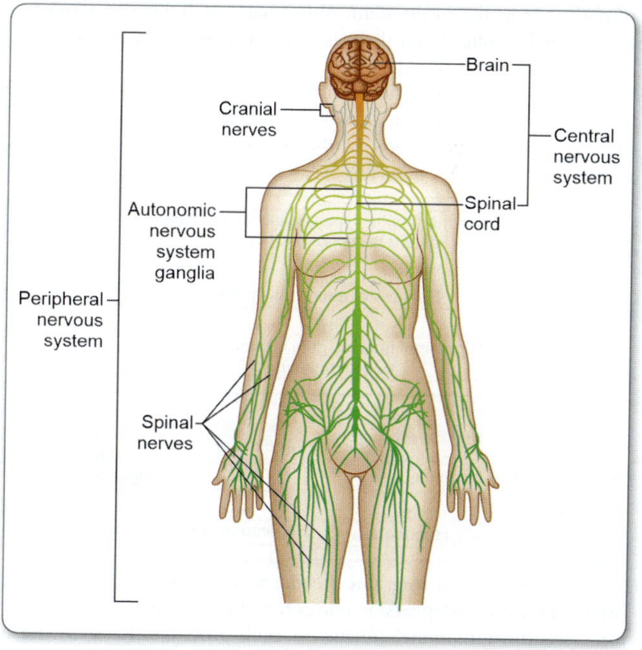

Fig. 1: Components of nervous system

The functions of nervous system include receiving sensory input from the environment, processing of the received information, and distributing the motor output. The sensory receptor neurons present in the PNS, respond to the physical stimuli like touch or temperature, and then forward the signals to the CNS. The received sensory information is then processed by the CNS, mainly by the brain.

After the processing of information, signals from the motor neurons are returned to the muscles and glands of the PNS, which gives out the motor output.

The disease conditions related to nervous system ultimately disrupts the functions of receiving sensory input, processing and giving the motor output.

Let's review the major changes occurring in various disorders related to nervous system.

HEADACHE

The cerebral signs and symptoms of migraine result from dysfunction of pathways in the brain stem. Abnormal metabolism of serotonin plays a major role. When there is a rise in plasma concentration of serotonin, cerebral blood vessels are dilated, producing headache. There is no complete understanding of the exact mechanism of migraine pain but the cranial blood vessels, and their innervations, and the reflex connections in the brain stem are thought to be involved.

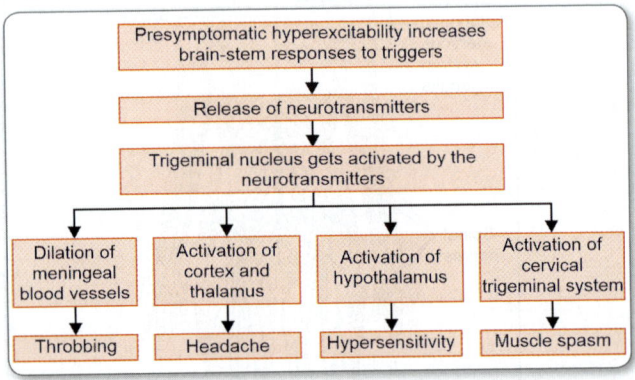

The triggers of migraine headache may be menstrual cycle, bright light, stress, depression and certain foods containing tyramine, monosodium glutamate, nitrites or milk products. Food in these categories include aged cheese and many processed foods. Use of oral contraceptives may be associated with increased frequency and severity of attacks in some women.

Emotional or physical stress may cause contraction of the muscles in the neck and scalp, resulting in tension headache. The pathophysiology of cluster headache is not fully understood.

HEAD INJURIES

Damage to the brain from traumatic injury can be either primary or secondary. An initial damage to the brain resulting from the trauma is known as **primary injury**, which may result from contusions, lacerations, impact injury, or penetration of foreign object. **secondary injury** results in few hours to days after an initial injury and is primarily due to swelling of brain or ongoing bleeding.

Skull is a rigid closed compartment that do not allow the expansion of cranial contents. Thus any bleeding or swelling within the skull increases the volume of contents within the cranium causing increased intracranial pressure (ICP). The result is restricted blood supply to brain, thereby decreasing the amount of oxygen available and inability to remove waste material. Anoxia of brain cells takes place, leading to improper metabolism, further causing ischemia and infarction of brain cells ultimately causing death of brain cells and tissues.

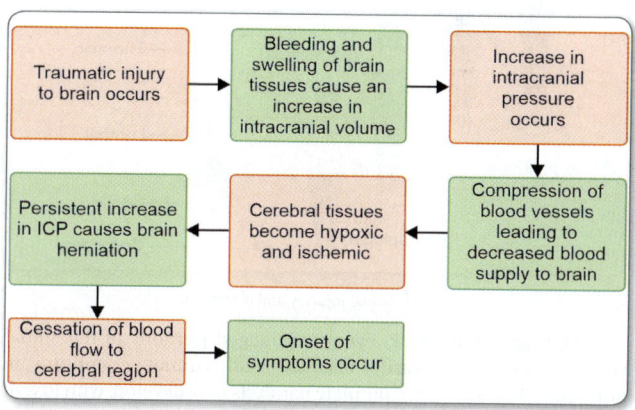

Abbreviation: ICP, intracranial pressure

Increased Intracranial Pressure

Acute neurological conditions alter the intracranial volume and pressure leading to increased ICP. Although head injury is known to be a common cause for an elevated ICP but it, also, may be seen as a secondary effect in conditions like brain tumors, subarachnoid hemorrhage and infectious conditions of the brain. Increased ICP decreases cerebral perfusion, stimulates edema, and causes shifting of brain tissues through opening in the rigid dura, resulting in **herniation** of brain.

SPINAL INJURIES—PARAPLEGIA, HEMIPLEGIA

Spinal cord injuries may be primary or secondary. Primary spinal cord injuries arise from mechanical disruption, transection, or distraction of neural elements. Penetrating injuries due to bullets or weapons may also cause primary spinal cord injury. Spinal cord compression occurs from an acute impact injury when a mass occupies the space in the spinal cord causing an increase in parenchymal pressure. Rapid or a critical degree of compression will result in collapse of the venous side of the microvasculature, resulting in vasogenic edema. Vasogenic edema exacerbates parenchymal pressure, and may lead to rapid progression of dysfunction (Fig. 2).

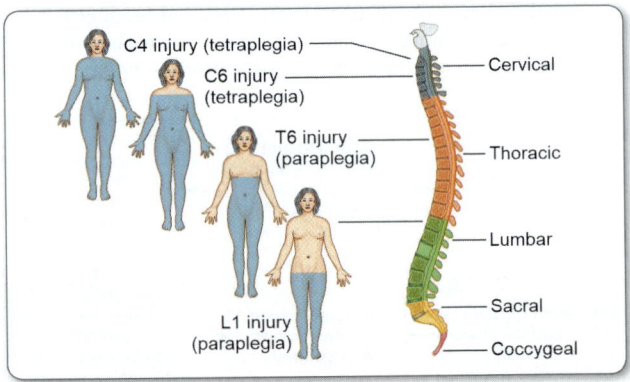

Fig. 2: Spinal injuries and its effects

During spinal shock, even undamaged portions of the spinal cord become temporarily disabled and cannot communicate normally with the brain. Complete paralysis may develop, with loss of reflexes and sensation in the limbs.

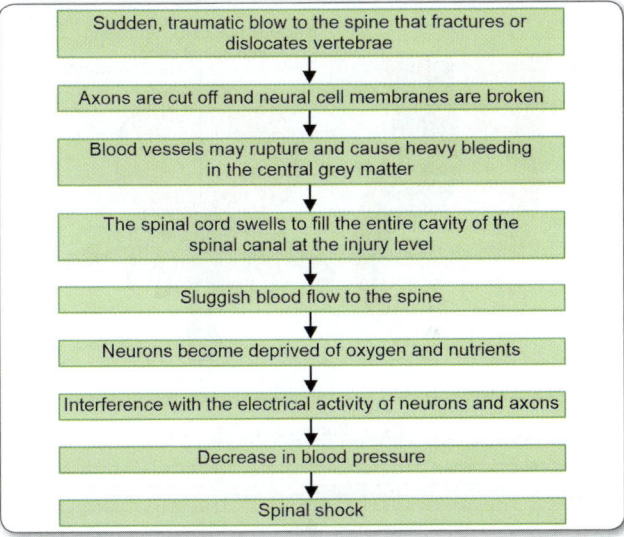

HERNIATION OF INTERVERTEBRAL DISC

The herniation of disc results from the protrusion of a part or whole of nucleus pulposus from the annulus fibrous. The degeneration of nucleus pulposus happens to be the most common cause of disc herniation where this part becomes dehydrated and weakens as a result of ageing leading to progressive disc herniation (Figs 3 and 4). The herniation may also be the result of trauma, disorders of connective tissues and certain congenital anomalies like short pedicles. The most common site is lumbar spine (Fig. 5). The cervical spine is also commonly affected by herniation of disc. The pathophysiology of herniated discs is believed to be a combination of the mechanical compression of the nerve by the bulging nucleus pulposus and the local increase in inflammatory chemokines.

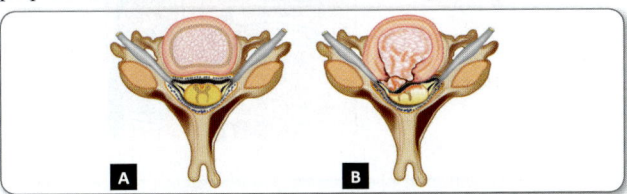

Figs 3A and B: A. Normal disc; **B.** Herniated disc

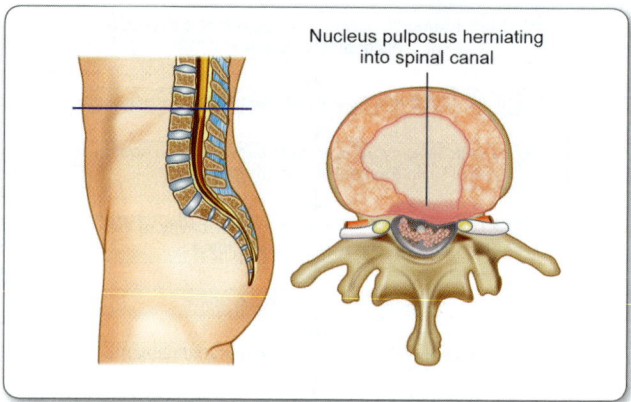

Nucleus pulposus herniating
into spinal canal

Fig. 4: Nucleus pulposus

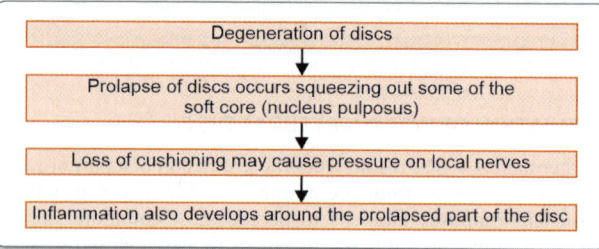

Degeneration of discs

↓

Prolapse of discs occurs squeezing out some of the
soft core (nucleus pulposus)

↓

Loss of cushioning may cause pressure on local nerves

↓

Inflammation also develops around the prolapsed part of the disc

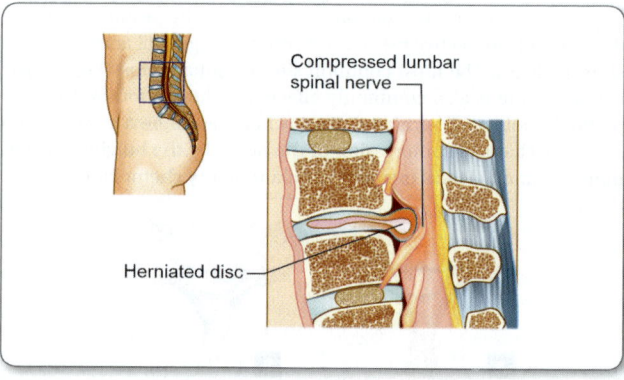

Compressed lumbar
spinal nerve

Herniated disc

Fig. 5: Compressed lumbar spinal nerve

CEREBRAL ANEURYSM

The ultimate cause of a brain aneurysm is an abnormal degenerative change in the arterial wall, and the effects of pressure from the pulsations of blood being pumped forward through the arteries in the brain. Certain locations of an aneurysm may create greater pressure such as at a bifurcation. The repeated trauma of blood flow against the vessel wall creates pressure against the point of weakness and causes the aneurysm to enlarge. Both high and low pressure of flowing blood can cause aneurysm and rupture (Fig. 6).

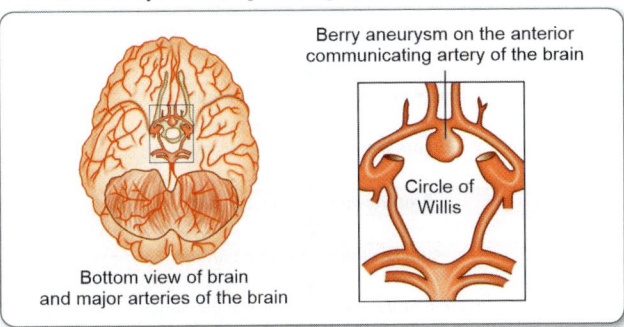

Berry aneurysm on the anterior communicating artery of the brain

Circle of Willis

Bottom view of brain and major arteries of the brain

Fig. 6: Berry aneurysm

Flow of changes leading to aneurysm formation and rupture are as follows:

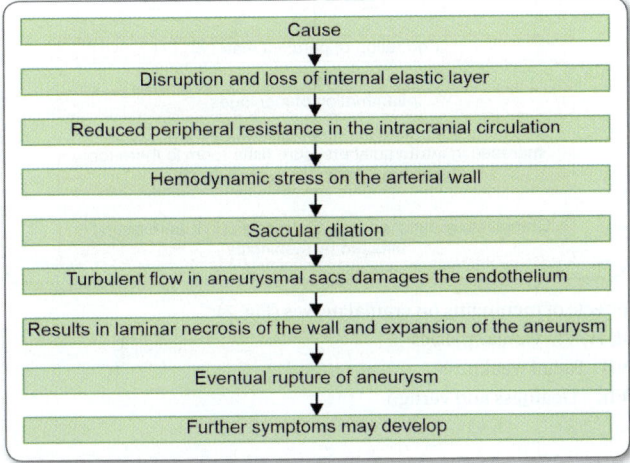

Cause
↓
Disruption and loss of internal elastic layer
↓
Reduced peripheral resistance in the intracranial circulation
↓
Hemodynamic stress on the arterial wall
↓
Saccular dilation
↓
Turbulent flow in aneurysmal sacs damages the endothelium
↓
Results in laminar necrosis of the wall and expansion of the aneurysm
↓
Eventual rupture of aneurysm
↓
Further symptoms may develop

MENINGITIS

The bacteria get engulfed into the cerebrospinal fluid (CSF) and grow rapidly in this compartment leading to inflammation in the CSF and the adjacent brain tissue. Initiation of the systemic inflammatory response occurs, further leading to migration of leukocytes into the subarachnoid space, an increased resistance to flow of CSF, and brain edema, ultimately causing an increase in intracranial pressure (ICP). Neuronal injury results from the attack of immune cells stimulated by the proinflammatory bacterial compounds.

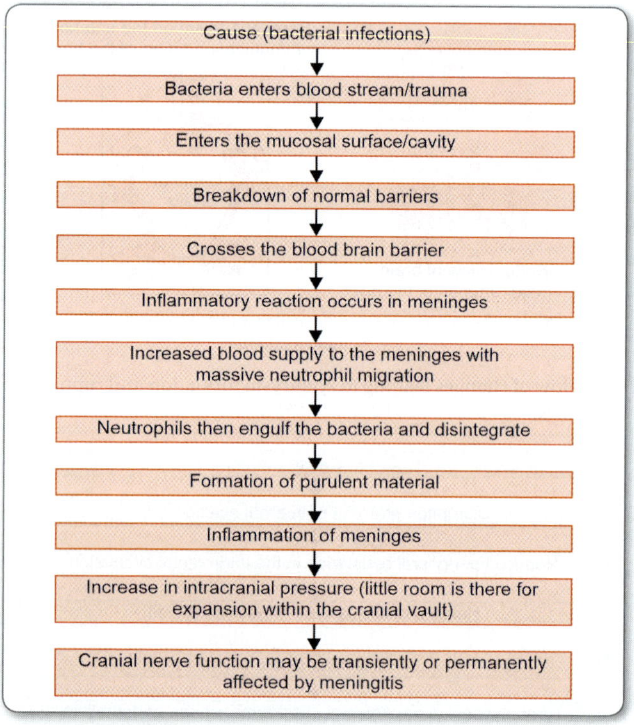

```
Cause (bacterial infections)
            ↓
Bacteria enters blood stream/trauma
            ↓
Enters the mucosal surface/cavity
            ↓
Breakdown of normal barriers
            ↓
Crosses the blood brain barrier
            ↓
Inflammatory reaction occurs in meninges
            ↓
Increased blood supply to the meninges with
massive neutrophil migration
            ↓
Neutrophils then engulf the bacteria and disintegrate
            ↓
Formation of purulent material
            ↓
Inflammation of meninges
            ↓
Increase in intracranial pressure (little room is there for
expansion within the cranial vault)
            ↓
Cranial nerve function may be transiently or permanently
affected by meningitis
```

Effects of meningitis on cranial nerves (Fig. 7):

II, IV, VI - Ocular palsies

VII - Facial weakness

VIII - Deafness and vertigo

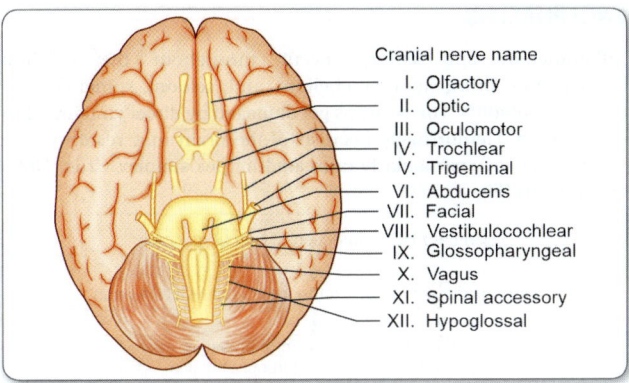

Cranial nerve name
- I. Olfactory
- II. Optic
- III. Oculomotor
- IV. Trochlear
- V. Trigeminal
- VI. Abducens
- VII. Facial
- VIII. Vestibulocochlear
- IX. Glossopharyngeal
- X. Vagus
- XI. Spinal accessory
- XII. Hypoglossal

Fig. 7: Cranial nerves

BRAIN ABSCESS

Brain abscesses develop in response to a parenchymal infection with pyogenic bacteria, beginning as a localized area of cerebritis and evolving into a suppurative lesion surrounded by a well-vascularized fibrotic capsule.

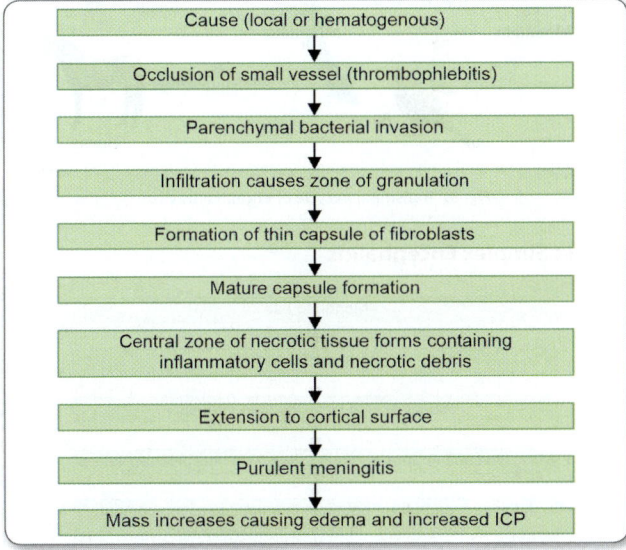

Cause (local or hematogenous)
↓
Occlusion of small vessel (thrombophlebitis)
↓
Parenchymal bacterial invasion
↓
Infiltration causes zone of granulation
↓
Formation of thin capsule of fibroblasts
↓
Mature capsule formation
↓
Central zone of necrotic tissue forms containing inflammatory cells and necrotic debris
↓
Extension to cortical surface
↓
Purulent meningitis
↓
Mass increases causing edema and increased ICP

Abbreviation: ICP, intracranial pressure

151

ENCEPHALITIS

Inflammation and edema occur throughout the cerebral hemispheres, brain stem, cerebellum, and, seldom, spinal cord in acute encephalitis. The neurons get damaged by direct viral invasion of the brain. Hemorrhagic necrosis of the brain may result from a severe infection, particularly untreated herpes simplex virus (HSV) encephalitis (Fig. 8).

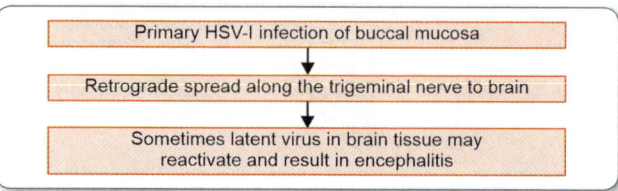

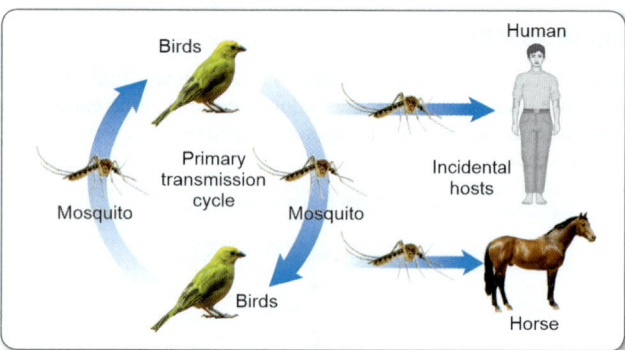

Fig. 8: Transmission cycle of encephalitis virus

Herpes Simplex Encephalitis

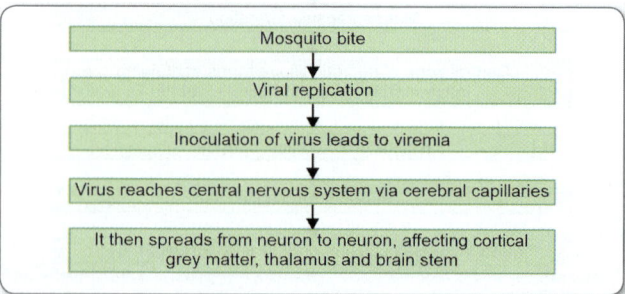

Fungal Encephalitis

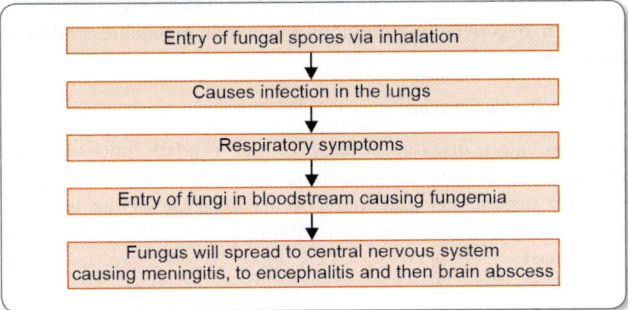

Neurocysticercosis is the result of accidental ingestion of eggs of *Taenia solium* (i.e., pork tapeworm), usually due to contamination of food by people with taeniasis. The embryos develop from the eggs, penetrating the small intestine mucosa and entering the circulation and subsequently different tissues and organs where cysticerci, small tissue larvae, are developed. Cysticerci have specific affinity for the central nervous system, eyes and striated muscles what is accounted for high concentration of glucose or glycogen in these organs.

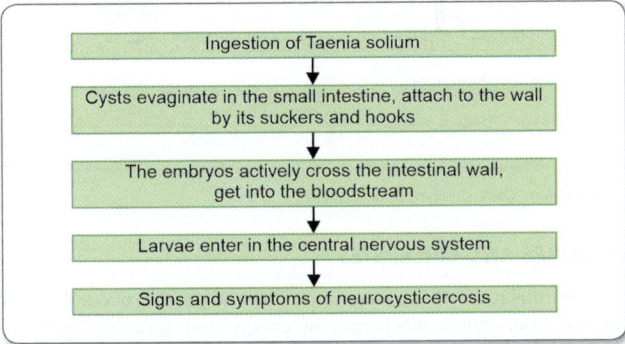

MOVEMENT DISORDERS—CHOREA

Chorea is a type of movement disorder that is caused by an injury to basal ganglia. There are sudden and brief involuntary muscle contractions of various parts of the body. Damage to striatum and subthalamic nucleus is responsible for the occurrence of chorea. The disorders associated with chorea may be infectious conditions of the brain, degenerative conditions and certain metabolic conditions as well.

Huntington's Chorea

In Huntington disease, atrophy of the caudate nucleus takes place, and the inhibitory medium spiny neurons in the corpus striatum degenerate, and there occurs decrease in the levels of the neurotransmitters gamma-aminobutyric acid (GABA) and substance P.

Huntington's disease results from gene mutation. Early and severe onset disease occurs with a greater number of coronary angiogram (CAG) repeats. The number of CAG repeats can increase with successive generations when the father transmits the mutation and, over time, can lead to increasingly severe phenotypes within a family.

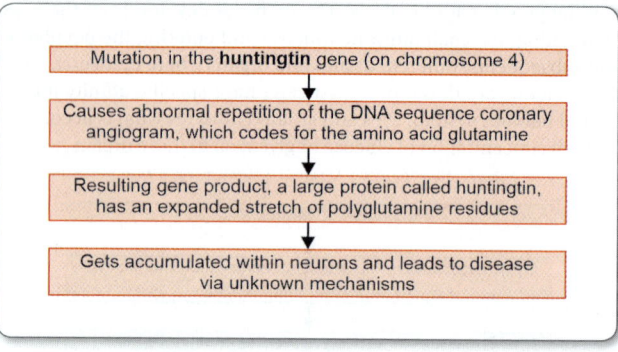

Abbreviation: DNA, deoxyribonucleic acid

SEIZURES AND EPILEPSIES

The neurons carry the messages from the body, which occur through the electrochemical discharges of energy and generally increase during a period of activity in the nerve cells. Seizures occur when an unwanted discharge from the nerve cells, leading to unpredictable movements in the body parts takes place. This dysfunction may be a mild episode but can even become debilitating causing unconsciousness. The repeated occurrence of these uncontrolled, abnormal discharges is known as an epileptic syndrome (Fig. 9).

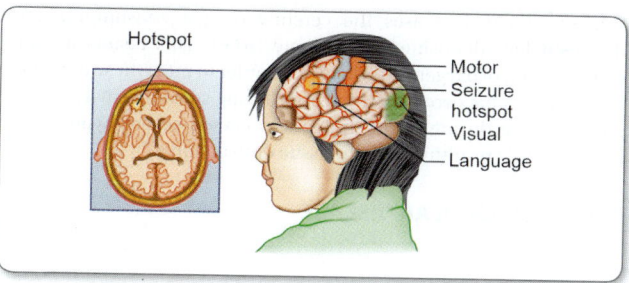

Fig. 9: Epilepsy

Figures 10A and B shows partial seizure and primary generalized seizure.

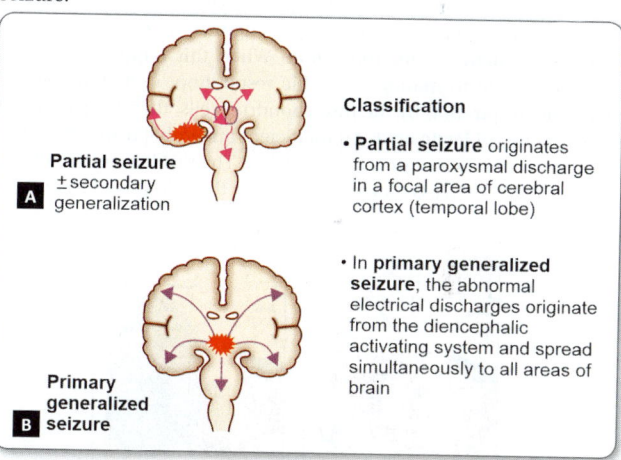

Classification

- **Partial seizure** originates from a paroxysmal discharge in a focal area of cerebral cortex (temporal lobe)

- In **primary generalized seizure**, the abnormal electrical discharges originate from the diencephalic activating system and spread simultaneously to all areas of brain

Figs 10A and B: **A.** Partial seizure; **B.** Primary generalized seizure

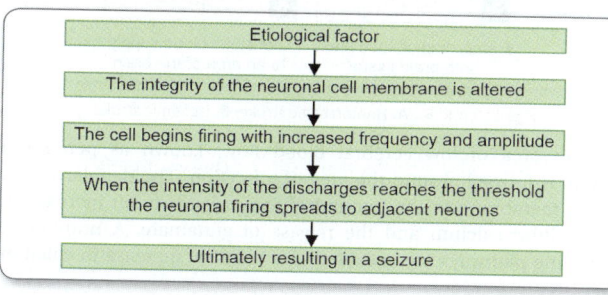

Seizure activity increases the cerebral oxygen consumption and the need for adenosine triphosphate (ATP). This results in rapid consumption of oxygen and glucose. In order to meet these demands, blood flow to the cerebrum increases during seizure activity. An ongoing seizure during status epilepticus causes severe hypoxia and lactic acidosis resulting in brain tissue destruction.

CEREBROVASCULAR DISEASE

Ischemic Stroke

An obstruction of cerebral blood vessels occurs leading to the disruption of the cerebral blood flow, which is the characteristic feature in an ischemic brain attack. The obstruction in the blood flow leads to an onset of a complex series of cellular metabolic events known as an ischemic cascade, beginning with a decrease in blood flow to less than 25 mL/100 g/min. When this happens, neurons become unable to maintain aerobic respiration, switching over to anaerobic respiration by the mitochondrial cells, thereby generating large amount of lactic acid. An inefficient anaerobic respiration also leads to an insufficient production of ATP. The result is an imbalance of electrolytes and cessation of functions of the cells (Figs 11A and B).

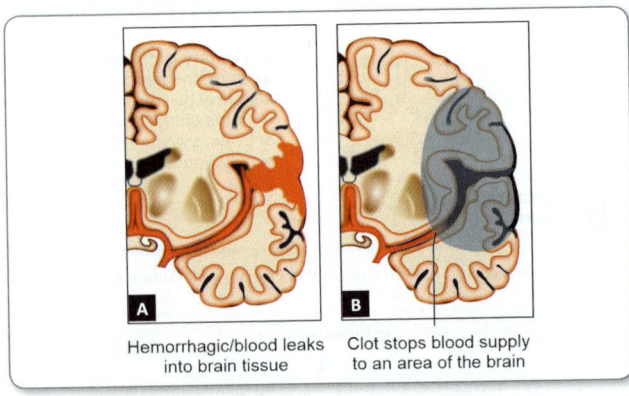

Hemorrhagic/blood leaks into brain tissue

Clot stops blood supply to an area of the brain

Figs 11A and B: **A.** Hemorrhagic stroke; **B.** Ischemic stroke

An area of low cerebral blood flow, known as penumbra region, is formed around the area of infarction. The depolarization of cell membrane in the penumbra region leads to an increase in intracellular calcium and the release of glutamate. A number of damaging pathways are activated as a result of increase in calcium and glutamate, causing destruction of the cell membrane, and generation of free radicals. All these events cause an enlargement in the area of infarction extending the stroke further (Fig. 12).

Each step into the ischemic cascade represents an opportunity for intervention to limit the extent of secondary brain damage caused by a stroke. Medications that protect the brain from secondary injury are called neuroprotectants. A number of clinical trials are focusing on calcium channel antagonists that block the calcium influx, glutamate antagonists, antioxidants, and other neuroprotectant strategies that help prevent secondary complications.

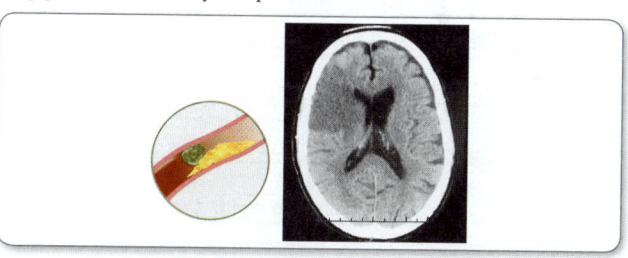

Fig. 12: Ischemic stroke

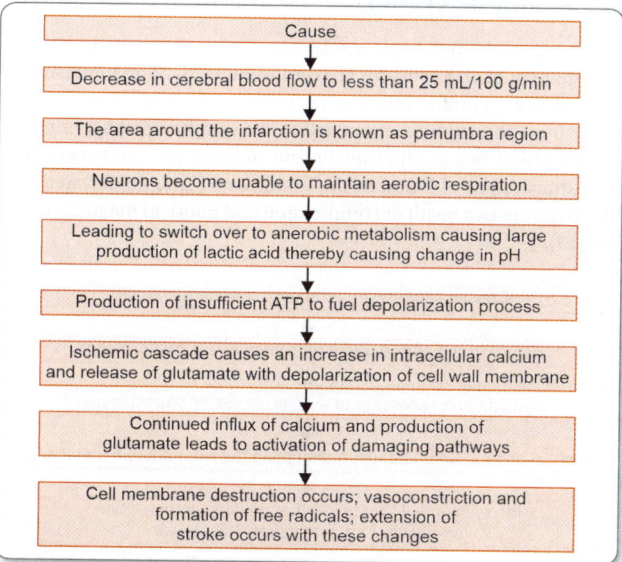

Abbreviation: ATP, adenosine triphosphate

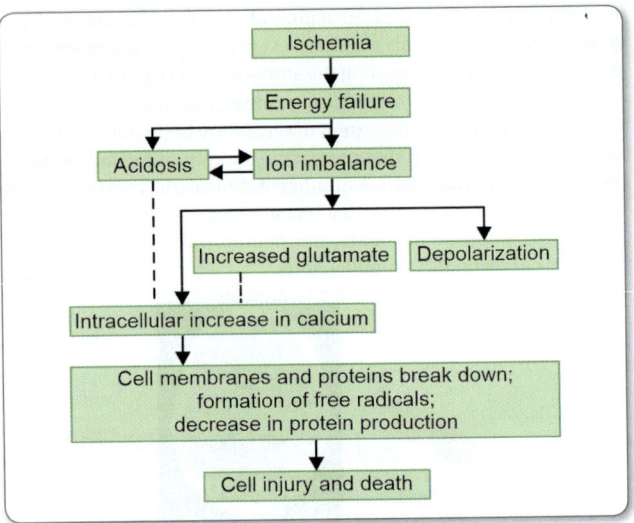

HEMORRHAGIC STROKE

Symptoms in hemorrhagic stroke are produced when there is an enlargement of an aneurysm or arteriovenous malformation causing compression of brain tissues and cranial nerves. The symptoms also result from the rupture of aneurysm causing hemorrhage into the subarachnoid space. The metabolism of brain gets disturbed from the extravasation of blood in the brain tissues and an elevated ICP, which occurs as a result of compression and injury to the brain tissue (Fig. 13).

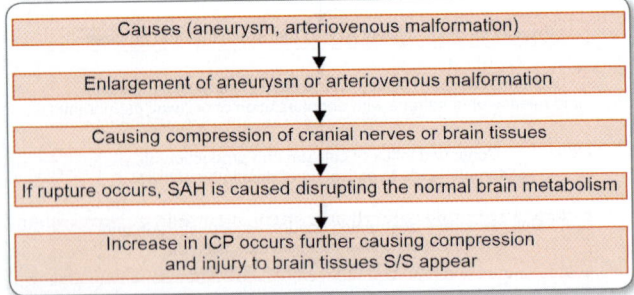

Abbreviations: ICP, intracranial pressure; SAH, subarachnoid hemorrhage

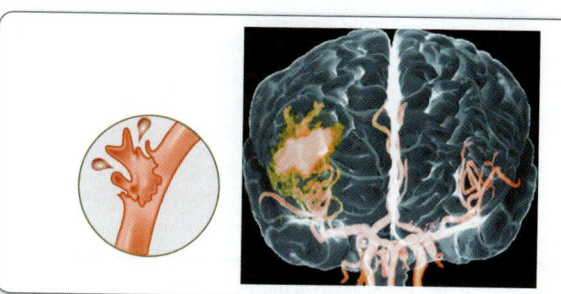

Fig. 13: Hemorrhagic stroke

BELL'S PALSY

Facial nerve passes through a portion of temporal bone known as the facial canal. Inflammation of geniculate ganglion (a group of fibers and sensory neurons of facial nerve located in the facial canal of the head) leads to compression within this bony canal.

This can in turn block the transmission of neural signals, result in ischemia and demyelination, and cause facial paralysis or Bell's palsy.

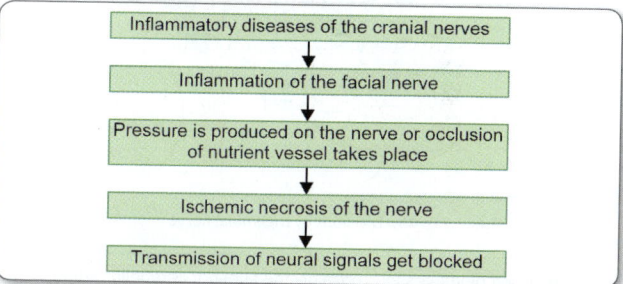

TRIGEMINAL NEURALGIA

There are three branches of the trigeminal nerve: (1) ophthalmic, (2) maxillary, and (3) mandibular. The pain of trigeminal neuralgia occurs almost exclusively in the maxillary and mandibular divisions (Fig. 14).

Classic trigeminal neuralgia is associated with neurovascular compression in the trigeminal root entry zone, which can lead to demyelination and a dysregulation of voltage-gated sodium channel expression in the membrane. These alterations may be responsible for pain attacks in trigeminal neuralgia patients.

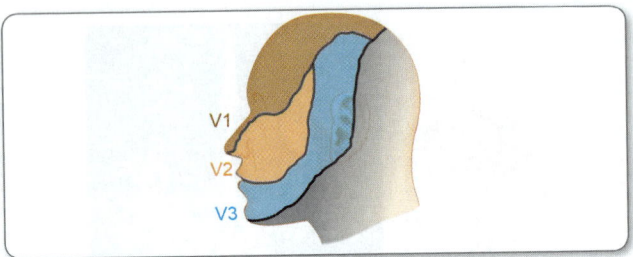

Fig. 14: Branches of trigeminal nerve

Figure 15 shows divisions of trigeminal nerve. Figures 16A to C also can be referred.

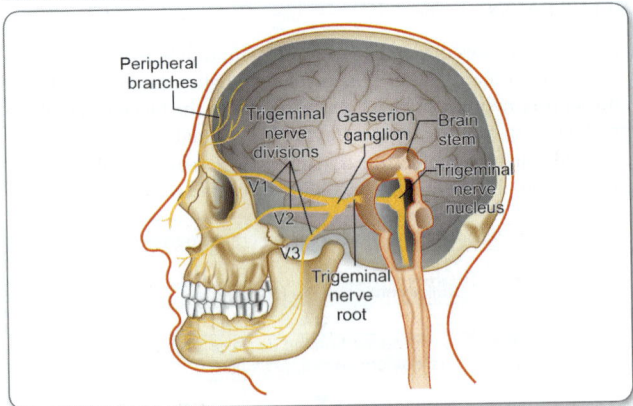

Fig. 15: Divisions of trigeminal nerve

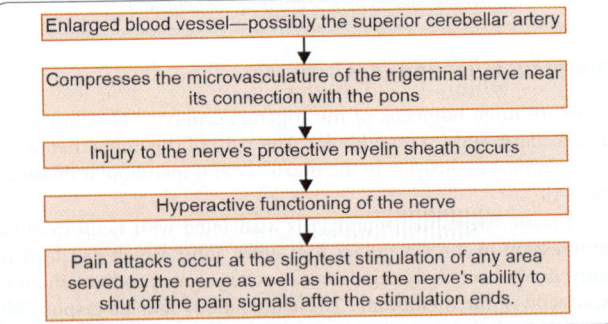

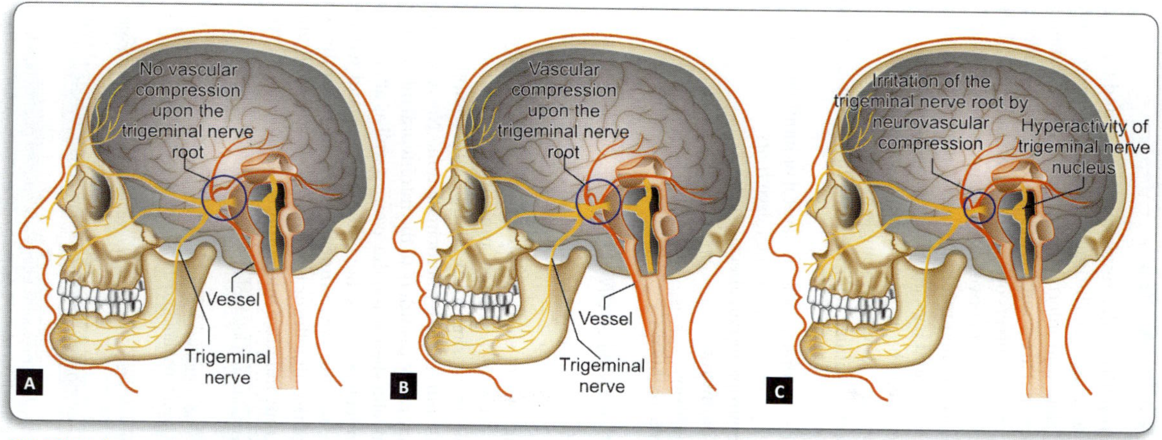

Figs 16A to C: A. In people without trigeminal nerve, there is usually no vascular compression upon the trigeminal nerve root; **B.** In most sufferers of typical trigeminal neuralgia, vessels compress the trigeminal nerve root; **C.** The generation of trigeminal nerve pain is thought to result from peripheral pathophysiology (i.e., neurovascular compression) and central pathophysiology (i.e., hyperactivity of the trigeminal nerve nucleus)

Understanding Pathophysiology of Diseases

PERIPHERAL NEUROPATHIES

Peripheral neuropathy is the result of disease conditions causing damage to the cranial nerves. The brain and spinal cord are connected to the muscles, skin, and internal organs by a complex network of peripheral nerves, that are arranged as dermatomes. Whenever, there is a damage to nerves, it affects one or more dermatomes, which then interrupts communication between the brain and other parts of the body. This leads to an impairment in muscle movement and normal sensation in the arms and legs, and also causes pain.

- Neuropathies might be acute or chronic
- Mononeuropathy—affecting a single nerve
- Polyneuropathy—diffuse, symmetrical disease usually starting peripherally.
- Mononeuritis multiplex—affects several or multiple nerves.
- Radiculopathy—disease affecting nerve roots
- Peripheral neuropathy can affect:
  - Sensory pathways
  - Motor pathways
  - Autonomic pathways

CARPAL TUNNEL SYNDROME

The entrapment neuropathy combines phenomena of compression and traction.

The compressive element of the pathophysiology includes a detrimental cycle of increased pressure, obstruction of overall venous outflow, increasing local edema, and compromise to the median nerve's intraneural microcirculation. Nerve compression and traction may cause disorders of the intraneural microcirculation, lesions in the myelin sheath and the axon, as well as alterations in the supporting connective tissue. Repetitive traction and wrist motion exacerbate the negative environment, further injuring the nerve. In addition, any of the nine flexor tendons traveling through the carpal tunnel can become inflamed and compress the median nerve.

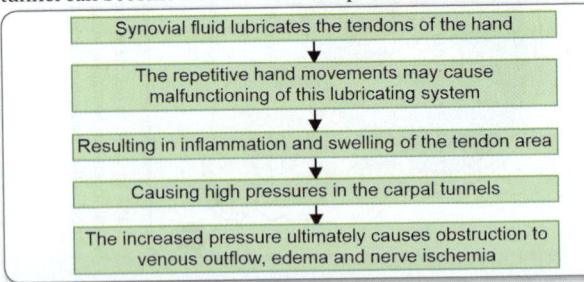

Synovial fluid lubricates the tendons of the hand
↓
The repetitive hand movements may cause malfunctioning of this lubricating system
↓
Resulting in inflammation and swelling of the tendon area
↓
Causing high pressures in the carpal tunnels
↓
The increased pressure ultimately causes obstruction to venous outflow, edema and nerve ischemia

ALZHEIMER'S DISEASE

Alzheimer's disease (AD) is a slowly progressive disease of the brain that is characterized by impairment of memory and eventually by disturbances in reasoning, planning, language, and perception.

Loss of synapses and neurons occur by the deposition of the beta-amyloid proteins and neurofibrillary tangles, resulting in gross atrophy of the affected areas of the brain (Fig. 17).

A complex cascade of events is triggered by this progressive accumulation of beta-amyloid and deficits in neurotransmitters, contributing to the clinical symptoms of dementia.

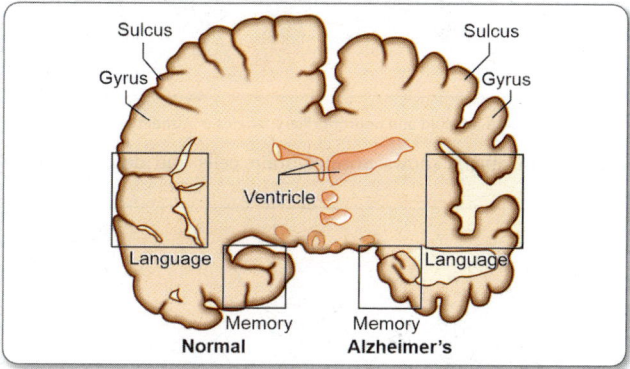

Fig. 17: Cross-section of brain showing normal and Alzheimer's disease

In **prion** diseases, the normal cell-surface protein of brain turns into a pathogenic form '**prion**'. The prion then causes other prion proteins to fold into an unusual structure, resulting in a marked increase in the number of abnormal proteins, leading to damage to the brain. The beta-amyloid and neurofibrillary tangles are believed to possess prion-like properties or replicating by self, leading to the onset of Alzheimer's disease (Fig. 18).

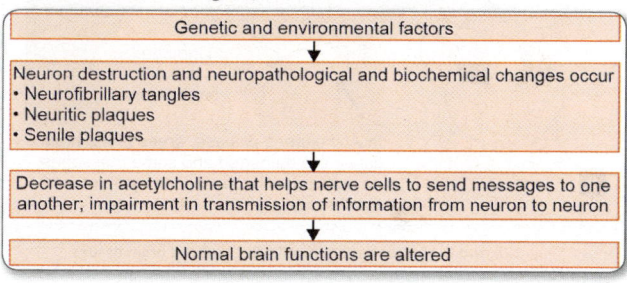

Normal
Alzheimer's
Neuron
Neurofibrillary tangles
Amyloid plaques

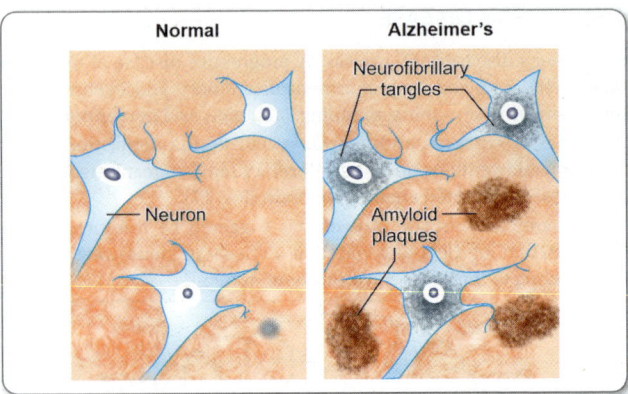

Fig. 18: Beta-amyloid and neurofibrillary tangles in Alzheimer's disease

Figures 19A and B shows normal brain cells and damaged brain tissues.

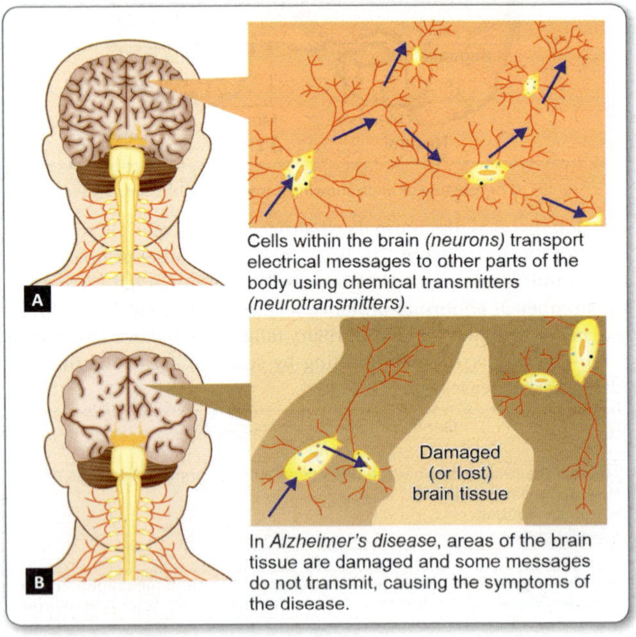

Cells within the brain *(neurons)* transport electrical messages to other parts of the body using chemical transmitters *(neurotransmitters)*.
A
Damaged (or lost) brain tissue
In *Alzheimer's disease*, areas of the brain tissue are damaged and some messages do not transmit, causing the symptoms of the disease.
B

Figs 19A and B: **A.** Normal brain cells; **B.** Damaged brain tissues

PARKINSON'S DISEASE

Parkinson's disease is primarily related to less production of dopamine that occurs because of gradual loss of cells in the substantia nigra. Dopamine is required for coordinated activity within the brain by transmitting signals between substantia nigra and corpus striatum. The deficiency of dopamine in the striatum causes an uncontrolled firing of the nerve cells, leading to uncontrolled movements. With the progression of disease, degeneration of other areas of brain occurs leading to a more profound movement disorder. Both genetic and environmental factors are believed to be responsible for the loss of cells.

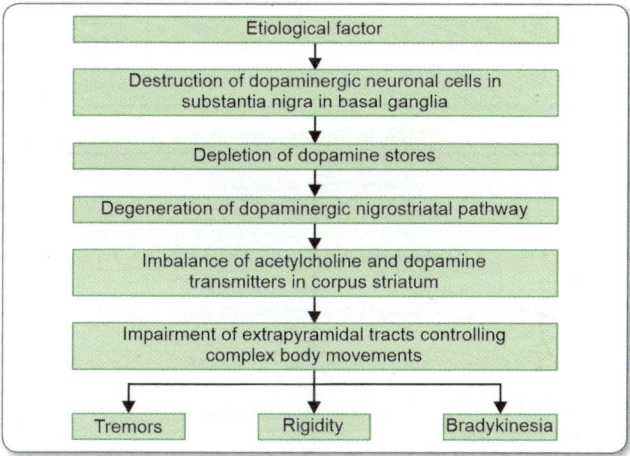

GUILLAIN-BARRÉ SYNDROME

The GBS is considered to be an autoimmune disease triggered by a preceding bacterial or viral infection. In the acute motor axonal neuropathy (AMAN) form of GBS, the infecting organisms probably share homologous epitopes to a component of the peripheral nerves (molecular mimicry) and, therefore, the immune responses cross-react with the nerves causing axonal degeneration. In the acute inflammatory demyelinating polyneuropathy (AIDP) form, immune system reactions against target epitopes in Schwann cells or myelin result in demyelination (Fig. 20).

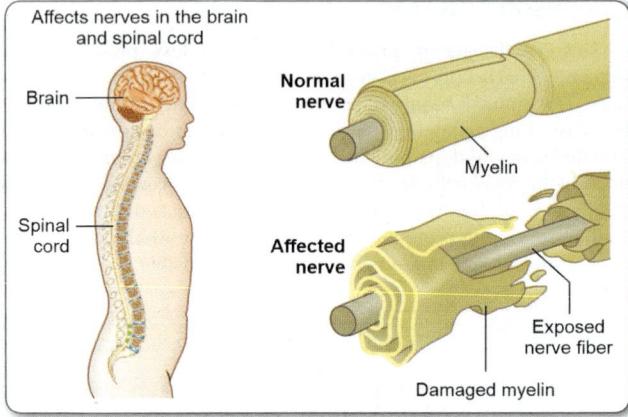

Fig. 20: Guillain-Barré syndrome

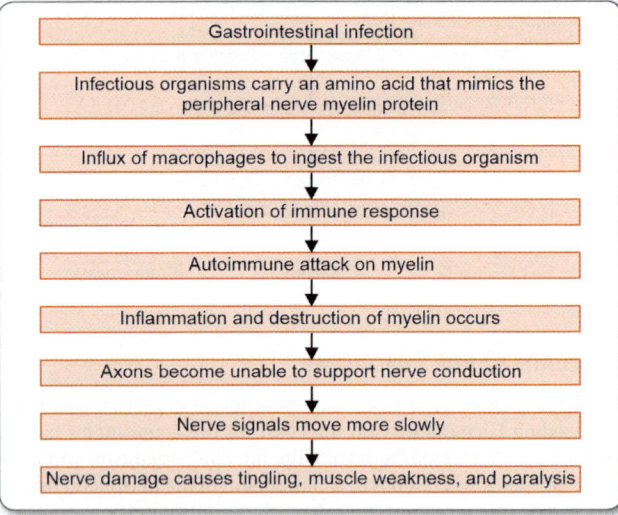

MYASTHENIA GRAVIS

A defect in the transmission of nerve impulses to muscles is responsible for causing weakness of muscles. Normally a muscle contraction is generated by the activation of acetylcholine receptors when acetylcholine released from the nerve endings, binds to these receptors. When a normal communication between the nerve and muscle is interrupted at the neuromuscular junction, it leads to the onset of symptoms in Myasthenia gravis.

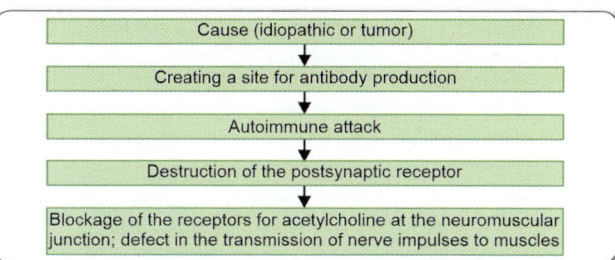

MULTIPLE SCLEROSIS

Multiple sclerosis occurs mostly in people who have a genetic susceptibility to environmental factors and events, which ultimately trigger the process of disease. It is thought that peripheral immune cells get mobilized and enter the CNS through the impaired blood-brain barrier in the subarachnoid space, and migration of a number of macrophages, T cells and B cells as well as plasma cells occur. Demyelination is mostly localized to focal lesions, whereas other areas of white matter appear normal. Over time, T cell and B cell infiltration becomes more diffuse and an extensive axonal injury takes place, leading to self-perpetuating atrophy in both white and gray matter (Fig. 21).

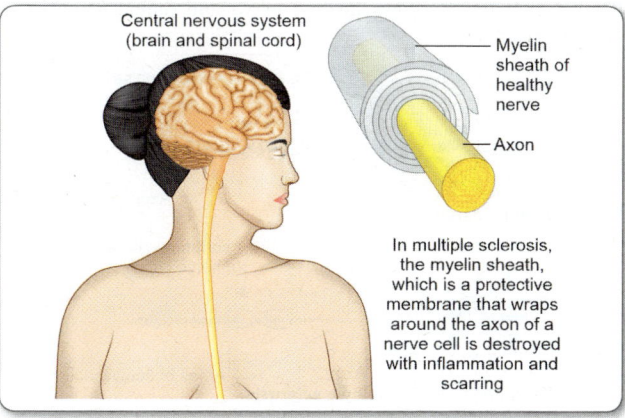

Fig. 21: Multiple sclerosis

Figure 22 shows a comparison between normal axon, disintegration of myelin and disruption of axon function.

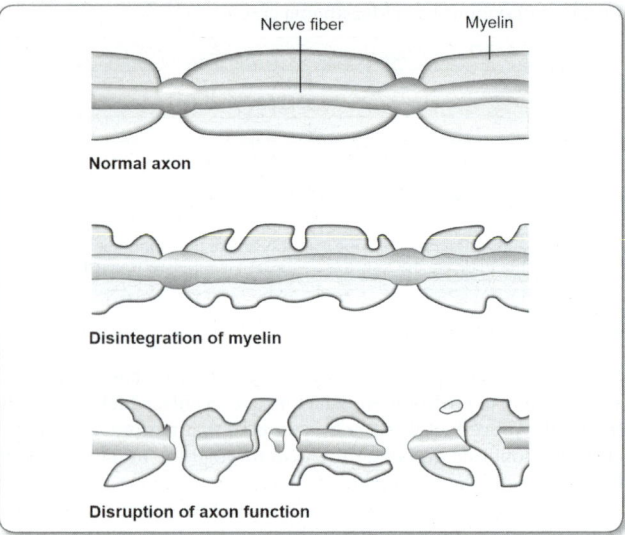

Fig. 22: Comparison between normal axon, disintegration of myelin and disruption of axon function

Process of Demyelination

Figures 23A and B shows healthy nerve and damaged nerve in multiple sclerosis

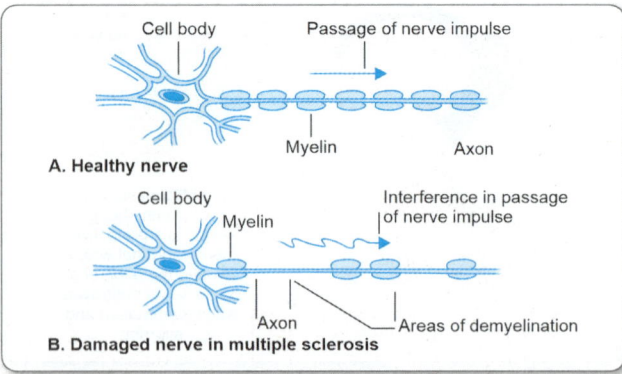

Figs 23A and B: **A.** Healthy nerve; **B.** Damaged nerve in multiple sclerosis

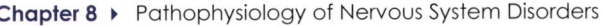

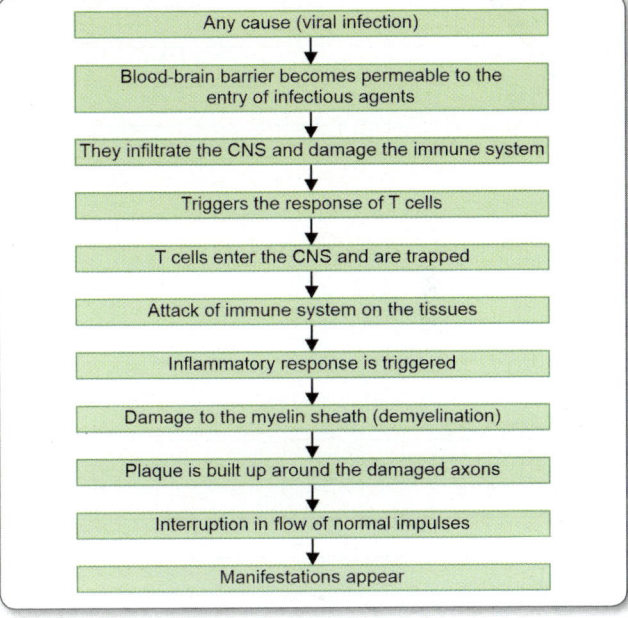

Abbreviation: CNS, central nervous system

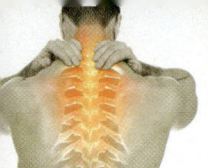

Pathophysiology of Musculoskeletal Disorders

INTRODUCTION

Bones, muscles, joints, cartilage, ligaments, tendons, and connective tissues make up the musculoskeletal system (Fig. 1).

The primary functions of musculoskeletal system are to support the body, allow movements, and protect the vital organs.

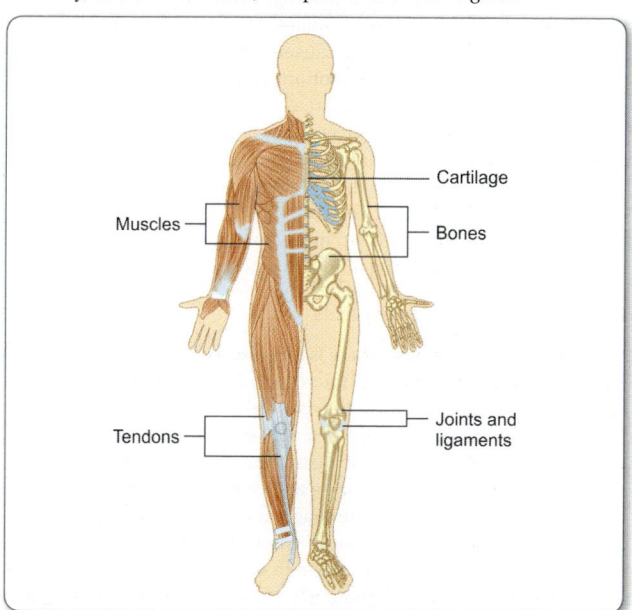

Fig. 1: Musculoskeletal system

The bones keep body stable. Muscles hold the bones in place and help in their movement. Articulating joints connected to different bones allow movement and cartilage functions as a cushion to the bone ends to prevent the direct rubbing onto each other.

The muscular system includes all types of muscles in the body. Skeletal muscles act on the joints of the body to produce movements. Tendons attach the muscles to the bones. The main component of skeletal system is bone. The articulation of bones occurs at the joints. The accessory structures of the skeletal system like articular cartilage, ligaments and bursae support the bones and joints.

SOFT-TISSUE INJURIES

These are classified as contusions (bruises), sprains, tendonitis, bursitis, stress injuries and strains.

A contusion (bruise) is an injury to the soft tissue often produced by a blunt force, such as a kick, fall, or blow. This results in pain, swelling, and discoloration because of bleeding into the tissue. A sprain is a partial ligament tear caused by a wrench or twist. It often affects wrists, knees or ankles. Inflammation of the tendon is called tendonitis. It is often caused by an overuse injury in the affected area due to repetitive motion. Wrist, hand, elbow, shoulder, hip, knee, ankle, and foot are the areas, which are commonly affected. A fluid-filled sac that provides a cushion between bones and muscles or tendons is called Bursa and its inflammation is known as bursitis. A small crack in a bone in the weight-bearing bones of the lower extremities caused by overuse and increase in physical activity is often called a stress fracture. An injury to a muscle or tendon caused due to overuse, or stretching is known as a strain.

Healing of Soft-tissue Injuries

In the inflammatory phase, there is an increased interaction between leukocytes and the injured microvascular endothelium. Platelet aggregation occurs as a result of exposure of subendothelial collagen structures by trauma. These release serotonin, adrenaline, and thromboxane-A, causing vasoconstriction and producing cytokines. Vasoconstriction and thrombocyte aggregation contribute to clotting and are an important part of the coagulation process to stop bleeding. The proliferative phase begins when fibroblasts, followed by endothelial cells, migrate into the area of the wound and proliferate. This is stimulated by mitogenic growth factors. These cells have a series of growth factor receptors on their surfaces and release several cytokines and synthesize structural proteins of the extracellular matrix, such as collagen. In the reparative phase, new capillaries are formed by the proliferation of endothelial cells. At the end of the reparative phase, water content is reduced and the collagen initially formed is replaced by cross-linked collagen type III.

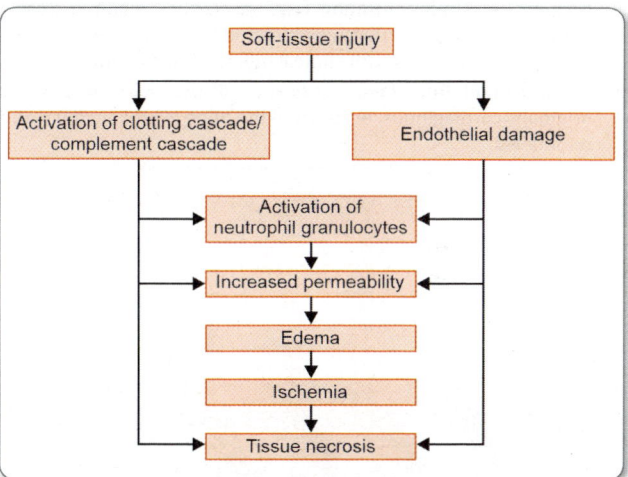

Fig. 2: Pathophysiological changes in soft-tissue injury

FRACTURE

Decreased bone strength that occurs with an injury leads to fractures. Thus, the pathophysiology of fractures encompasses multiple factors that determine bone strength (bone mass, bone quality, age, skeletal geometry) and the frequency, nature and effects of injuries. These factors become more prevalent with advancing age, resulting in an increase in the occurrence of osteoporosis in the elderly individuals.

Healing Process

Bone healing depends on the age and coexisting disorders of the patient. For example, healing rate is much faster in children than in adults; healing is slow in disorders that impair peripheral circulation (e.g., diabetes, peripheral vascular disease).

Fractures heal in three overlapping stages:

1. In the **inflammatory stage**, hematoma is formed at the fracture site, and resorption of the small amount of bone in the distal fracture fragments occurs. If a fracture line is not visible initially, one typically becomes visible about one week after the injury because of this resorption of small amount of bone.

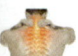
2. A callus is formed during the **reparative stage**. New blood vessels are developed to enable the cartilage to be formed across the fracture line. Immobilization (e.g., casting) is required during the first two stages so that new blood vessels can be grown. The reparative phase ends with clinical union of the fracture.

3. In the **remodeling stage**, ossification of the callus, which was originally cartilaginous, occurs and the bone is broken down and remodeled.

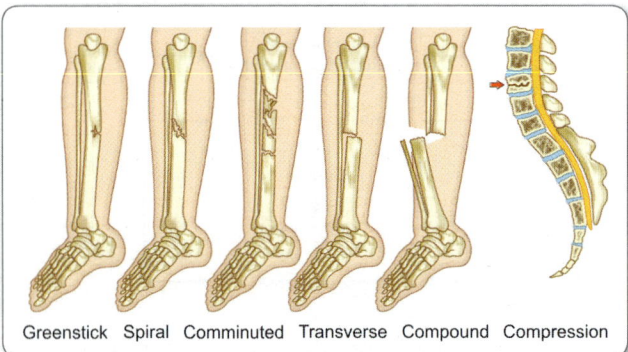

Greenstick   Spiral   Comminuted   Transverse   Compound   Compression

Fig. 3: Typical bone fractures

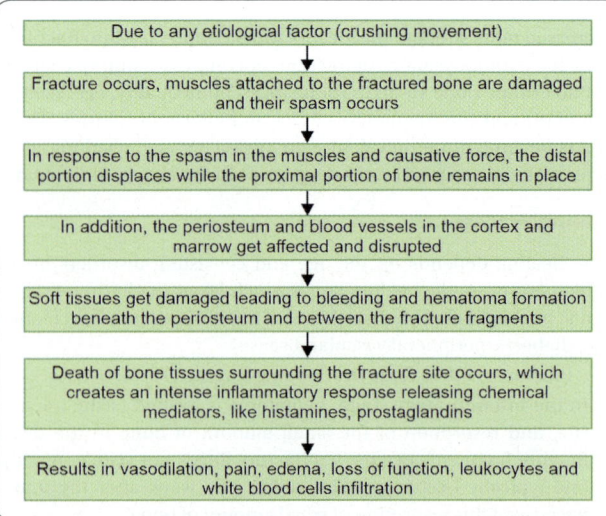

Due to any etiological factor (crushing movement)
↓
Fracture occurs, muscles attached to the fractured bone are damaged and their spasm occurs
↓
In response to the spasm in the muscles and causative force, the distal portion displaces while the proximal portion of bone remains in place
↓
In addition, the periosteum and blood vessels in the cortex and marrow get affected and disrupted
↓
Soft tissues get damaged leading to bleeding and hematoma formation beneath the periosteum and between the fracture fragments
↓
Death of bone tissues surrounding the fracture site occurs, which creates an intense inflammatory response releasing chemical mediators, like histamines, prostaglandins
↓
Results in vasodilation, pain, edema, loss of function, leukocytes and white blood cells infiltration

OSTEOMYELITIS

About 70–80% of bone infections are caused by *Staphylococcus aureus*. Other causes are *Proteus, Pseudomonas* species and *Escherichia coli*.

Inflammation, increased vascularity, and edema occur as an initial response to infection. After two to three days, thrombosis of the blood vessels occurs in the area, resulting in ischemia with bone necrosis. The infection extends into the medullary cavity and under the periosteum and may spread into adjacent soft tissues and joints. A bone abscess forms if the infective process is not treated promptly. The resulting abscess cavity contains dead bone tissues (the **sequestrum**), which does not easily liquefy and drain. Therefore, the cavity cannot collapse and heal, as occurs in soft tissue abscesses. New bone growth (the **involucrum**) forms and surrounds the sequestrum. Although healing appears to take place, a chronically infected sequestrum remains and produces recurring abscesses throughout the patient's life. This is referred to as chronic osteomyelitis (Figs 4A to C).

Invasion of bacteria into bone and surrounding soft tissues
↓
Activation of inflammatory response
↓
Thrombosis of blood vessels occurs within 2–3 days
↓
Ischemia (decreased blood flow)
↓
Bone tissues become necrotic
↓
Healing process is retarded and causes more infection
↓
Infection extends into medullary cavity and under periosteum and may spread into adjacent soft tissues and joints
↓
Bone abscess forms containing sequestrum
↓
Cavity cannot heal
↓
New bone growth (involucrum) forms surrounding sequestrum
↓
Recurring abscess
↓
Chronic osteomyelitis

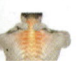

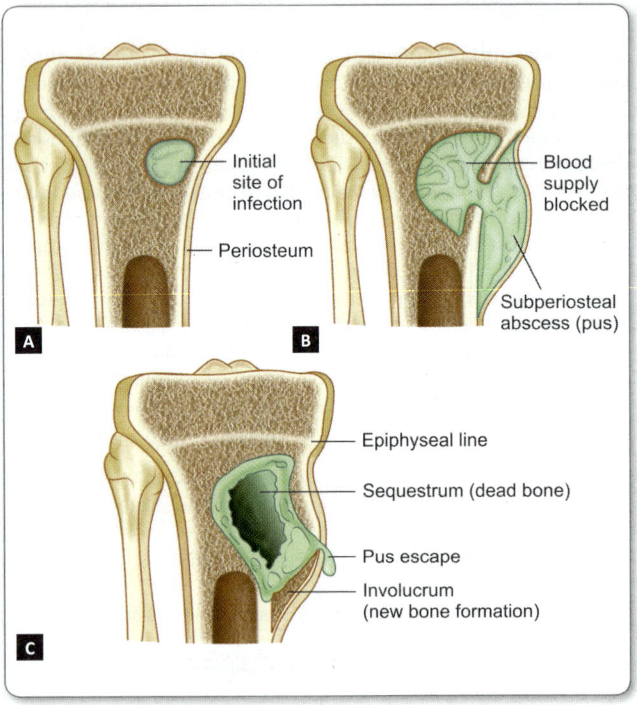

Initial
site of
infection

Periosteum

Blood
supply
blocked

Subperiosteal
abscess (pus)

A

B

Epiphyseal line

Sequestrum (dead bone)

Pus escape

Involucrum
(new bone formation)

C

Figs 4A to C: A. Initial infection; **B.** First stage; **C.** Second stage

OSTEOARTHRITIS

Osteoarthritis is characterized by the **progressive loss of articular cartilage** and **remodeling of the underlying bone**.

The pathophysiological changes of osteoarthritis involve degradation of cartilage and remodeling of bone due to an active response given by chondrocytes in the articular cartilage and the inflammatory cells present in the surrounding tissues. Enzymes released from these cells break down the collagen and proteoglycans thereby causing damage to the articular cartilage. Sclerosis of the underlying subchondral bone occurs, followed by remodeling changes leading to the formation of osteophytes and subchondral cysts of bone. There is a progressive loss of joint space over time (Fig. 5).

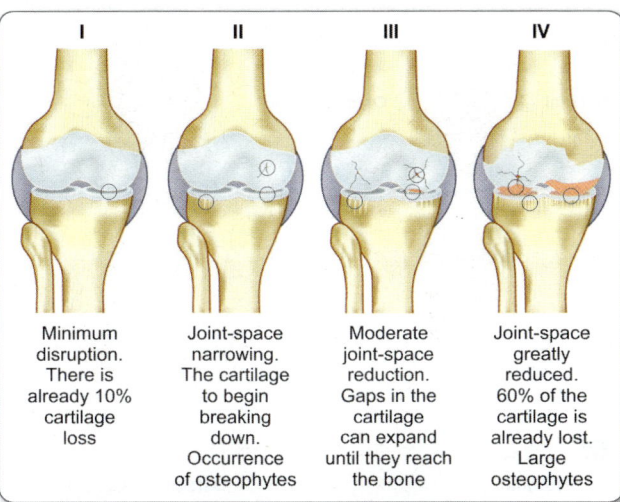

I	II	III	IV
Minimum disruption. There is already 10% cartilage loss	Joint-space narrowing. The cartilage to begin breaking down. Occurrence of osteophytes	Moderate joint-space reduction. Gaps in the cartilage can expand until they reach the bone	Joint-space greatly reduced. 60% of the cartilage is already lost. Large osteophytes

Fig. 5: Osteoarthritis (progressive loss of joint space)

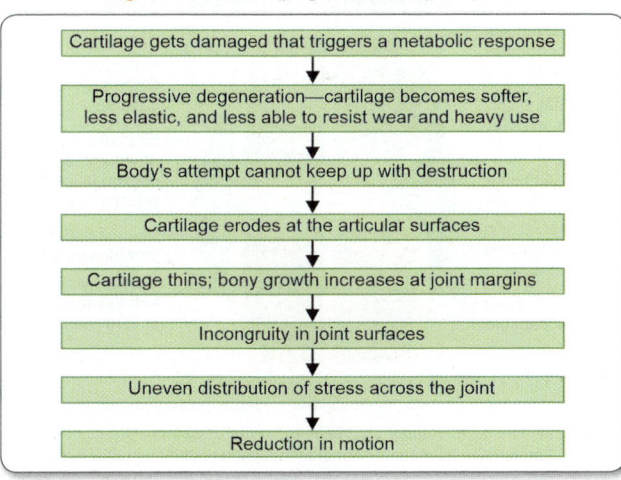

Cartilage gets damaged that triggers a metabolic response

↓

Progressive degeneration—cartilage becomes softer, less elastic, and less able to resist wear and heavy use

↓

Body's attempt cannot keep up with destruction

↓

Cartilage erodes at the articular surfaces

↓

Cartilage thins; bony growth increases at joint margins

↓

Incongruity in joint surfaces

↓

Uneven distribution of stress across the joint

↓

Reduction in motion

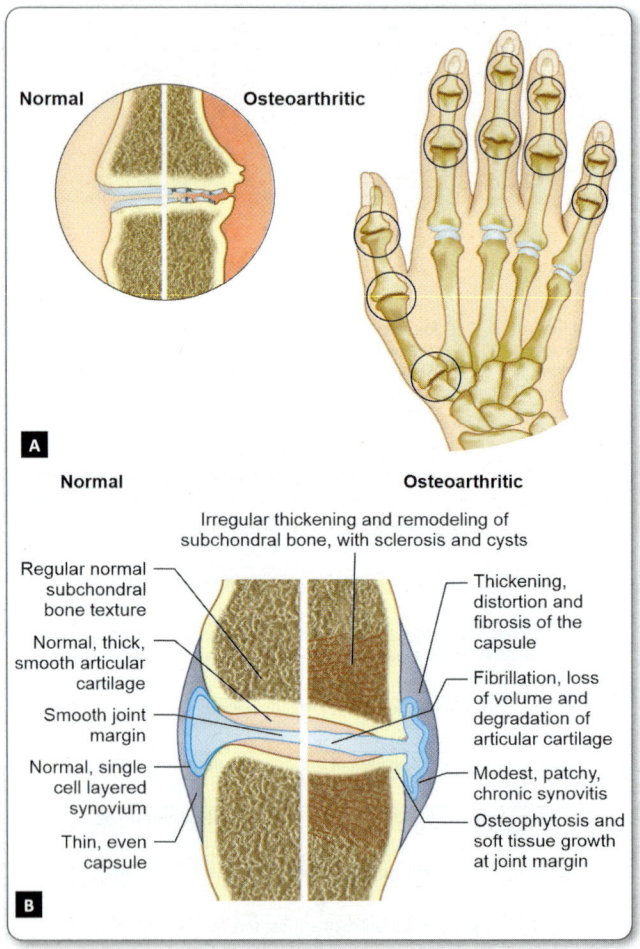

Figs 6A and B: **A.** Comparison between normal and osteoarthritis bone; **B.** Comparison between a normal and an osteoarthritic synovial joint

RHEUMATOID ARTHRITIS

Rheumatoid arthritis (RA) is a chronic autoimmune disease. When the immune system is functioning normally, it recognizes things like harmful bacteria and viruses, and responds by creating an 'army' of antibodies that seek out and fight them off. In an autoimmune disease, the immune system mistakenly thinks that normal tissues or organs of the body are harmful, leading to inflammation and damage. Although, the pathophysiology of RA is not completely understood, the process generally involves deregulated inflammation, with antigen presentation, T cell activation, and autoantibody production all serving as mediators in the inflammatory process.

Genetic or environmental factors

↓

Infiltration of synovial membrane with inflammatory cells, like macrophages, lymphocytes, plasma cells and dendritic cells

↓

Thickening of synovial lining and formation of lymphoid follicles within the synovial membrane

↓

Activation of T cells and production of cytokines and autoantibodies

↓

Production of proinflammatory cytokines by synovial macrophages activated by immune complexes

↓

Proinflammatory cytokines act on synovial fibroblasts to promote swelling of synovial membrane and damage to soft tissues and cartilage

↓

Activation of osteocytes and chondroblasts lead to destruction of bone and cartilage. The joint with rheumatoid arthritis becomes hypoxic leading to neoangiogenesis

↓

The inflammatory granulation tissue (pannus) forms, which spreads over and under the articular cartilage and progressively gets eroded and destroyed

↓

Destruction of articular cartilage and subchondrial bone produces bony ankylosis

↓

Atrophy of muscles adjacent to inflamed joints may occur along with infiltration with lymphocytes

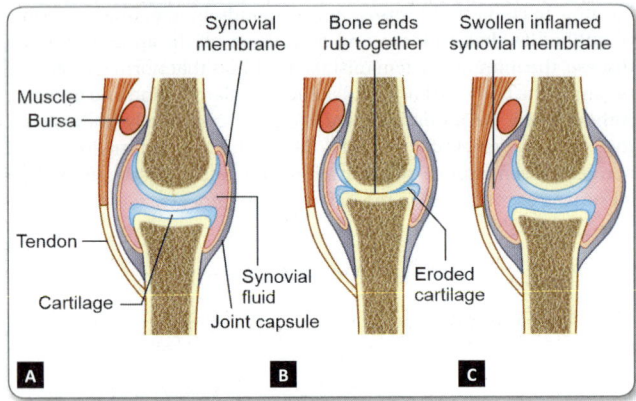

Figs 7A to C: **A.** Normal bone; **B.** Osteoarthritis bone;
C. Rheumatoid arthritis bone

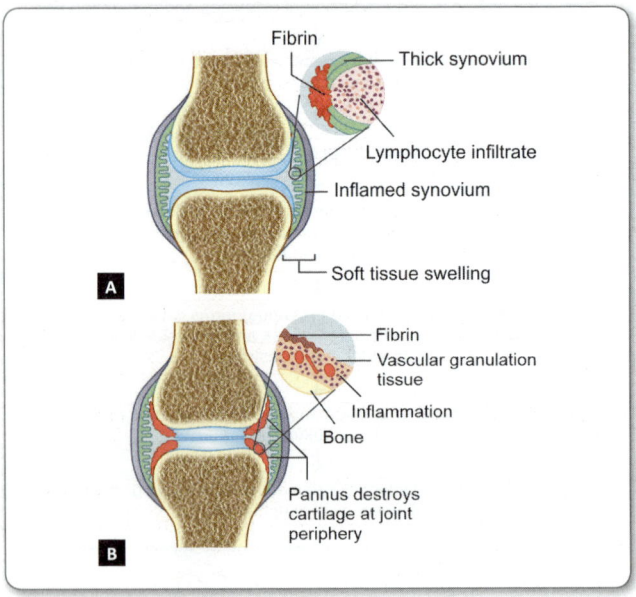

Figs 8A and B:

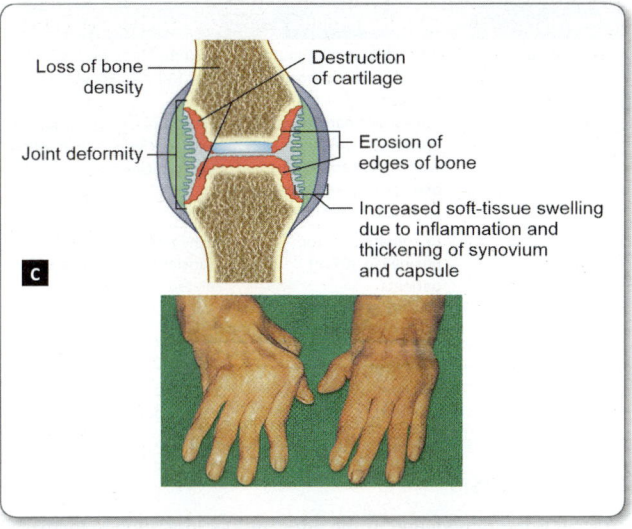

Figs 8A to C: **A.** Rheumatoid synovitis; **B.** Articular cartilage destruction; **C.** Focal destruction of bone

Table 1: Differences between rheumatoid arthritis and osteoarthritis

Parameter	Rheumatoid arthritis	Osteoarthritis
Age at onset	Young to middle age	Usually >40 years of age
Gender	Female/male ratio is 2:1 or 3:1; less marked gender difference after age 60	Before age 50, more men than women; after age 50, more women than men
Weight	Lost or maintained weight	Often overweight
Disease	Systemic disease with exacerbations and remissions	Localized disease with variable, progressive course
Affected joints	Small joints first (PIPs, MCPs, MTPs), wrists, elbows, shoulders, knees; usually bilateral, symmetric	Weight-bearing joints (knees, hips), MCPs, DIPs, PIPs, cervical and lumbar spine; often asymmetric
Stiffness	1 hour to all day	On arising but usually subsides after 30 minutes
Effusions	Common	Uncommon
Nodules	Present, especially on extensor surfaces	Heberden's (DIPs) and Bouchard's (PIPs) nodes

Contd...

Parameter	Rheumatoid arthritis	Osteoarthritis
Synovial fluid	• White blood cells count >2000/ μL with mostly neutrophils	• White blood cells <2000/ μL (mild leukocytosis)
X-rays	• Joint space narrowing, erosion, subluxation with advanced disease; osteoporosis related to corticosteroid use	• Joint space narrowing, p1 osteophytes, subchondral cysts, sclerosis
Laboratory findings	• Rheumatoid factor positive in 80% of patients • Elevated ESR, CRP indicative of active inflammation	RF negative Transient elevation in ESR related to synovitis

Abbreviations: CRP, c-reactive protein; DIP, distal interphalangeal joints; ESR, erythrocyte sedimentation rate; MCP, metacarpophalangeal; MTP, metatarsophalangeal; PIP, proximal interphalangeal

OSTEOPOROSIS

Normal bone remodeling in the adult results in gradually increased bone mass until the early 30s. Gender, race, genetics, aging, low body weight and body mass index, nutrition, lifestyle choices (e.g., smoking, caffeine and alcohol consumption), and physical activity influence peak bone mass and the development of osteoporosis (Fig. 9).

Bone is a living tissue that is constantly breaking down and being replaced. Osteoporosis happens when growth of new bone does not keep up with the breaking down of old bone. This makes the bones very brittle and fragile. Primary osteoporosis is a result of the normal aging process, while secondary osteoporosis is a result of another disease process.

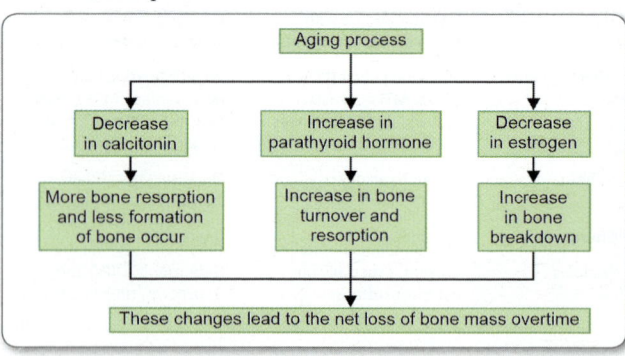

Bone resorption is caused due to the estrogen withdrawal at menopause and this continues during the postmenopausal years. Osteoporosis is developed more frequently and more extensively in women than men due to the lower peak bone mass and estrogen loss during menopause.

Secondary osteoporosis is associated with many nutritional deficiencies, other disease states, and medications.

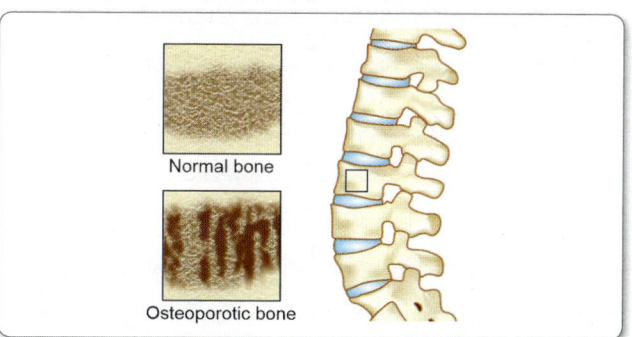

Fig. 9: Comparison between normal and osteoporotic bone

OSTEOMALACIA

Osteomalacia is mainly characterized by a deficiency of activated vitamin D (calcitriol), which is responsible for absorption of calcium from the gastrointestinal tract and facilitates mineralization of bone. Without adequate vitamin D, calcium and phosphate are not moved to calcification sites in bones.

Osteomalacia may result from failed calcium absorption (e.g., malabsorption syndrome) or from excessive loss of calcium from the body. Gastrointestinal disorders (e.g., celiac disease, chronic pancreatitis, small bowel resection) in which there is an inadequate absorption of fat may cause osteomalacia due to loss of vitamin D and calcium. Additionally, as liver and kidney convert vitamin D to its active form, thus, diseases of liver and kidney can cause lack of vitamin D.

Reduction in serum phosphorus level and demineralization of bone occur because of chronic glomerulonephritis, obstructive uropathies and heavy metal poisoning.

Hyperparathyroidism results in skeletal decalcification by increasing phosphate excretion in urine

- Prolonged use of antiseizure medication
- Insufficient exposure to sunlight

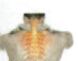

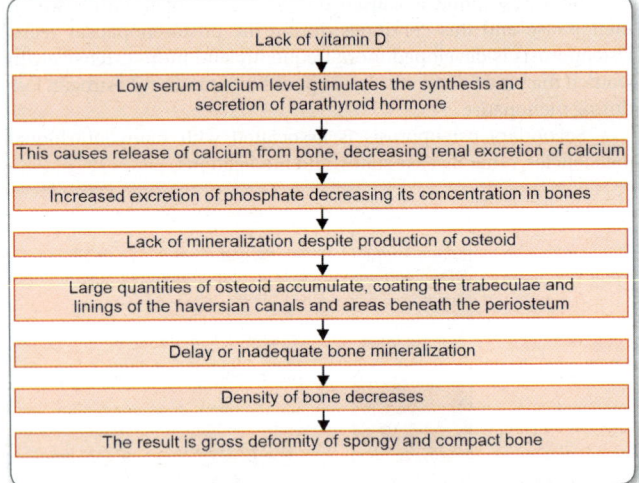

Lack of vitamin D

↓

Low serum calcium level stimulates the synthesis and secretion of parathyroid hormone

↓

This causes release of calcium from bone, decreasing renal excretion of calcium

↓

Increased excretion of phosphate decreasing its concentration in bones

↓

Lack of mineralization despite production of osteoid

↓

Large quantities of osteoid accumulate, coating the trabeculae and linings of the haversian canals and areas beneath the periosteum

↓

Delay or inadequate bone mineralization

↓

Density of bone decreases

↓

The result is gross deformity of spongy and compact bone

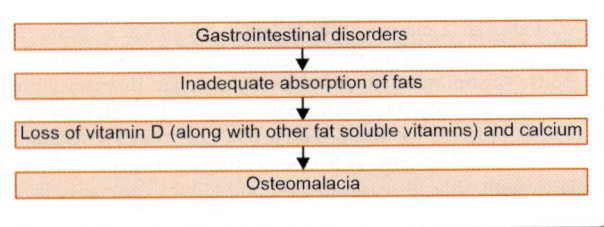

Failed calcium absorption or excessive loss of calcium from body

↓

Osteomalacia

Gastrointestinal disorders

↓

Inadequate absorption of fats

↓

Loss of vitamin D (along with other fat soluble vitamins) and calcium

↓

Osteomalacia

Liver and kidney diseases produce

↓

Osteomalacia

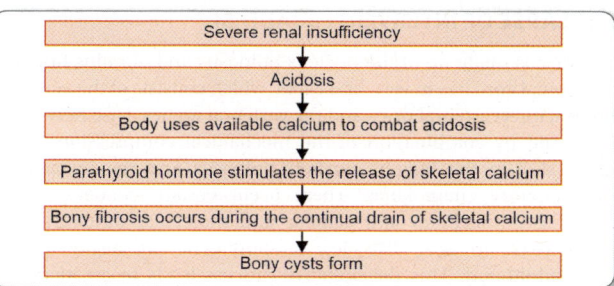

Severe renal insufficiency
↓
Acidosis
↓
Body uses available calcium to combat acidosis
↓
Parathyroid hormone stimulates the release of skeletal calcium
↓
Bony fibrosis occurs during the continual drain of skeletal calcium
↓
Bony cysts form

PAGET'S DISEASE

Paget's disease of the bone is a skeletal disorder, which results in increased and disorganized bone remodeling, leading to dense but fragile and expanding bones. The normal architecture of bones gets disrupted by such abnormalities leading to various complications like bone pain, pathological fracture and deformity of bones. Genetic factors are thought to play an important role in Paget's disease and the mutations that occur in four genes (TNFRSF11A, TNFRSF11B, VCP and SQSTM1) that disrupts the signaling pathway of RANK-NFKB, thereby causing osteoclast activation leading to onset of disease process.

The pathology of Paget's disease is separated into active and inactive phases. Early in the active phase (lytic phase), there is an excessive resorption of osteoclasts. Later in the active phase (mixed phase), compensatory bone formation is evident. In very late phase (sclerotic phase), formation of osteoblasts predominates. Occasionally, an inactive phase can occur in which in the absence of excessive bone-cell activity, a sclerotic lesion may remain present.

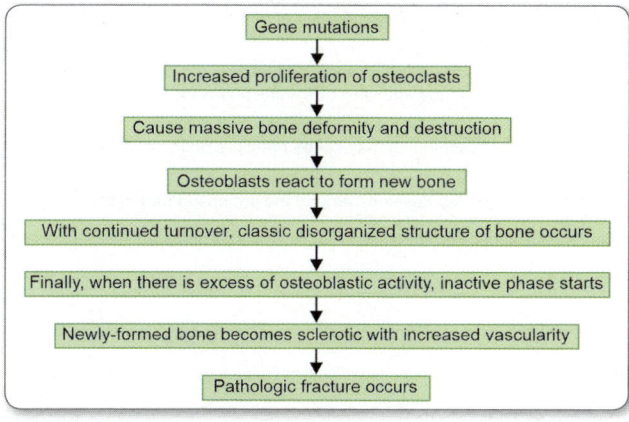

Gene mutations
↓
Increased proliferation of osteoclasts
↓
Cause massive bone deformity and destruction
↓
Osteoblasts react to form new bone
↓
With continued turnover, classic disorganized structure of bone occurs
↓
Finally, when there is excess of osteoblastic activity, inactive phase starts
↓
Newly-formed bone becomes sclerotic with increased vascularity
↓
Pathologic fracture occurs

PROLAPSE OF INTERVERTEBRAL DISC

The disc is made up of the nucleus pulposus and annulus fibrosus. The spinal cord lies in vertebral canal, which consists of the vertebral bodies, intervertebral discs and the vertebral arches. Disc herniation is caused by combination of the mechanical compression of the nerve due to the bulging nucleus pulposus and the increase in inflammatory chemokines. There occur certain changes in the vascularity, nutrition, and cellular and molecular structure with an increase in age. Disc degeneration generally begins in the early adulthood. This degenerative process leads to an increased inability of the disc to withstand physiologic loading. This can precipitate annular tearing and subsequent herniation of the disc (Figs. 10A and B).

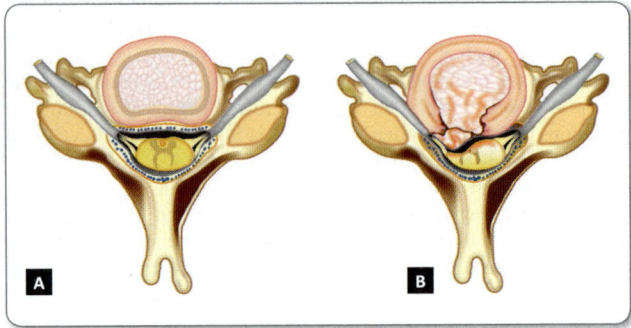

Figs 10A and B: **A.** Normal disc; **B.** Herniated disc

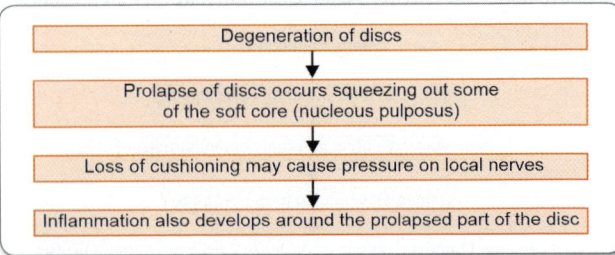

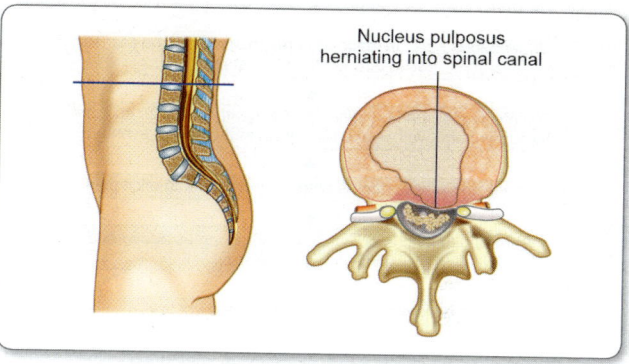

Fig. 11: Herniated nucleus pulposus

POTT'S SPINE/DISEASE

Pott's disease is usually caused by hematogenous spread and extraspinal source of infection. The anterior aspect of the vertebral body is usually affected. Tuberculosis may reach to the adjacent intervertebral discs. Abscesses, granulation tissue, or direct invasion of dura can lead to the narrowing of the spinal canal, which causes spinal cord compression and neurologic deficits (Fig. 12).

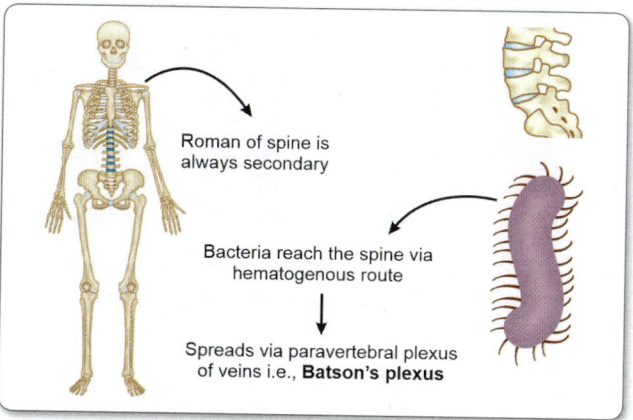

Fig. 12: Pott's disease

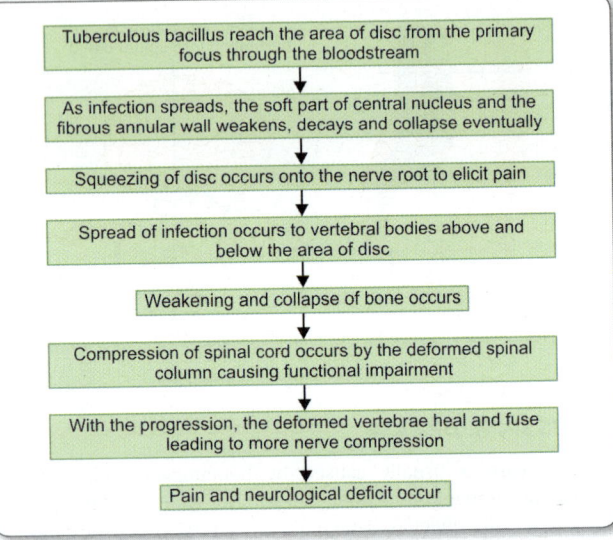

Tuberculous bacillus reach the area of disc from the primary focus through the bloodstream

↓

As infection spreads, the soft part of central nucleus and the fibrous annular wall weakens, decays and collapse eventually

↓

Squeezing of disc occurs onto the nerve root to elicit pain

↓

Spread of infection occurs to vertebral bodies above and below the area of disc

↓

Weakening and collapse of bone occurs

↓

Compression of spinal cord occurs by the deformed spinal column causing functional impairment

↓

With the progression, the deformed vertebrae heal and fuse leading to more nerve compression

↓

Pain and neurological deficit occur

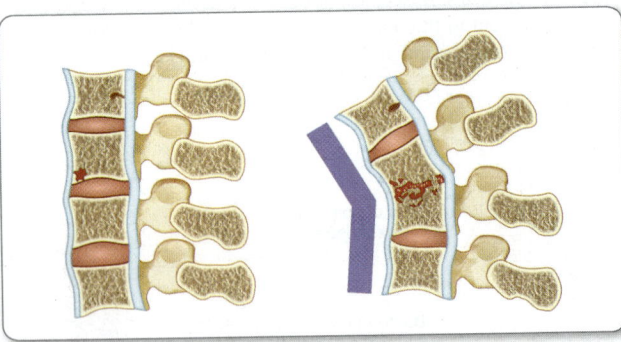

Fig. 13: Tuberculous spondylitis (Pott's disease)

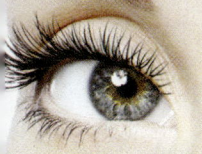

Pathophysiology of Eye Disorders

INTRODUCTION

The human eye, the organ responsible for the sense of sight, is a very complex structure. We use our vision in almost every activity, so eye is an important organ in human body (Fig. 1).

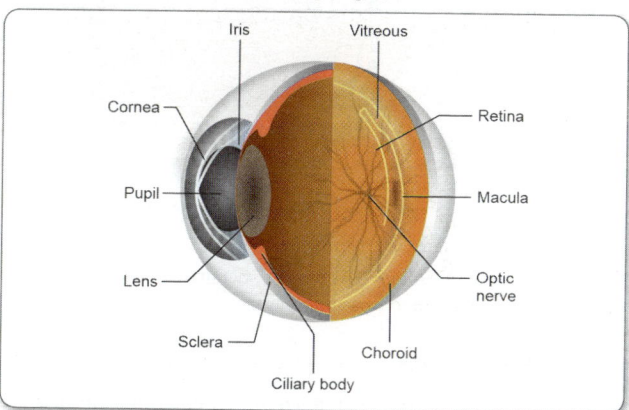

Fig. 1: Parts of an eye

VISION

We see when light rays from an object enter the eye through the cornea. The cornea's refractive power bends the light rays in such a way that they pass freely through the pupil.

The iris has the ability to enlarge and shrink, depending upon the amount of light entering in the pupil from the environment.

The light rays strike the lens after passing through the iris. The lens functions just like a camera; focusing light rays properly by adjusting its width.

After exiting the back of the lens, the light rays pass through the vitreous humor that maintains the spherical shape of the eye. Finally, the light rays reach up to a sharp focusing point on the retina.

Retina is responsible for capturing all of the light rays, processing them into light impulses through millions of tiny nerve endings, and then sending these light impulses through over a million nerve fibers to the optic nerve.

The optic nerve is an extension of the brain. The light impulses travel through this nerve fiber to the brain, where they are interpreted as an image (Fig. 2).

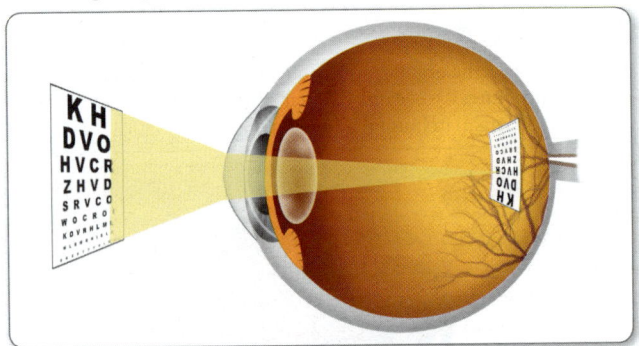

Fig. 2: Vision

The pathophysiological changes occurring in various eye disorders are discussed in this chapter.

REFRACTIVE ERRORS

In the emmetropic (normally refracted) eye, entering light rays are focused on the retina by the cornea and the lens, creating a sharp image that is transmitted to the brain. The lens is more elastic, in younger people. During accommodation, the ciliary muscles adjust lens shape to properly focus images. Refractive errors are failure of the eye to focus images sharply on the retina, causing blurred vision. Four common refractive errors are:

1. **Myopia**, or nearsightedness—clear vision closes up but blurry in the distance.
2. **Hyperopia**, or far-sightedness—clear vision in the distance but blurry close up.
3. **Presbyopia**—inability to focus close up as a result of aging.
4. **Astigmatism**—focus problems caused by the cornea.

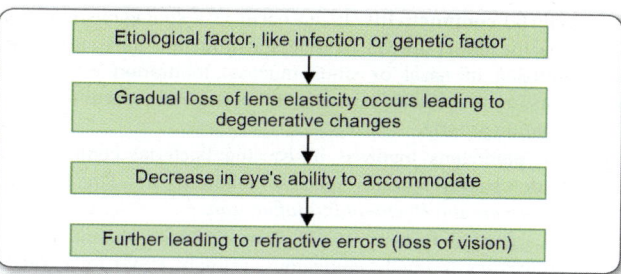

BLEPHARITIS

Blepharitis is inflammation of the eyelids. Blepharitis usually affects both eyes along the edges of the eyelids.

Blepharitis commonly occurs when tiny oil glands near the base of the eyelashes become clogged, causing irritation and redness. Blepharitis can be divided anatomically into anterior and posterior blepharitis. Anterior blepharitis refers to inflammation mainly centered around the skin, eyelashes, and lash follicles, while the posterior variant involves the meibomian gland orifices, meibomian glands, tarsal plate, and blepharo-conjunctival junction.

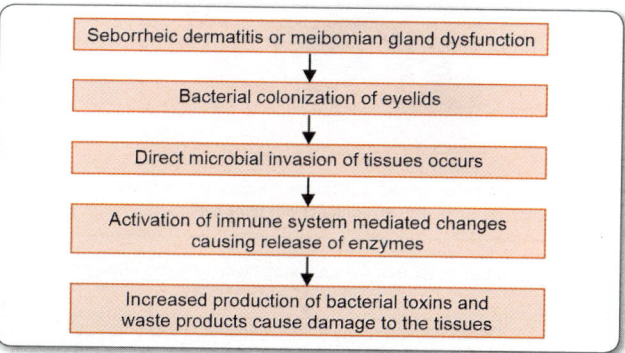

CONJUNCTIVITIS

The conjunctiva is a thin, transparent, mucus membrane that lines the inner surfaces of the eyelid and the anterior sclera and it provides defense against infection and trauma. Inflammation or infection of the conjunctiva is characterized by dilatation of the conjunctival vessels, resulting in hyperemia and edema of the conjunctiva that occurs along with discharge (Fig. 3).

- **Bacterial conjunctivitis:** It can occur as a contagious infection or by the direct spread of infection from the microorganisms colonizing in nasal or sinus mucosa. Infiltration of bacteria occurs in the epithelial layer of conjunctiva and sometimes in the substantia propria.

  The pathogens involved in causing bacterial conjunctivitis include staphylococcal species, followed by *Streptococcus pneumoniae* and *Haemophilus influenzae.*

- **Viral conjunctivitis:** Viral conjunctivitis secondary to adenoviruses is highly contagious. Primary HSV-l infection in humans occurs as a nonspecific upper respiratory tract infection. HSV spreads from infected skin and mucosal epithelium via sensory nerve axons to establish latent infection in associated sensory 5th cranial nerve.

- **Allergic conjunctivitis:** Allergic conjunctivitis is an inflammation of the ocular surface in response to a transient allergen (e.g., pollen in seasonal allergic conjunctivitis), or a persistent allergen (e.g., house dust mite in perennial allergic conjunctivitis).

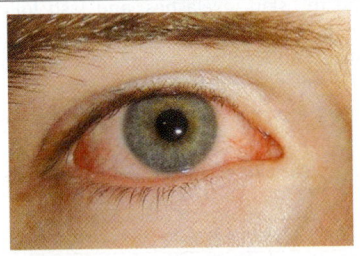

Fig. 3: Conjunctivitis (Pink eye)

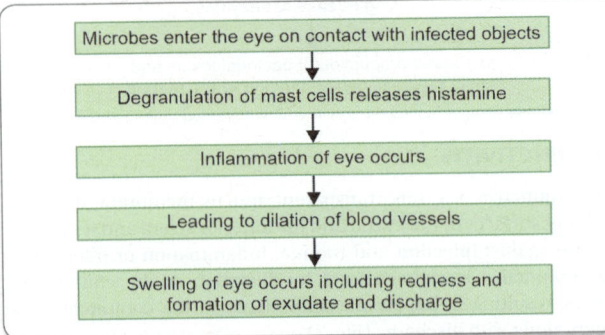

Microbes enter the eye on contact with infected objects

↓

Degranulation of mast cells releases histamine

↓

Inflammation of eye occurs

↓

Leading to dilation of blood vessels

↓

Swelling of eye occurs including redness and formation of exudate and discharge

CORNEAL ULCER/KERATITIS

Ulcers are characterized by corneal epithelial defects with underlying inflammation and necrosis of the corneal stroma. Corneal ulcers tend to heal with scar tissue, resulting in opacification of the cornea and decreased visual acuity. Uveitis, corneal perforation with iris prolapse, pus in the anterior chamber (hypopyon), panophthalmitis, and destruction of the eye may occur without treatment (Figs 4 and 5).

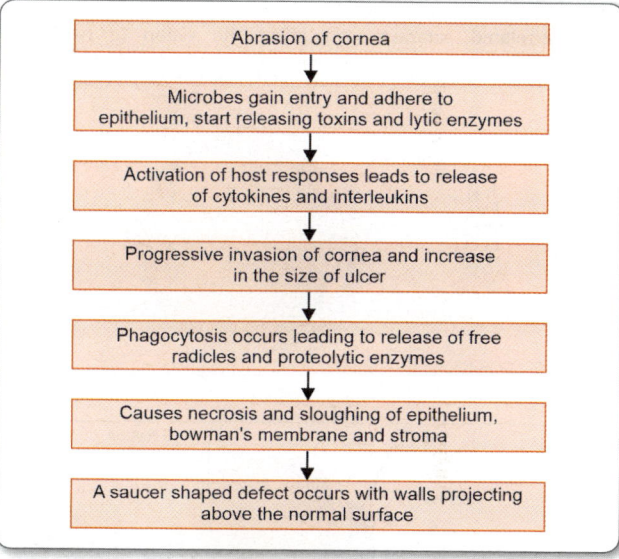

Abrasion of cornea
↓
Microbes gain entry and adhere to epithelium, start releasing toxins and lytic enzymes
↓
Activation of host responses leads to release of cytokines and interleukins
↓
Progressive invasion of cornea and increase in the size of ulcer
↓
Phagocytosis occurs leading to release of free radicles and proteolytic enzymes
↓
Causes necrosis and sloughing of epithelium, bowman's membrane and stroma
↓
A saucer shaped defect occurs with walls projecting above the normal surface

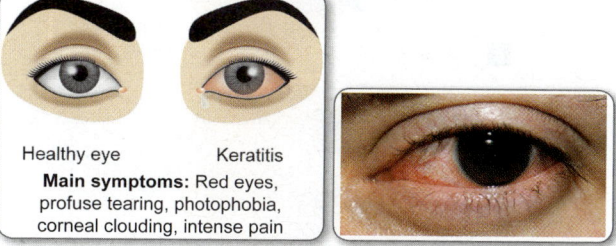

Healthy eye   Keratitis
Main symptoms: Red eyes, profuse tearing, photophobia, corneal clouding, intense pain

Fig. 4: Comparison between healthy eye and keratitis eye

Fig. 5: Bacterial keratitis

CATARACT

The lens lies behind the iris and the pupil. It works much like a camera lens. It focuses light onto the retina at the back of the eye, where an image is recorded. The lens also adjusts the eye's focus, letting us see things clearly both up close and far away.

The lens is made up of mostly water and protein. The protein is arranged in a precise way that keeps the lens clear and lets light pass through it.

Age-related cataracts can affect the vision in two ways (Figs 6 and 7):

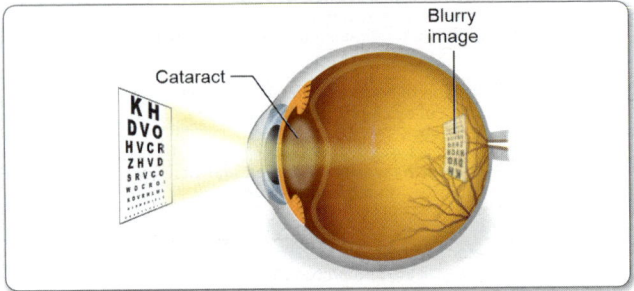

Fig. 6: Cataract

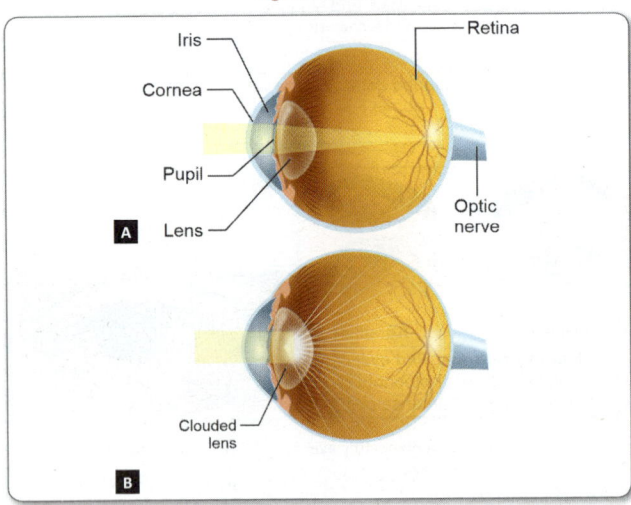

Figs 7A and B: A. Normal lens; **B.** Lens affected by cataract

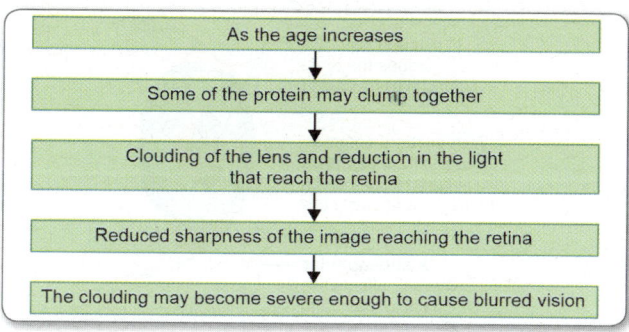

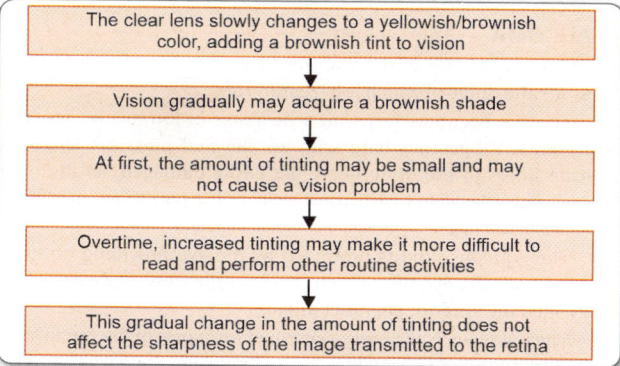

Types of Cataracts

The three most common types of age-related cataracts are defined by their location in the lens: nuclear, cortical, and sub capsular. The extent of visual impairment depends on the size, density and location in the lens (Fig. 8).

1. Myopia will lead to **nuclear cataract** and as it progresses, it will further cause blurred vision.

2. A **cortical cataract** involves anterior, posterior or equatorial cortex of the lens. A cataract in the equator or periphery does not interfere with the passage of light through the center of lens and has little effect on vision. Vision is worse in bright light.

3. **Posterior subcapsular cataract** occurs in front of posterior capsule. This develops in younger people and is associated with prolonged corticosteroid use, inflammation or trauma. The eye is extremely sensitive to glare from bright light.

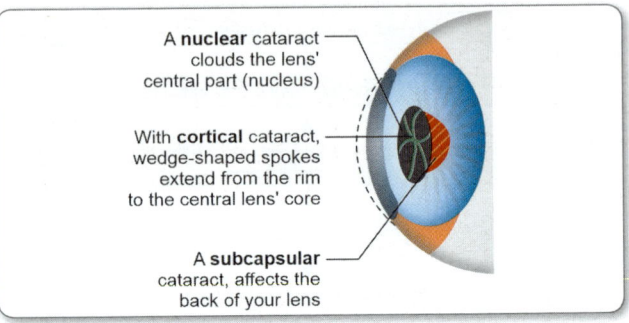

A **nuclear** cataract clouds the lens' central part (nucleus)

With **cortical** cataract, wedge-shaped spokes extend from the rim to the central lens' core

A **subcapsular** cataract, affects the back of your lens

Fig. 8: Types of cataracts

GLAUCOMA

The tone and shape of the eye are maintained by the intraocular pressure, the range of which is 8–22 mm Hg.

The eye becomes soft with a decrease in intraocular pressure (IOP) while it becomes hard with an elevated pressure. Since the delicate fibers of the optic nerve get easily damaged, so the optic nerve is considered to be the most susceptible part to an increase in pressure of the eye.

The aqueous fluid is produced by the eye providing nutrition to it. It leaves the eye through channels at the front of the eye in an area called the anterior chamber angle.

The following is the cross-section of front part of the eye to show the drainage angle. The angle is located between the cornea and the iris. The arrow shows the flow of the aqueous fluid from the ciliary body, through the pupil, and into the drainage channels (Fig. 9).

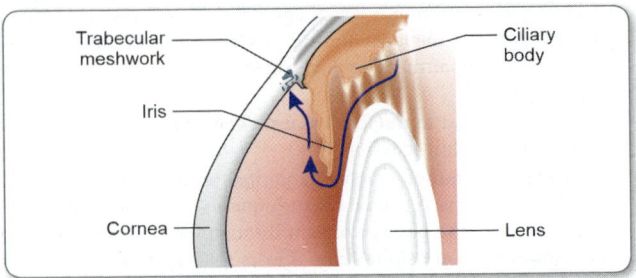

Trabecular meshwork

Iris

Cornea

Ciliary body

Lens

Fig. 9: Cross-section of eye showing the drainage angle

The aqueous fluid drains into capillaries into the main bloodstream, after exiting through the trabecular meshwork in the drainage angle.

Anything that slows or blocks the flow of this fluid out of the eye will cause pressure to build up in the eye. This pressure is called intraocular pressure (IOP). In most cases of glaucoma, this pressure is high and causes damage to the major nerve in the eye, called the optic nerve (Fig. 10).

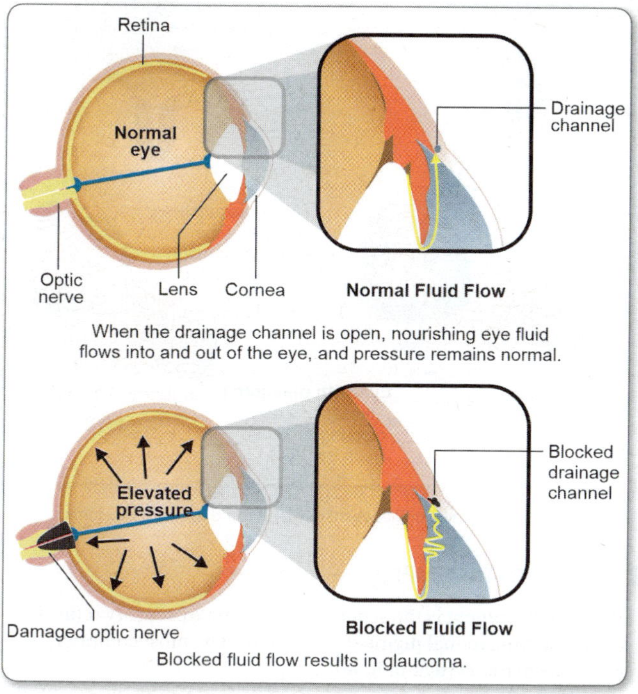

Retina

Normal eye

Optic nerve

Lens Cornea

Drainage channel

Normal Fluid Flow

When the drainage channel is open, nourishing eye fluid flows into and out of the eye, and pressure remains normal.

Elevated pressure

Damaged optic nerve

Blocked drainage channel

Blocked Fluid Flow

Blocked fluid flow results in glaucoma.

Fig. 10: Comparison between normal fluid flow and blocked fluid flow

This process of producing and removing the fluid from the eye is similar to that of a sink with the faucet always turned on, producing and draining the water (Fig. 11).

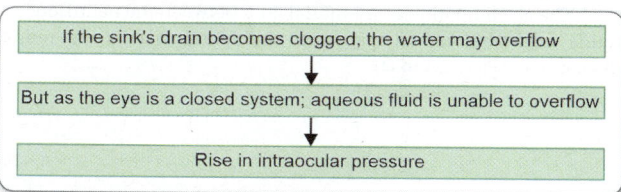

If the sink's drain becomes clogged, the water may overflow

But as the eye is a closed system; aqueous fluid is unable to overflow

Rise in intraocular pressure

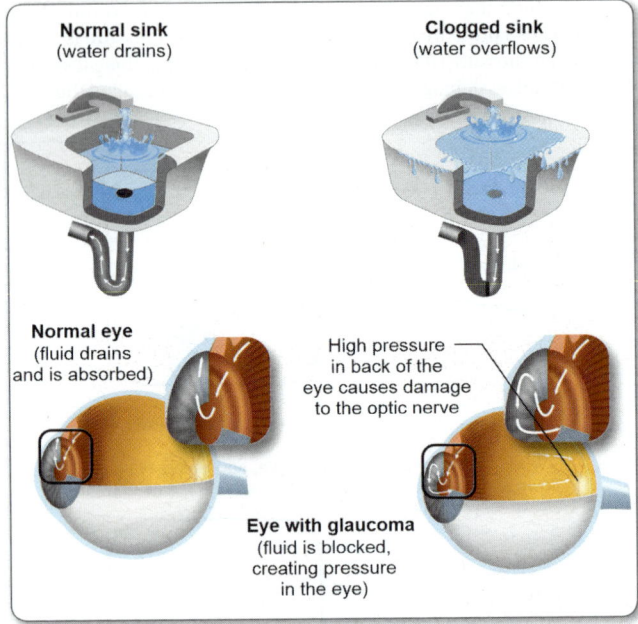

Normal sink
(water drains)

Clogged sink
(water overflows)

Normal eye
(fluid drains
and is absorbed)

High pressure
in back of the
eye causes damage
to the optic nerve

Eye with glaucoma
(fluid is blocked,
creating pressure
in the eye)

Fig. 11: Comparison between normal eye and eye with glaucoma

RETINAL DETACHMENT

Retinal detachment is the separation of the neurosensory retina from the underlying retinal pigment epithelium. The most common cause is a break in retina (tear or hole).

Normally, the adhesion of retinal pigment epithelium with the overlying neurosensory retina occurs through certain mechanisms that include active transport of subretinal fluid. These mechanisms are dazed in case of retinal detachment leading to separation of the neurosensory retina from the retinal pigment epithelial layer.

The accumulation of subretinal fluid between the neurosensory retina and the retinal pigment epithelium occurs in retinal detachment (Figs 12A to D).

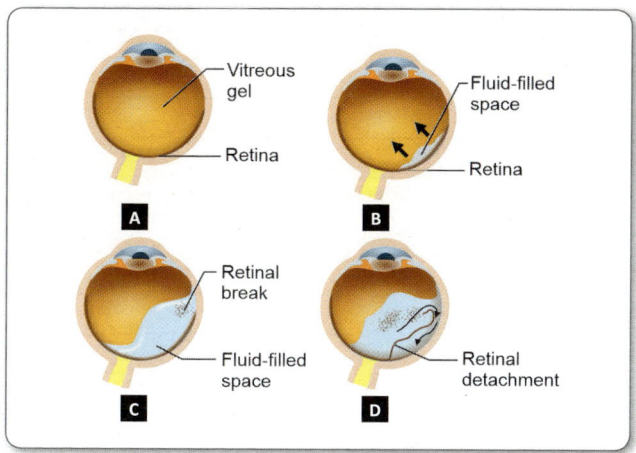

Figs 12A to D: Retinal detachment

A break in the retina allows the vitreous to enter the subretinal space directly, known as a **rhegmatogenous** retinal detachment.

Another factor is the proliferative membranes that can pull on the neurosensory retina causing a physical separation between the neurosensory retina and retinal pigment epithelium, called as **traction** retinal detachment. Next, the inflammatory mediators or exudation of fluid from a mass lesion causes accumulation of subretinal fluid, and is known as a **serous** or **exudative** retinal detachment.

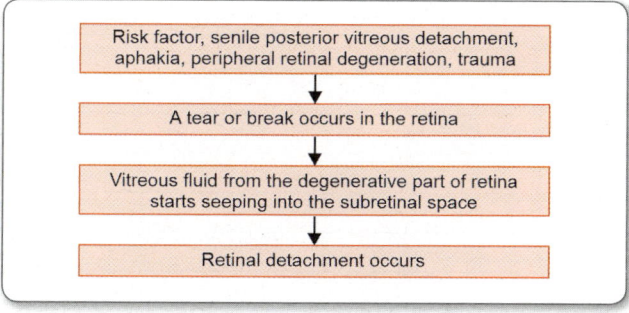

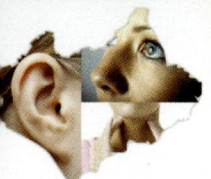

Pathophysiology of Ear, Nose and Throat Disorders

EAR

The **ear** is the organ of hearing. The ear has three parts—the outer ear, middle ear and the inner ear. The outer ear consists of the pinna and the ear canal. The tympanic cavity and the three ossicles form the middle ear. The inner ear is surrounded by the bony labyrinth, the semicircular canals, which enable balance and eye tracking when moving; the utricle and saccule, which enable balance when stationary; and the cochlea, which enables hearing. The ear may be affected by an infection or traumatic damage. Diseases of the ear may lead to hearing loss, tinnitus and balance disorders such as vertigo, although many of these conditions may also be affected by damage to the brain or neural pathways leading from the ear.

Hearing starts with the outer ear. When a sound is made outside the outer ear, the sound waves, or vibrations, travel down the external auditory canal and strike the tympanic membrane. The vibration of eardrum occurs by this striking. These vibrations further are passed to the ossicular chain in the middle ear. The amplification of sound occurs by the ossicles and then these sound waves are sent to the inner ear and into the fluid-filled hearing organ (cochlea). The sound waves after reaching the inner ear are converted into electrical impulses, which are sent to the brain by the auditory nerve. The brain then translates these electrical impulses as sound.

NOSE

The function of our nose is to smell. It is located in the middle of the face. It consists of:

- **External meatus:** Located in the center of the face. It is triangular in shape.
- **External nostrils:** Two chambers separated by the septum.
- **Septum:** Consists of cartilage and bone. It is covered by mucus membranes.

- **Nasal passages:** Lined with mucus membranes and tiny hairs (cilia) that filter the air.
- **Sinuses:** Air-filled cavities lined with mucus membranes.

Sinuses are of four different types (Fig. 1):

1. **Ethmoid sinus:** Located around the area of the bridge of the nose. It is present at the time of birth, and continues to grow.
2. **Maxillary sinus:** Located around the area of the cheeks. It is also present at birth, and continues to grow.
3. **Frontal sinus:** Located in the area of the forehead. It is developed after around seven years of age.
4. **Sphenoid sinus:** Located behind the nose. It develops after adolescence.

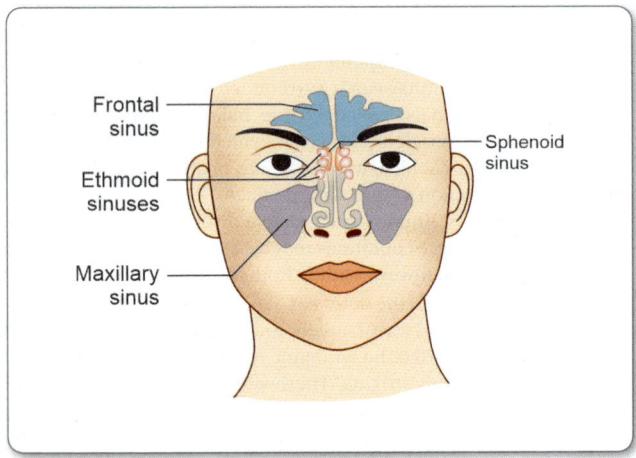

Fig. 1: Types of sinuses

THROAT

The throat is a passageway for air, food, and liquid. It is a ring-like muscular tube, which helps in speech formation too. It consists of:

- **Larynx:** Also called the voice box. It is a cylindrical grouping of muscles, cartilage, and soft tissue, which contains the vocal cords.
- **Epiglottis:** A flap of soft tissues present just above the vocal cords. It folds down on the vocal cords to prevent irritants and food from entering the lungs.

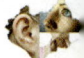

- **Tonsils and adenoids:** Located at the back and the sides of the mouth. They consist of lymph tissue and protect against infection. They generally have little purpose beyond childhood.

Let us now discuss the pathophysiological changes occurring in the disease conditions related to ear, nose and throat.

DISORDERS OF EXTERNAL EAR

Foreign Body in the Ear

Foreign bodies may stay unobserved until they aggravate an inflammatory response, which may cause pain, itching, infection, and foul-smelling, purulent drainage.

Generally, foreign body that appears easy to grasp can be removed with alligator forceps by most practitioners. Whereas, round and smooth objects are pushed deeper into the canal by the forceps. For removing smooth, rounded foreign body, the best way is to reach behind it and roll it out with a small, blunt hook (Fig. 2).

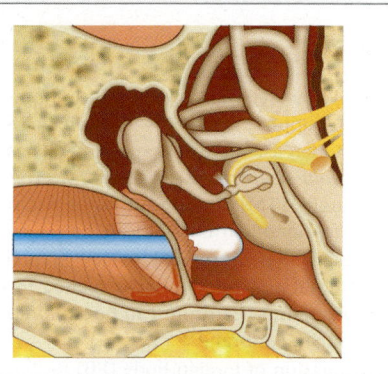

Fig. 2: Foreign body in the ear

DISORDERS OF MIDDLE EAR

Cerumen Impaction

In humans, cerumen production is a normal process. It moisturizes and softens the skin of the external auditory canal and protects it from infection by providing a barrier for insects and water. It is spont-aneously expelled from the ear canal through natural jaw movement. However, this self-cleaning mechanism fails in some individuals, cerumen gets impacted. This cerumen impaction may obstruct the canal or lead to pressure against the tympanic membrane, which potentially cause ear discomfort, itching and conductive hearing loss.

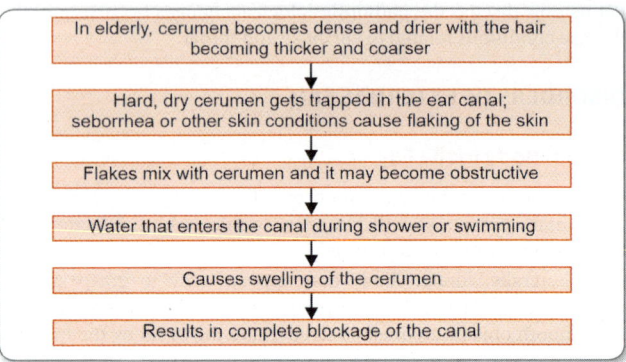

Insects may fly or crawl into the ear and cause blockage in the ear canal.

Tympanic Membrane Perforation

The pathophysiology of tympanic membrane perforation depends on the etiology of the rupture. With acute otitis media (AOM), recurrent episodes of AOM increase the risk of spontaneous perforation. Non-typeable *Hemophilus influenzae* causes AOM. The risk factors of tympanic membrane (TM) rupture are prior ear surgeries, severe otitis externa, and prior or current otitis media.

For example, large or rapid changes in pressure gradients between the external and middle ear is related to the perforation secondary to barotrauma. Eardrum can be ruptured because of the difference across the membrane.

Direct penetration of foreign body (FB) to the eardrum or ear cleaning leads to TM perforation. The pars tensa is usually affected area. It is the largest and thinnest area of the TM.

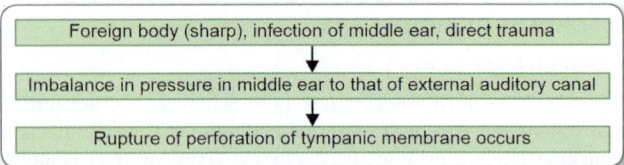

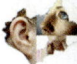

Acute Otitis Media

Dysfunctional eustachian tube
↓
Entry of pathogens in the sterile ear
↓
Exudate formation in middle ear
↓
Blockage of eustachian tube
↓
Negative pressure is created
↓
Conductive hearing loss

Chronic Otitis Media

Cause
↓
Microorganisms enter the ear canal
↓
Inflammatory response is initiated
↓
Exudate formation (pus) in middle ear
↓
Blockage of eustachian tube
↓
Negative pressure is created
↓
Damage to tympanic membrane and ossicles
↓
Tissue necrosis will take place
↓
Conductive hearing loss
↓
Extension of infection
↓
Involvement of mastoid
↓
Mastoiditis

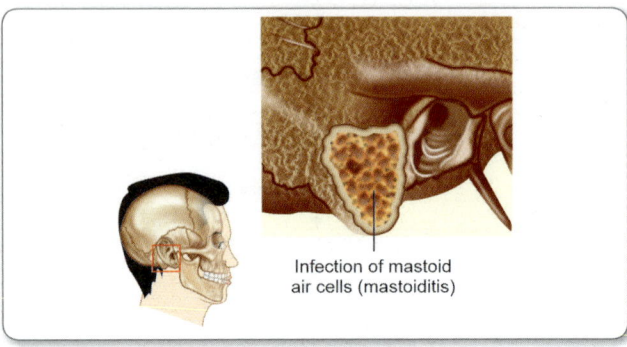

Fig. 3: Mastoiditis

DISORDERS OF INTERNAL EAR

Meniere's Disease (Figs 4A and B)

Disturbance in the fluid physiology in the ear resulting either from increased production or decreased absorption

↓

Increased pressure within the labyrinth

↓

Increased pressure causes episodes of vertigo and tinnitus

↓

Repeated episodes kill hair cells in the inner ear frequently resulting in unilateral functional deafness

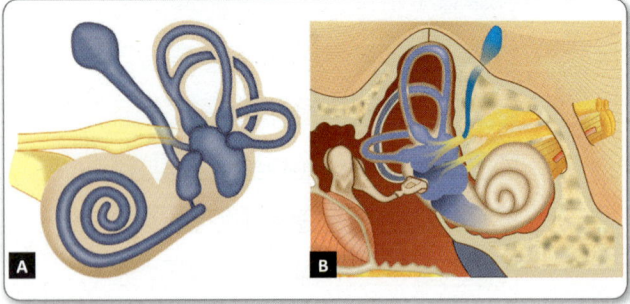

Figs 4A and B: A. Swelling in the canals due to increased fluid; **B.** Dilated membranous labyrinth in Meniere's disease

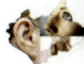

Labyrinthitis (Figs 5A and B)

- Infections arising in the middle ear can spread to the inner ear through the oval or round window.
- Inflammation or infectious agents can spread from the inner ear into the internal auditory canal.
- Infection in the membranous labyrinth may result in a significant inflammatory response with resultant intraluminal fibrosis and possible ossification.
- The membranous labyrinth is surrounded by dense bone formed.

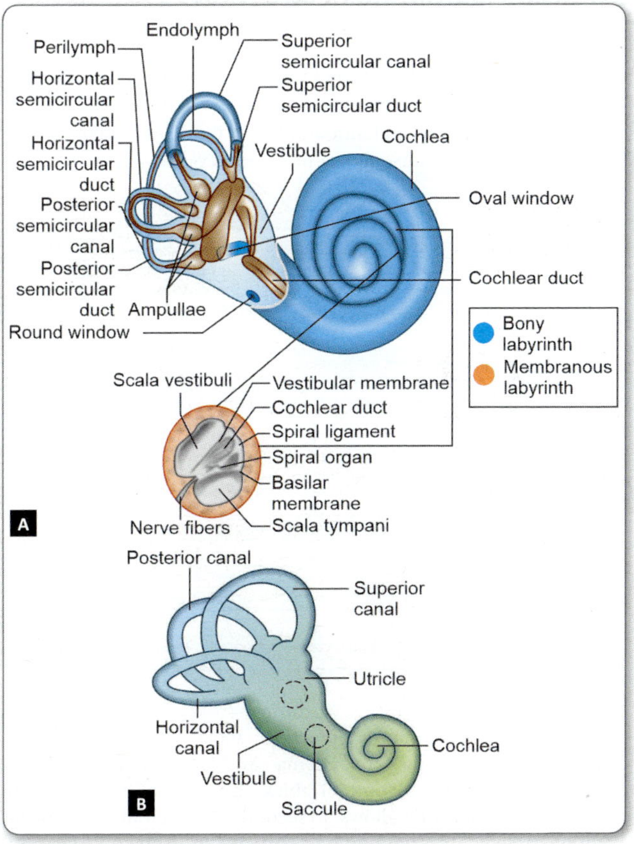

Endolymph
Perilymph
Horizontal semicircular canal
Horizontal semicircular duct
Posterior semicircular canal
Posterior semicircular duct
Round window
Superior semicircular canal
Superior semicircular duct
Cochlea
Vestibule
Oval window
Cochlear duct
Ampullae

Scala vestibuli
Nerve fibers
Vestibular membrane
Cochlear duct
Spiral ligament
Spiral organ
Basilar membrane
Scala tympani

● Bony labyrinth
● Membranous labyrinth

A

Posterior canal
Superior canal
Utricle
Horizontal canal
Vestibule
Saccule
Cochlea

B

Figs 5A and B: **A.** Parts of inner ear; **B.** Swelling of semicircular canals

Ototoxicity

- A variety of medications may have adverse effects on the cochlea, vestibular apparatus, or cranial nerve VIII.
- All but a few, such as aspirin and quinine, cause irreversible hearing loss. At high doses, aspirin toxicity can produce bilateral tinnitus.
- IV medications, especially the aminoglycosides, are the most common causes of ototoxicity which destroy the hair cells in the organ of Corti.

UPPER RESPIRATORY TRACT INFECTIONS

Rhinitis

Rhinitis is a reaction that occurs in the eyes, nose and throat when airborne irritants (allergens) trigger the release of histamine.

Histamine causes inflammation and fluid production in the fragile linings of nasal passages, sinuses, and eyelids.

Common Cold

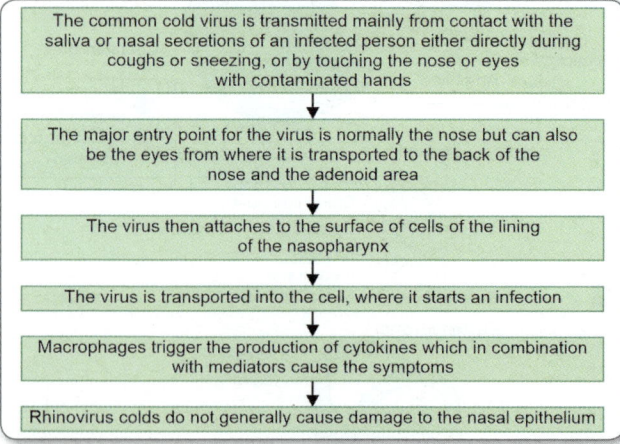

The common cold virus is transmitted mainly from contact with the saliva or nasal secretions of an infected person either directly during coughs or sneezing, or by touching the nose or eyes with contaminated hands

↓

The major entry point for the virus is normally the nose but can also be the eyes from where it is transported to the back of the nose and the adenoid area

↓

The virus then attaches to the surface of cells of the lining of the nasopharynx

↓

The virus is transported into the cell, where it starts an infection

↓

Macrophages trigger the production of cytokines which in combination with mediators cause the symptoms

↓

Rhinovirus colds do not generally cause damage to the nasal epithelium

Sinusitis

A viral upper respiratory infection most commonly causes rhinosinusitis secondary to edema and inflammation of the nasal lining and production of thick mucus that obstructs the paranasal **sinuses** and allows a secondary bacterial overgrowth. Pathophysiology and symptoms of **sinusitis** are shown in Figure 6 and Figure 7 respectively.

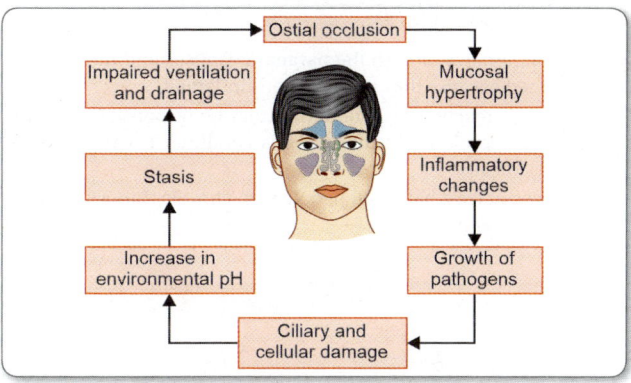

Fig. 6: Pathophysiology of sinusitis

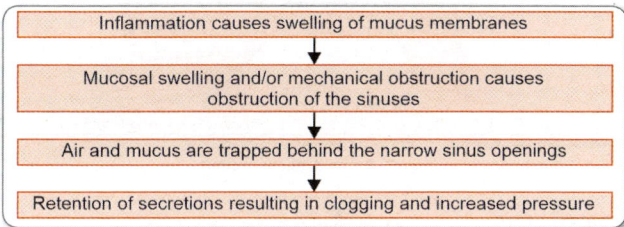

Inflammation causes swelling of mucus membranes

Mucosal swelling and/or mechanical obstruction causes obstruction of the sinuses

Air and mucus are trapped behind the narrow sinus openings

Retention of secretions resulting in clogging and increased pressure

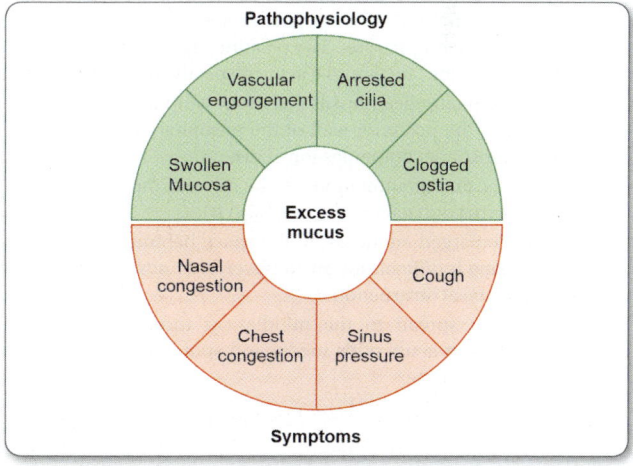

Fig. 7: Symptoms of sinusitis

Chronic Sinusitis (Fig. 8)

- The membranes of both the paranasal sinuses and the nose are thickened because they are constantly inflamed.
- An allergic reaction to certain fungi may be responsible for some cases of chronic rhinosinusitis; this condition is called allergic fungal sinusitis.
- However, at least half of all people with chronic rhinosinusitis do not have allergies.

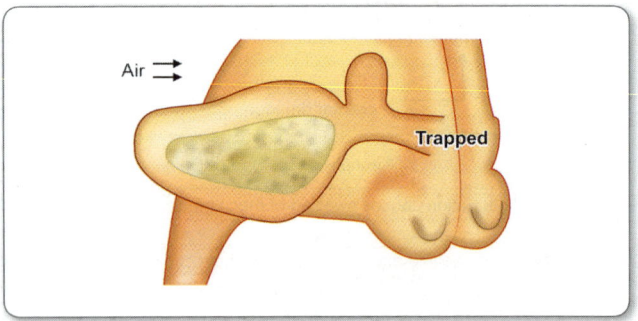

Fig. 8: Trapped mucus in sinus

TONSILLITIS

- Tonsils are composed of lymphatic tissues and are located on each side of the oropharynx. The palatine and lingual tonsils are located behind the fauces and tongue respectively (Fig. 9).
- Adenoids or pharyngeal tonsils consist of lymphatic tissues near the center of the posterior wall of the nasopharynx. Infection of adenoids mostly accompanies tonsillitis.
- Tonsillitis is an inflammation of the tonsils most commonly caused by virus or bacteria (Figs 10A and B).
- Unusually enlarged adenoids fill the space behind the posterior nares, making it difficult for air to travel from nose to the throat resulting in nasal obstruction.
- Infection can spread to the middle ear through Eustachian tube resulting in acute otitis media and spontaneous rupture of tympanic membrane.

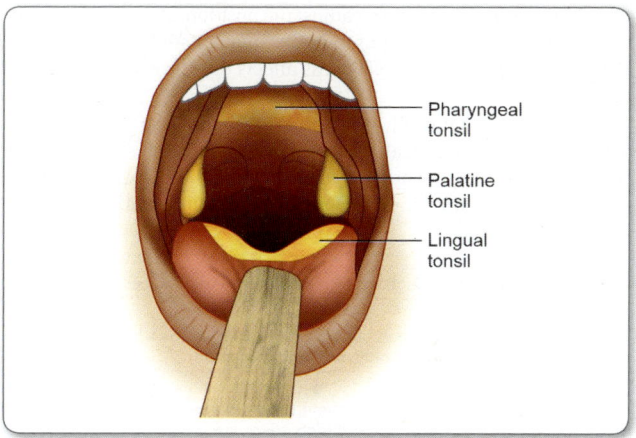

Fig. 9: Types of tonsils

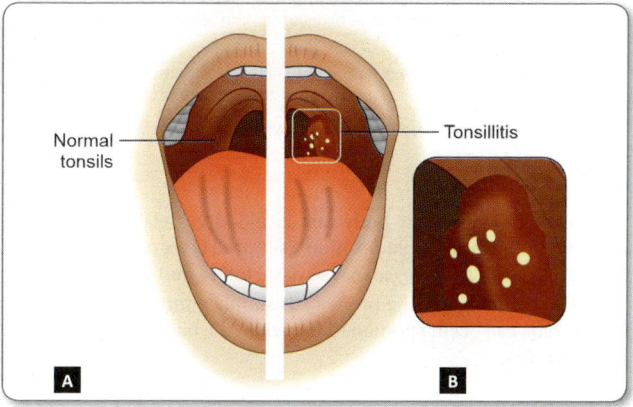

Figs 10A and B: A. Normal tonsils; **B.** Tonsillitis

LARYNGITIS

Larynx is the voice box consisting of vocal cords located at the junction of mouth and trachea and has a flap-like covering called the epiglottis, which prevents food and saliva from entering the larynx during swallowing.

Muscles inside the larynx adjust the position, shape, and tension of the vocal cords, allowing us to make different sounds. Any change in the airflow across the vocal cords affects the voice and the quality of the sound.

Laryngitis may result from prolonged straining of voice, may occur as an isolated local infection or as a part of another, more serious underlying disorder (pneumonia, tuberculosis). In most cases, however, it is a minor ailment and clears up on its own within a few days or weeks.

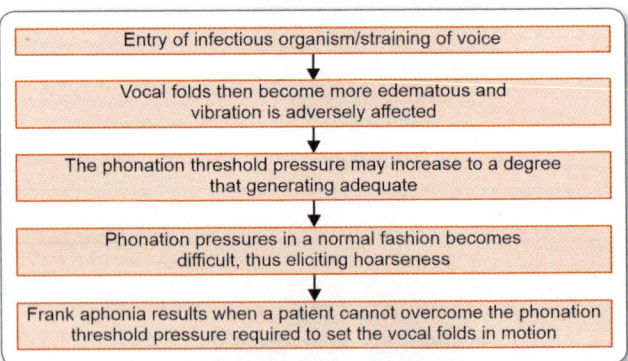

Entry of infectious organism/straining of voice

↓

Vocal folds then become more edematous and vibration is adversely affected

↓

The phonation threshold pressure may increase to a degree that generating adequate

↓

Phonation pressures in a normal fashion becomes difficult, thus eliciting hoarseness

↓

Frank aphonia results when a patient cannot overcome the phonation threshold pressure required to set the vocal folds in motion

EPISTAXIS

The nose is a part of the body rich in blood vessels (vascular) and is situated in a vulnerable position as it protrudes on the face. As a result, trauma to the face can cause nasal injury and bleeding.

The bleeding may be profuse, or simply a minor complication. Nosebleeds can occur spontaneously when the nasal membranes dry out and crack.

NASAL OBSTRUCTION

Congestion, blockage or stuffiness of the nose is known as nasal obstruction, which is a crucial symptom in allergic rhinitis (AR). It may affect quality of life as well as sleep. It may be caused due to both the early and late-phase-allergic reactions. A complex network of inflammatory and neurogenic phenomena including the subepithelial accumulation of inflammatory cells, especially mast cells and eosinophils, and the release of neuropeptides are related to chronic nasal obstruction.

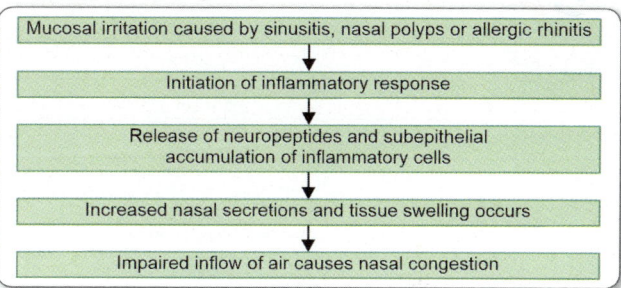

Mucosal irritation caused by sinusitis, nasal polyps or allergic rhinitis

↓

Initiation of inflammatory response

↓

Release of neuropeptides and subepithelial accumulation of inflammatory cells

↓

Increased nasal secretions and tissue swelling occurs

↓

Impaired inflow of air causes nasal congestion

LARYNGEAL OBSTRUCTION

An airway obstruction is a blockage in any part of the airway. The airway is a complex system of tubes that conveys inhaled air from the nose and mouth into the lungs. An obstruction may partially or totally prevent air from getting into the lungs.

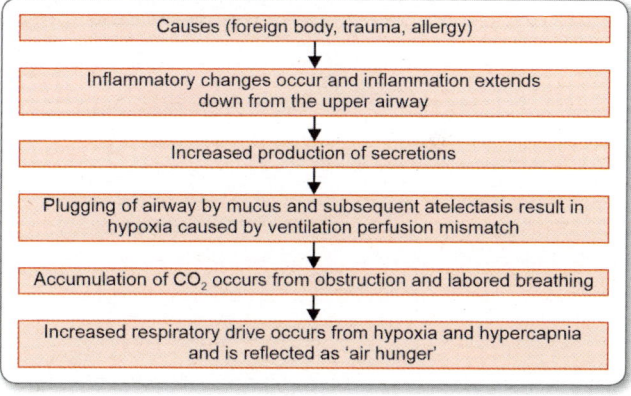

Causes (foreign body, trauma, allergy)

↓

Inflammatory changes occur and inflammation extends down from the upper airway

↓

Increased production of secretions

↓

Plugging of airway by mucus and subsequent atelectasis result in hypoxia caused by ventilation perfusion mismatch

↓

Accumulation of CO_2 occurs from obstruction and labored breathing

↓

Increased respiratory drive occurs from hypoxia and hypercapnia and is reflected as 'air hunger'

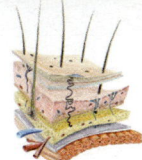

Pathophysiology of Integumentary System

INTRODUCTION

The skin is considered to be the largest organ of the body that protects the underlying tissues, helps to regulate the temperature of body, and permits the sensations of touch, heat, and cold. The three layers of skin are:

1. **Epidermis:** It provides a waterproof barrier and maintains tone of skin
2. **Dermis:** It contains connective tissues, hair follicles and sweat glands
3. **Hypodermis (deep subcutaneous tissue):** It is made up of fat and connective tissues. The melanocytes present in epidermis provide color to the skin (Fig. 1).

The skin is connected to the muscles by the subcutaneous tissue. The insulation from cold to the heat is provided by the hair present on the scalp. Whereas the hair present on eyelashes and eyebrows protect the eyes from dirt and sweat. Similarly, dust is kept out of the nasal cavities by the hair in the nostrils.

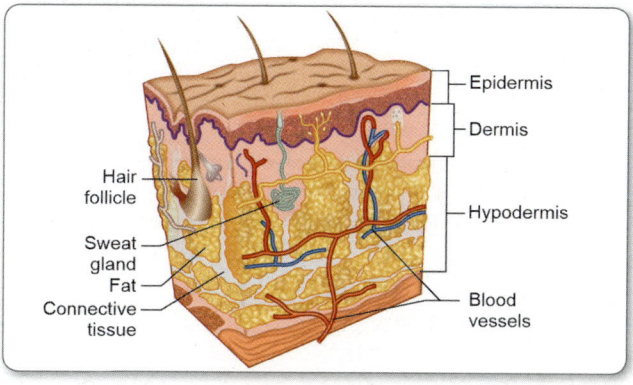

Fig. 1: Skin

The glands in the integumentary system are:

- **Sudoriferous glands:** Sweat producing glands that help to maintain temperature of the body.
- **Sebaceous glands**: Oil producing glands, which prevent bacterial invasion, and prevent drying out of hair and skin.
- **Ceruminous glands**: Produce earwax, which maintains flexibility of eardrum and also prevents drying of ear canal.
- **Mammary glands**: Produce milk.

Let us now discuss the pathophysiological changes in the major disease conditions associated with integumentary system.

SYSTEMIC LUPUS ERYTHEMATOSUS

The disruption of normal disease fighting function of immune system results in lupus. There is a global loss of self-tolerance that occurs with an activation of autoreactive B and T cells causing production of autoantibodies, which are pathogenic in nature. The antigen-antibody complex forms and builds up in the tissues causing inflammation. These mechanisms lead to tissue injury (Fig. 2).

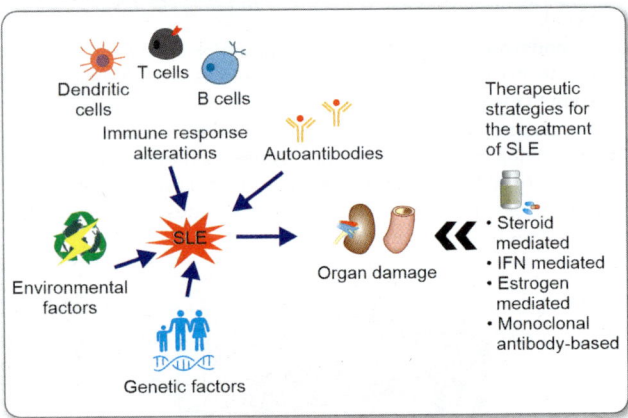

Fig. 2: Systemic lupus erythematosus

Abbreviations: IFN, interferons; SLE, systemic lupus erythematosus

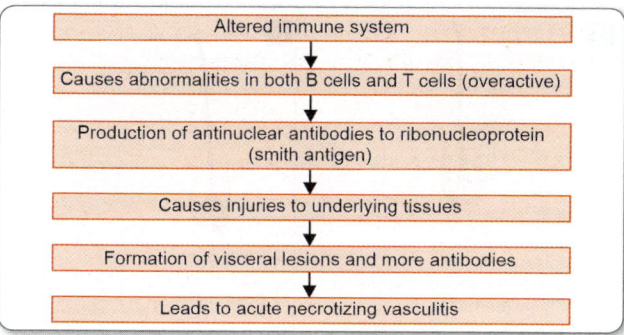

Altered immune system
↓
Causes abnormalities in both B cells and T cells (overactive)
↓
Production of antinuclear antibodies to ribonucleoprotein (smith antigen)
↓
Causes injuries to underlying tissues
↓
Formation of visceral lesions and more antibodies
↓
Leads to acute necrotizing vasculitis

ACNE VULGARIS

- During puberty, sebaceous glands are stimulated by the androgens, causing enlargement and making them to secrete sebum that rises up to the top level of hair follicle and then flows out on the surface of skin.
- When acne is developed, stimulation of androgens leading to heightened response in the sebaceous glands, plugging the pilosebaceous ducts by this accumulated sebum.
- Comedones are formed as a result of this accumulation (Figs 3A to D).

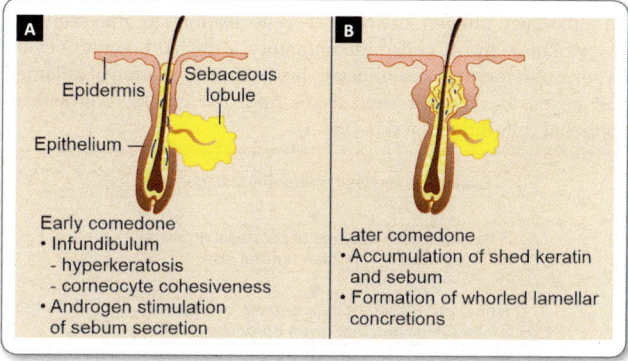

A
Epidermis
Sebaceous lobule
Epithelium

Early comedone
• Infundibulum
 - hyperkeratosis
 - corneocyte cohesiveness
• Androgen stimulation of sebum secretion

B
Later comedone
• Accumulation of shed keratin and sebum
• Formation of whorled lamellar concretions

Figs 3A and B:

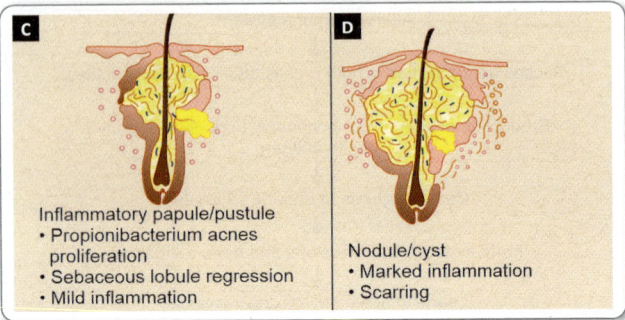

Figs 3A to D: Pathogenesis of acne

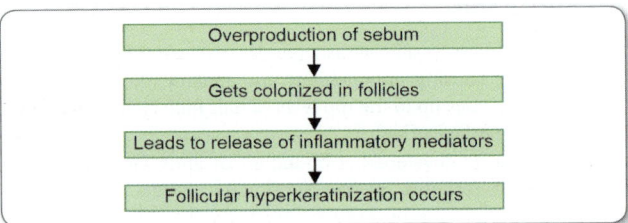

PSORIASIS

An unknown antigen activates T cells leading to the secretion of cytokines by T cells, inflammatory cells and keratinocytes. Hyperproliferation of keratinocytes leads to the formation of inflamed and raised lesions that shed flakes from the excessive growth of epithelial cells lining the skin (Fig. 4).

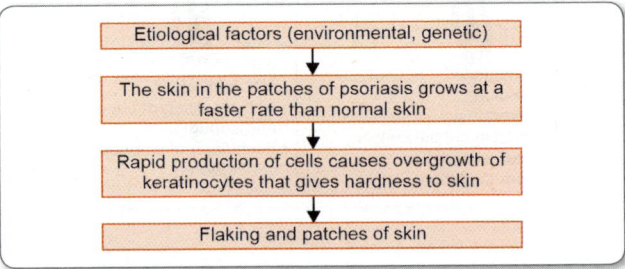

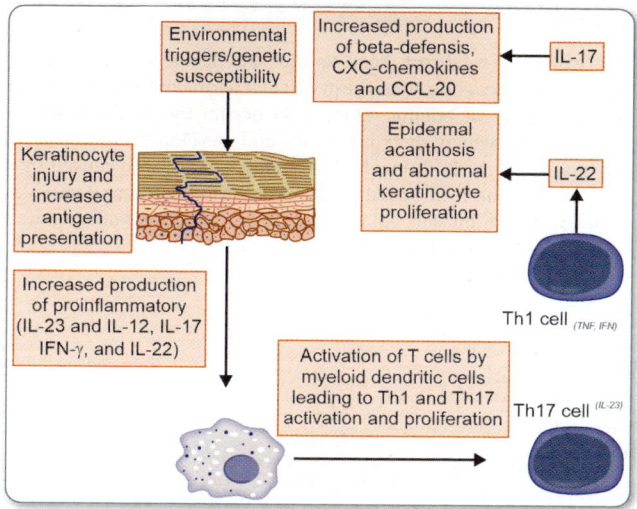

Fig. 4: Psoriasis

MALIGNANT MELANOMA

Melanomas grow in two phases as radial and vertical. The malignant cells grow in a radial pattern in the epidermis in the radial growth phase. With the progression of disease, the melanomas take up the vertical phase of growing, develop their ability to metastasize and invade the dermis.

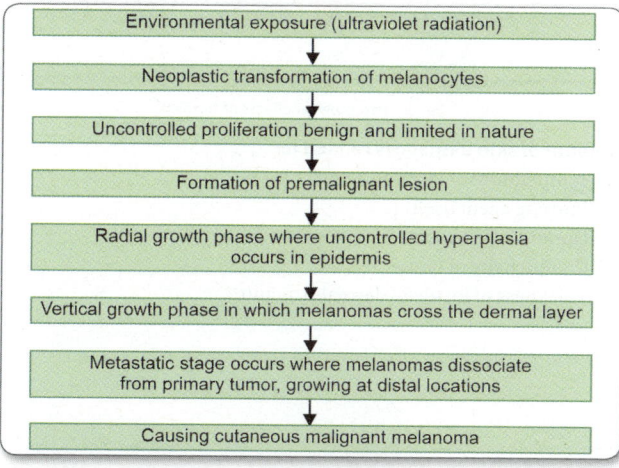

BURNS

The exposure to direct heat to the skin leads to the onset of inflammatory reaction, increase in vascular permeability, vasodilation and formation of edema. There also occurs the denaturation of protein cells, which then coagulate and develops thrombosis in the blood vessels. Both local and systemic changes are caused by a burn injury. The local reaction increases vasodilation and vascular permeability in the skin. All internal organ systems get affected as a systemic response to burns (Fig. 5).

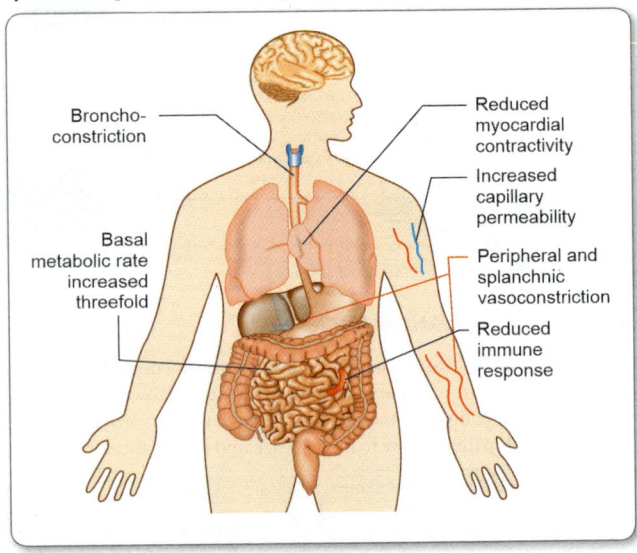

Fig. 5: Pathological effects of burns

Amount of skin damage is related to:

- Temperature of burning agent
- Burning agent itself
- Duration of exposure
- Conductivity of tissue
- Thickness of involved dermal structure

Pathophysiology

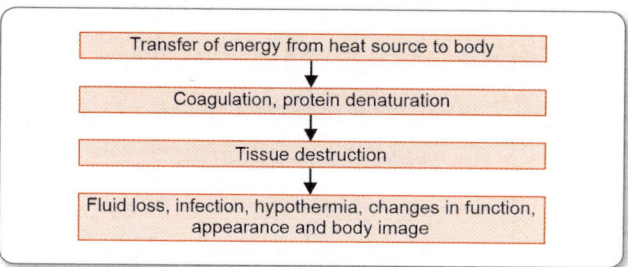

Transfer of energy from heat source to body
↓
Coagulation, protein denaturation
↓
Tissue destruction
↓
Fluid loss, infection, hypothermia, changes in function, appearance and body image

Local and Systemic Response to Burns

Cardiovascular Response

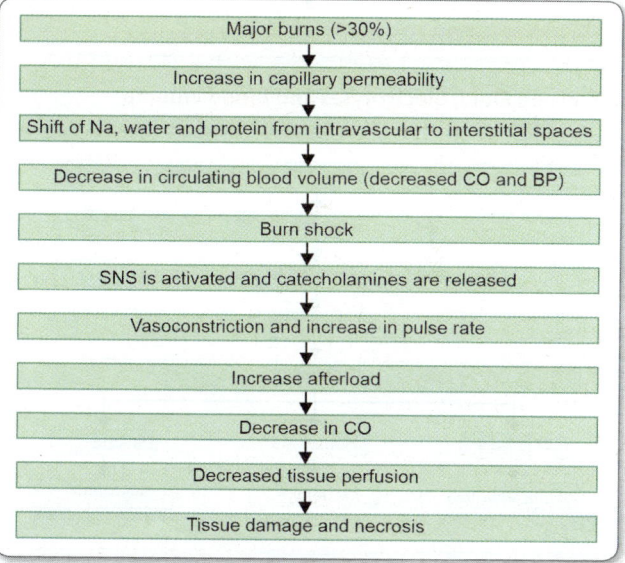

Major burns (>30%)
↓
Increase in capillary permeability
↓
Shift of Na, water and protein from intravascular to interstitial spaces
↓
Decrease in circulating blood volume (decreased CO and BP)
↓
Burn shock
↓
SNS is activated and catecholamines are released
↓
Vasoconstriction and increase in pulse rate
↓
Increase afterload
↓
Decrease in CO
↓
Decreased tissue perfusion
↓
Tissue damage and necrosis

Abbreviations: BP, blood pressure; CO, cardiac output; SNS, sympathetic nervous system

BURN EDEMA

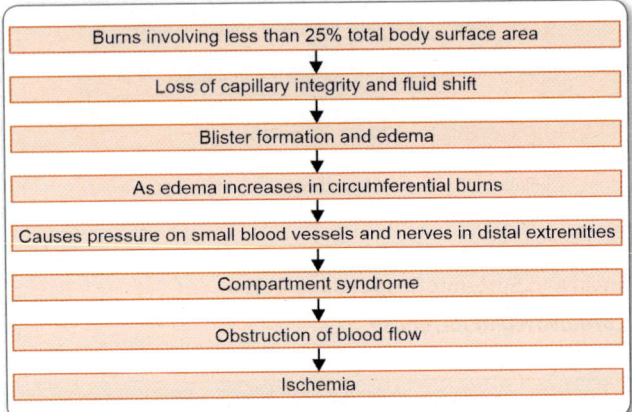

Burns involving less than 25% total body surface area
↓
Loss of capillary integrity and fluid shift
↓
Blister formation and edema
↓
As edema increases in circumferential burns
↓
Causes pressure on small blood vessels and nerves in distal extremities
↓
Compartment syndrome
↓
Obstruction of blood flow
↓
Ischemia

Effects on Fluid, Electrolytes and Blood Volume

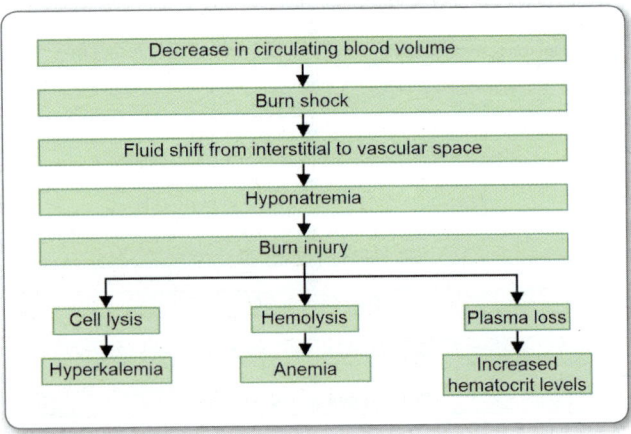

Decrease in circulating blood volume
↓
Burn shock
↓
Fluid shift from interstitial to vascular space
↓
Hyponatremia
↓
Burn injury
↓

Cell lysis	Hemolysis	Plasma loss
Hyperkalemia	Anemia	Increased hematocrit levels

Pulmonary Response

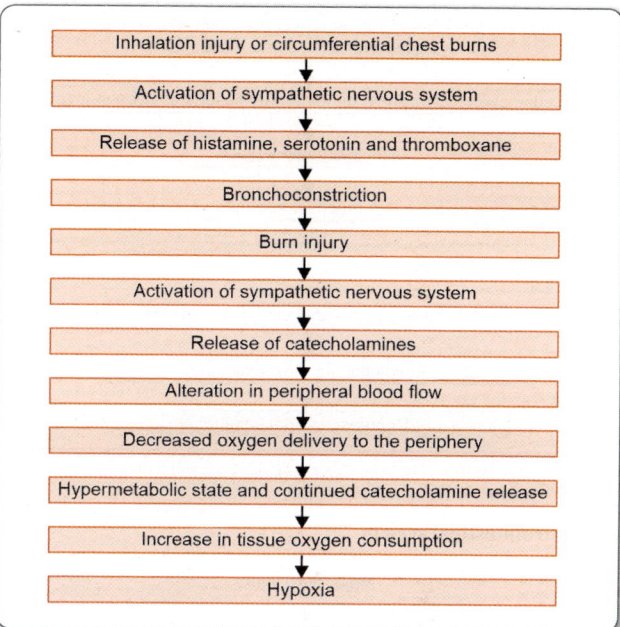

Inhalation injury or circumferential chest burns

↓

Activation of sympathetic nervous system

↓

Release of histamine, serotonin and thromboxane

↓

Bronchoconstriction

↓

Burn injury

↓

Activation of sympathetic nervous system

↓

Release of catecholamines

↓

Alteration in peripheral blood flow

↓

Decreased oxygen delivery to the periphery

↓

Hypermetabolic state and continued catecholamine release

↓

Increase in tissue oxygen consumption

↓

Hypoxia

- **Upper airway injury**

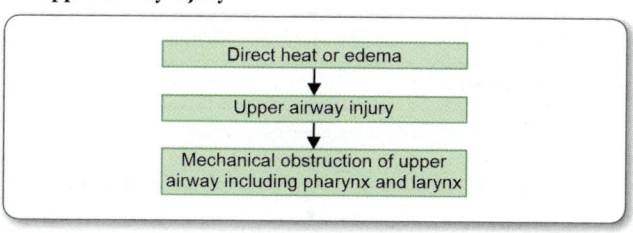

Direct heat or edema

↓

Upper airway injury

↓

Mechanical obstruction of upper airway including pharynx and larynx

- **Inhalation injury below the glottis**

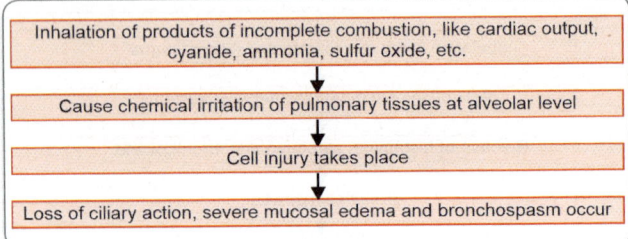

Inhalation of products of incomplete combustion, like cardiac output, cyanide, ammonia, sulfur oxide, etc.

↓

Cause chemical irritation of pulmonary tissues at alveolar level

↓

Cell injury takes place

↓

Loss of ciliary action, severe mucosal edema and bronchospasm occur

- **Restrictive defects**

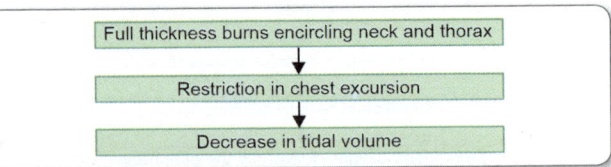

Full thickness burns encircling neck and thorax

↓

Restriction in chest excursion

↓

Decrease in tidal volume

Other Systemic Responses

- **Gastrointestinal system**

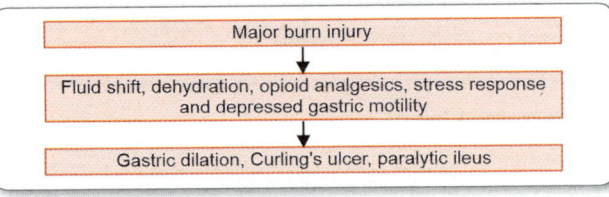

Major burn injury

↓

Fluid shift, dehydration, opioid analgesics, stress response and depressed gastric motility

↓

Gastric dilation, Curling's ulcer, paralytic ileus

- **Renal system:**

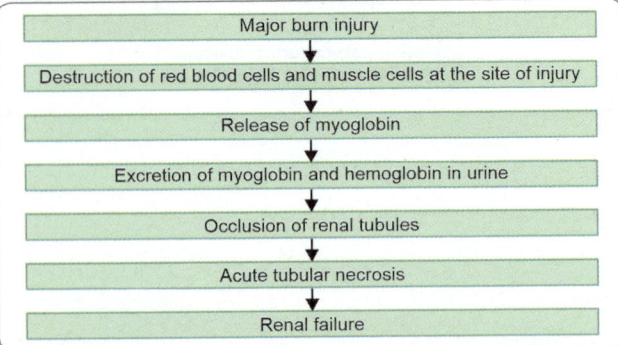

Major burn injury

↓

Destruction of red blood cells and muscle cells at the site of injury

↓

Release of myoglobin

↓

Excretion of myoglobin and hemoglobin in urine

↓

Occlusion of renal tubules

↓

Acute tubular necrosis

↓

Renal failure

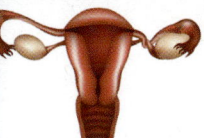

Disorders of Female Reproductive System

INTRODUCTION

The female reproductive system is mainly responsible for producing sex hormones, ova and maintaining the fertilized egg. The internal organs include uterus, fallopian tubes and ovaries. The uterus is responsible for holding the embryo that further develops into fetus. The secretions produced by uterus help in transporting sperms to the fallopian tubes. The external organs also known as genitals include vulva having labia, clitoris and vaginal opening. The uterus and vagina are connected at the cervix (Fig. 1).

The cycles of hormonal activity are experienced by the females of reproductive age, which repeat every month. An average menstrual cycle takes about 28 days and is divided into follicular, ovulation and luteal phase. Follicle stimulating hormone (FSH), luteinizing hormone (LH), estrogen and progesterone regulate the activity of cells involved in menstrual cycle.

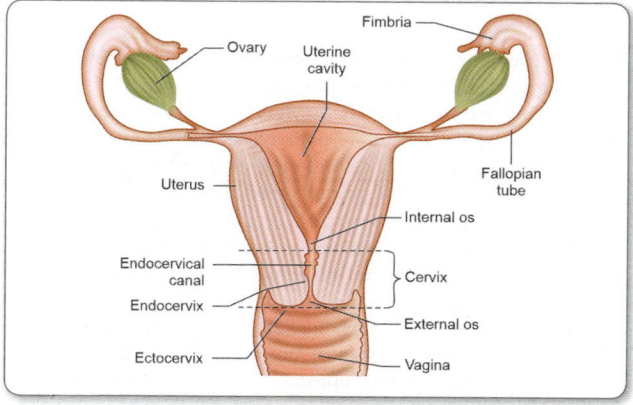

Fig. 1: Parts of female reproductive system

In this chapter, we will discuss the pathophysiological changes that take place in various disorders related to female reproductive system.

MENSTRUAL DISORDERS

Dysmenorrhea

An imbalance in the level of prostaglandins along with other factors like ovarian hormones, cervical factors and level of vasopressin, all contribute to hyperactivity of endometrium. This leads to frequent and dysrhythmic contractions of the uterus with an increase in active pressure and basal tone. The hypercontractility of uterus, reduced blood flow to uterus (due to vasoconstriction caused by vasopressin) and hypersensitivity of peripheral nerve lead to the onset of pain.

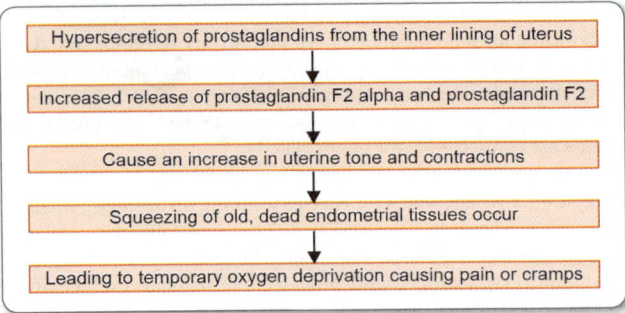

Amenorrhea

It can be classified as primary or secondary. Primary amenorrhea is the absence of initiation of menses whereas secondary amenorrhea occurs when menses stop in previously menstruating female of reproductive age. The basic pathophysiological mechanism of amenorrhea is related to disturbance in hormonal balance and functions or it can be due to any anatomic abnormalities.

During a normal menstrual cycle, hypothalamus releases gonadotropin releasing hormone that stimulates the pituitary to release follicle stimulating hormone and luteinizing hormone. Both these hormones further act on the ovaries to produce estrogen and progesterone, which then make the uterus to carry out the follicular and secretory phase of the menstrual cycle. In case of any malfunctioning in this normal cycle, dysfunction occurs in ovulation and also endometrial changes get disrupted, resulting in amenorrhea. Sometimes, amenorrhea can also be present in case of normal ovulatory function, which is actually the result of anatomic abnormalities in the genital structures in spite of having a normal secretion of hormones.

Premenstrual Syndrome

Premenstrual syndrome is triggered by the activity of hormones just after ovulation. The symptoms can begin in any stage of luteal phase and are not very specific to gonadal or nongonadal hormones.

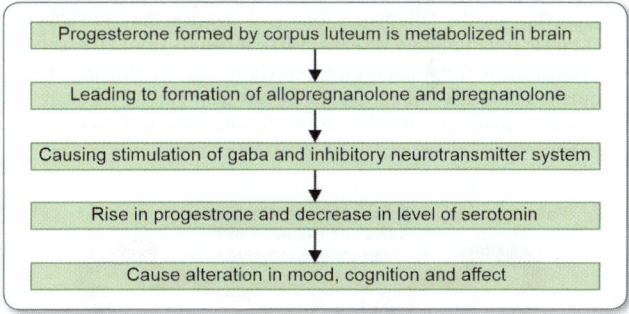

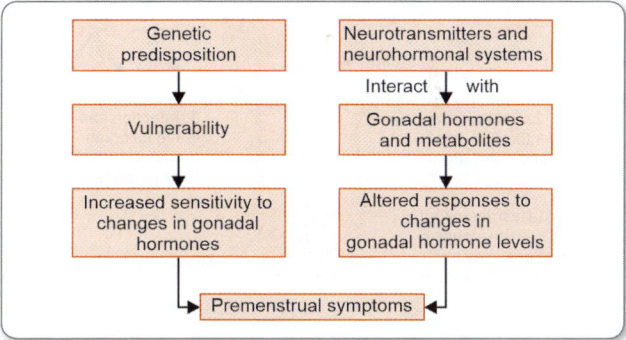

Abnormal Uterine Bleeding

It includes menstrual cycle irregularities such as frequency, duration, regularity and volume of flow. The blood to the uterus is supplied via the uterine and ovarian arteries forming into arcuate arteries. The functionalis and basalis layers of endometrium are supplied by the radial branches of the arcuate arteries. A decrease in the level of progesterone towards the end of menstrual cycle leads to breakdown of enzyme in the functionalis layer, leading to loss of blood and shedding of endometrium. The blood loss is controlled by the vasoconstriction of the arteries of endometrium along with normally functioning platelets and thrombin. Abnormal uterine bleeding occurs as a result of disturbance in uterine structure caused by hyperplasia or polyps, blood coagulopathies or imbalance of hormones.

PELVIC INFLAMMATORY DISEASE

The cervix, uterus, fallopian tubes and ovaries may be affected from pelvic inflammatory disease (PID). It results from an ascent of microorganisms from vagina and cervix to the endometrium and fallopian tubes. The microorganisms can also spread through the lymphatic system, e.g. infection caused by intrauterine device (Fig. 2).

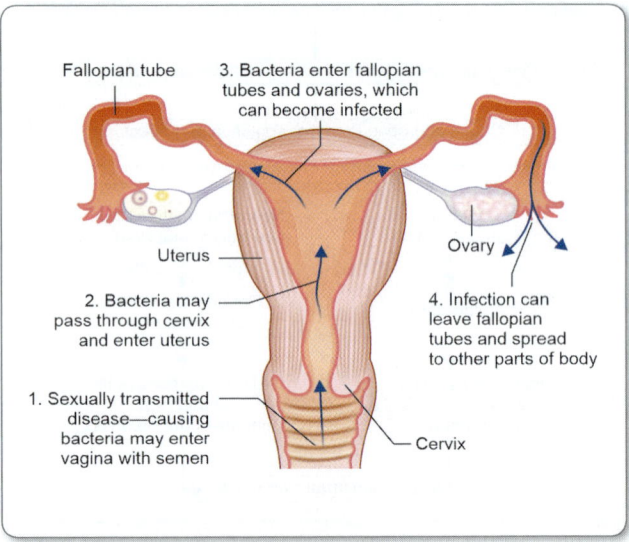

Fig. 2: Pathophysiology of pelvic inflammatory disease

POLYCYSTIC OVARIAN SYNDROME

It is mainly characterized by an excess of ovarian or adrenal secretion of androgens.

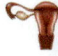

Pathophysiology of polycystic ovarian syndrome:

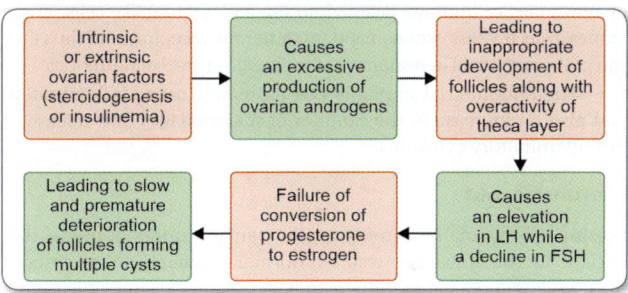

Abbreviations: LH, luteinizing hormone; FSH, follicle stimulating hormone

UTERINE AND CERVICAL DISORDERS

Endometriosis

It is an inflammatory condition that is estrogen dependent and can cause pelvic pain and infertility. During menstruation, the endometrial cells get transported from the uterine cavity through the fallopian tubes and are implanted in certain ectopic sites. This is known as retrograde menstruation as a result of which the endometrial cells adhere to the surface of pelvic organs, where they keep on growing and cause bleeding during each cycle of menstruation (Fig. 3).

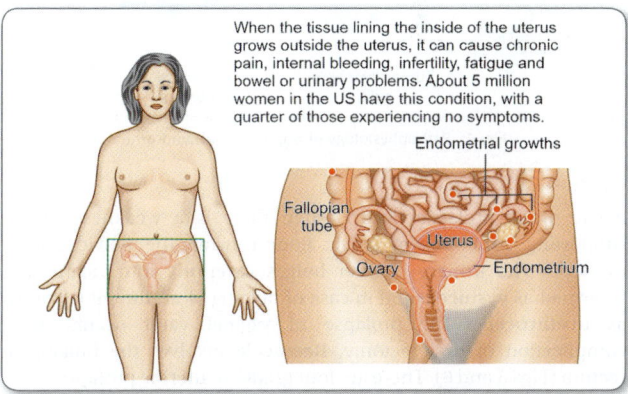

When the tissue lining the inside of the uterus grows outside the uterus, it can cause chronic pain, internal bleeding, infertility, fatigue and bowel or urinary problems. About 5 million women in the US have this condition, with a quarter of those experiencing no symptoms.

Endometrial growths

Fallopian tube

Uterus

Ovary

Endometrium

Fig. 3: Endometriosis

Endometrial tissue can also be transplanted during the surgical procedure through the surgical instruments, or the spread can also occur through the lymphatic or venous systems.

In some cases, there is a transformation of peritoneal cells promoted by hormones or immune factors into the endometrial like cells. These tissues/cells possess estrogen and progesterone receptors and thus they can grow, and bleed in response to the change in level of hormones.

The endometrial implants can ultimately cause inflammation and also an increase in the number of macrophages and release of proinflammatory cytokines.

Uterine Fibroid

Uterine leiomyoma or fibroids are the benign tumors of uterus that initiate in the muscular wall. Abnormal proliferation of smooth muscle cells and an alteration in angiogenesis are responsible for the formation of fibroids (Fig. 4).

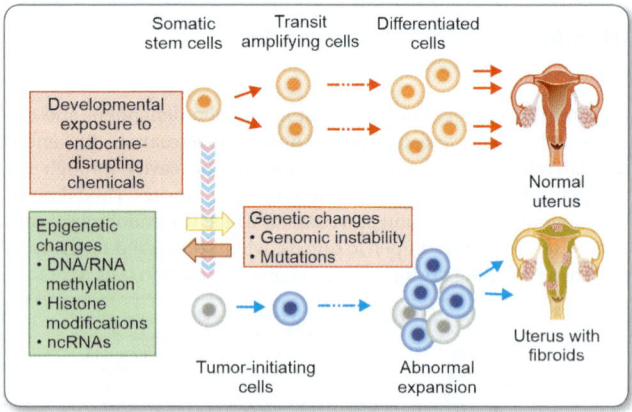

Fig. 4: Pathophysiology of premenstrual syndrome

Uterine Prolapse

Pelvic organ prolapse occurs when there is a weakness in the supporting structures of pelvic floor causing the pelvic viscera to slope. The urinary bladder bulges anteriorly into vagina and is termed as **cystocele** and in case of bulging of urethra, it is known as **urethrocele**. The prolapse of vaginal vault occurs as a complication of hysterectomy. **Rectocele** involves the bulging of rectum (Figs 5 and 6). There are four grades of uterine prolapse:

1. Descent of uterus above the hymen
2. Descent of uterus till hymen
3. Descent of uterus beyond hymen
4. Total prolapse

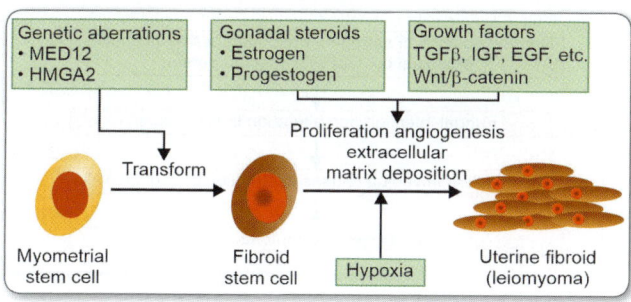

Fig. 5: Molecular pathogenesis of uterine fibroid development

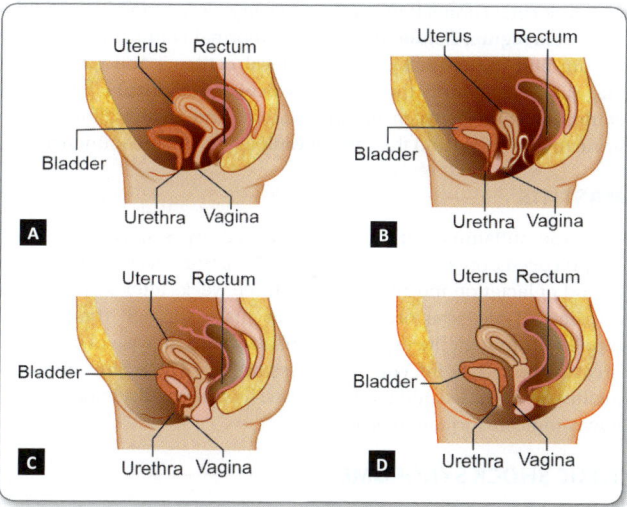

Figs 6A to D: A. Normal uterus; **B.** Uterine prolapse; **C.** Cystocele; **D.** Rectocele

VAGINAL DISORDERS

Vaginitis

The normal vaginal flora is maintained by a balance of vaginal secretions, cervical mucus and exfoliated cells. Lactobacillus, yeast and corynebacterial help balance this flora. Anything that changes the vaginal environment can cause alteration in the normal vaginal flora by the introduction of pathogens making them to multiply and cause infection and related symptoms.

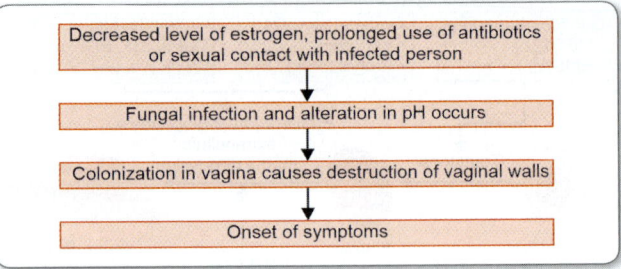

Decreased level of estrogen, prolonged use of antibiotics or sexual contact with infected person

↓

Fungal infection and alteration in pH occurs

↓

Colonization in vagina causes destruction of vaginal walls

↓

Onset of symptoms

Vaginal Fistulas

Any abnormal connection between two organs is termed as a fistula. In a **rectovaginal fistula**, there is an abnormal connection between rectum and vagina that causes the fecal contents and gas to pass into the vagina from the bowel. **Vesicovaginal fistula** involves a communication between urinary bladder and vagina allowing the urine to freely flow into the vaginal vault leading to incontinence.

MASTITIS

It is the inflammation of breast caused by staphylococcus or streptococcus organisms. Acute mastitis mainly occurs during the period of lactation mostly in the first three weeks after delivery. The invasion of bacterial organisms takes place through the cracked nipples or through the exposed lymphatic ducts. In case of overfilled breasts, the risk of infection increases further. The main symptoms include swollen, red and tender breasts. If purulent discharge occurs, it may indicate formation of abscess.

TOXIC SHOCK SYNDROME

Toxic shock syndrome (TSS) is caused by staphylococcus or streptococcus exotoxins. These toxins are systemically absorbed in patients who do not have a protective antitoxin antibody. A preexisting colonization of vagina by staphylococcus, and use of tampons and contraceptive devices like diaphragm predisposes the females to toxic shock syndrome. There is an enhanced production of exotoxins as a result of mechanical or chemical factors related to the use of tampons. These exotoxins gain access to the bloodstream via the uterus or a break in the mucosal layer. This syndrome is characterized by high fever, hypotension, rashes and a multiorgan failure that appears about 1–2 weeks after an initial onset of disease condition.

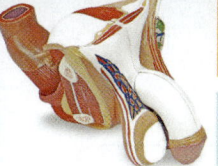

Disorders of Male Reproductive System

INTRODUCTION

The male reproductive system is responsible for promoting the formation, storage and ejaculation of sperm for the fertilization process. The testes produce both sperm and androgens for the development of males. The process of sperm maturity and transport to the penis is aided by various accessory organs and the penis then transfers the sperm to female reproductive tract (Fig. 1).

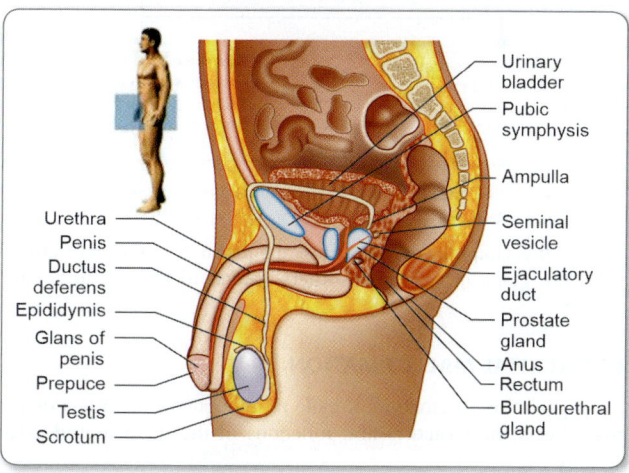

Urinary bladder
Pubic symphysis
Ampulla
Seminal vesicle
Ejaculatory duct
Prostate gland
Anus
Rectum
Bulbourethral gland

Urethra
Penis
Ductus deferens
Epididymis
Glans of penis
Prepuce
Testis
Scrotum

Fig. 1: Parts of male reproductive system

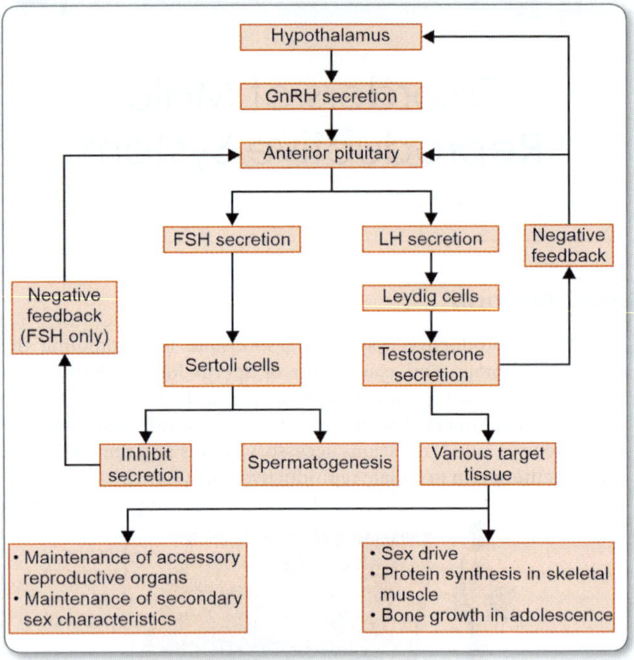

```
                    ┌─────────────────┐
                    │  Hypothalamus   │◄──────────────┐
                    └─────────────────┘               │
                            │                          │
                    ┌─────────────────┐               │
                    │ GnRH secretion  │               │
                    └─────────────────┘               │
                            │                          │
          ┌────────►┌─────────────────┐◄──────────────┤
          │         │Anterior pituitary│              │
          │         └─────────────────┘               │
          │            │         │                     │
          │   ┌────────┘         └──────┐      ┌──────────────┐
          │   ▼                         ▼      │  Negative    │
    ┌───────────┐              ┌─────────────┐ │  feedback    │
    │FSH secretion│            │LH secretion │ └──────────────┘
    └───────────┘              └─────────────┘        ▲
┌──────────┐  │                      │                │
│ Negative │  │               ┌─────────────┐         │
│ feedback │  │               │ Leydig cells│         │
│(FSH only)│  │               └─────────────┘         │
└──────────┘  │                      │                │
      ▲       ▼                ┌─────────────┐         │
   ┌──────────────┐            │ Testosterone│─────────┘
   │ Sertoli cells│            │  secretion  │
   └──────────────┘            └─────────────┘
        │     │                   │
   ┌────┘     └────┐         ┌─────┘
   ▼               ▼         ▼
┌────────┐  ┌──────────────┐ ┌──────────────┐
│Inhibit │  │Spermatogenesis│ │Various target│
│secretion│  └──────────────┘ │   tissue     │
└────────┘                    └──────────────┘
```

| • Maintenance of accessory reproductive organs
• Maintenance of secondary sex characteristics | • Sex drive
• Protein synthesis in skeletal muscle
• Bone growth in adolescence |

Abbreviations: FSH, follicle stimulating hormone; GnRH, gonadotropin-releasing hormone; LH, luteinizing hormone

In this chapter, we will discuss the pathophysiological changes that take place in various disorders related to male reproductive system.

CONGENITAL MALFORMATION

A congenital malformation of male reproductive system is a defect that affects the structure and functions of the male reproductive system.

Hypospadias

Hypospadias is a congenital malformation in which the opening of urethra is present on the ventral area of the shaft of the penis, proximal to the end of the glans penis. Types of hypospadias depend upon the location of meatus. It may be present anywhere from glans to the perineum (Fig. 2).

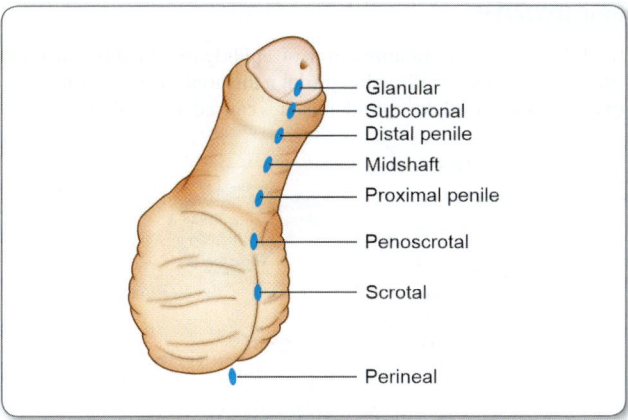

Glanular
Subcoronal
Distal penile
Midshaft
Proximal penile
Penoscrotal
Scrotal
Perineal

Fig. 2: Type of hypospadias

Epispadias

Epispadias is a condition in which the opening of the urethra is on the dorsum of the penis. The causes of **epispadias** are unknown. It may be related to improper development of the pubic bone (Fig. 3).

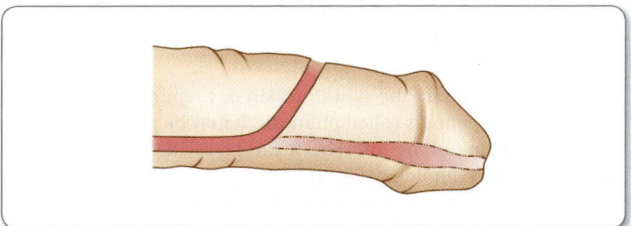

Fig. 3: Epispadias (dorsal)

CRYPTORCHIDISM

Failure of one or both testes to descend into the scrotum through the inguinal canal is called cryptorchidism. It is also known as undescended testis.

ORCHITIS

The inflammation of the testicles is called orchitis. It can be caused by either bacteria or a virus.

EPIDIDYMITIS

Epididymitis is the inflammation of epididymis. In this, infection spreads in an upward direction through the urethra, ejaculatory duct, vas deferens toward the epididymis. It is caused by *E. coli* (Fig. 4).

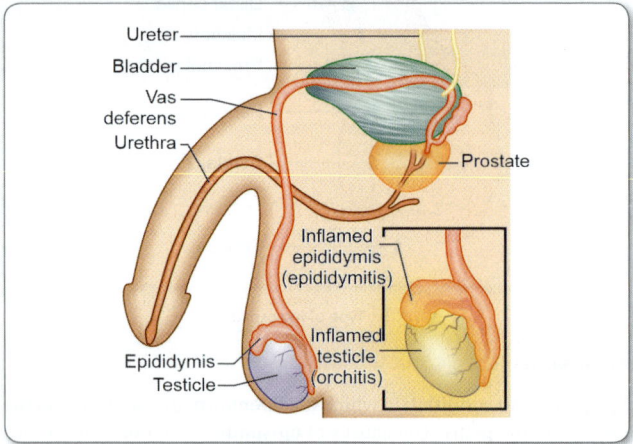

Fig. 4: Epididymitis

PHIMOSIS

The inability to retract the skin (foreskin or prepuce), which covers the glans of the penis, is called phimosis. It may be present as rubber band or tight ring of the foreskin. It can be divided into two types: physiologic and pathologic (Fig. 5).

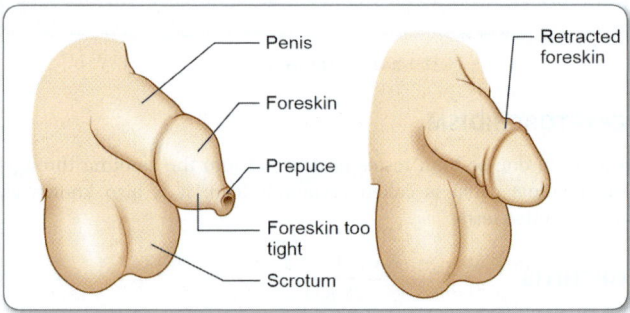

Fig. 5: Phimosis

Physiologic phimosis: In this type, tight foreskin is present at the time of birth and it separates naturally over the time.

Pathologic phimosis: In this type, scarring, infection or inflammation results in phimosis. Forceful foreskin retraction can cause bleeding, scarring, and psychological trauma to the child and parent.

SEXUAL DYSFUNCTION

Sexual disorders are the conditions which affect normal sexual functions. There are three phases in sexual disorders:

1. **Desire disorders:**
   - **Hyperactive sexual desire:** It is the abnormal regulation or lack of control over the sexual motivation. Examples are inadequate control of the sexual impulses, compulsive sexual behavior, and spontaneous sexual desire.
   - **Hypoactive sexual desire:** It is the decreased desire for sexual activity and deficiency or absence of sexual fantasies.
   - **Sexual aversion:** It is the active avoidance of genital sexual contact with the sexual partner.

2. **Arousal disorders:**
   - **Erectile dysfunction:** It is the inability to attain or to maintain an adequate erection until the sexual activity gets completed.
   - **Erectile dyspareunia:** Erectile dyspareunia is the painful sexual intercourse during erection of penis.
     - **Penile induration/Peyronie's disease:** It is the severe curvature of penis, which is caused by scarring in the tunica. It may cause pain during sexual intercourse.
     - **Balanitis:** It is the inflammation of the foreskin.
     - **Balanoposthitis:** It is the inflammation of prepuce and glans penis.
     - **Frenular tethering:** It is the scarring of frenulum, which causes loss of elasticity.
     - **Paraphimosis:** It is the condition in which the opening of foreskin is too small.
     - **Chordee:** It is the congenital curvature of the penis.
     - **Neurologic damage**

3. **Orgasm (ejaculatory) disorders:**
   - **Premature ejaculation:** Premature ejaculation is also called rapid ejaculation or early ejaculation. In this condition, with minimal sexual stimulation, the onset of orgasm and early ejaculation takes place.

- **Retarded ejaculation:** Retarded ejaculation is the delay or absence of orgasm after a normal sexual excitement phase.
- **Ejaculatory incompetence:** Ejaculatory incompetence is the consistent inability to reach orgasm irrespective of the type or duration of sexual stimulation.
- **Retrograde ejaculation:** Retrograde ejaculation is the backward ejaculation of all or part of the semen into the bladder.
- **Ejaculatory dyspareunia:** Ejaculatory dyspareunia is the pain during ejaculation.
  - ♦ **Prostatitis:** Prostatitis is the inflammation of the prostate. Acute or chronic infection of the prostate is often caused due to the bacteria entering from the urethra.
  - ♦ **Urethritis:** Urethritis is the inflammation of the urethra. It is often caused by the bacteria.
  - ♦ **Neurologic damage.**

GYNECOMASTIA

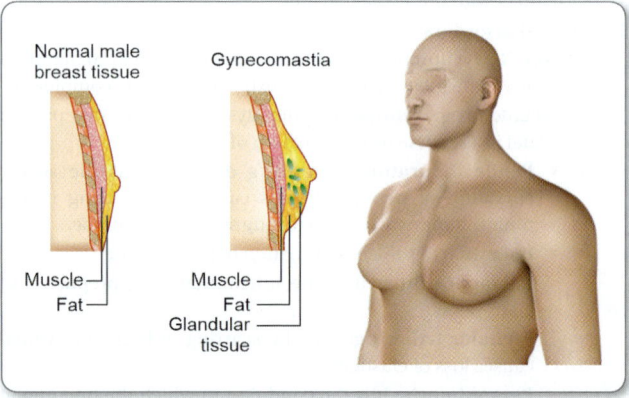

Fig. 6: Gynecomastia

Gynecomastia (Fig. 6) is the condition in which amount of breast gland tissue is increased in men. It is caused because of the imbalance in the level of estrogen and testosterone hormones. It can affect one breast or both breasts.

- **Gynecomastia in infants:** It is caused because of the effects of the mother's estrogen on infants. It generally gets resolved within two to three weeks after birth.

- **Gynecomastia during puberty:** It is caused by hormone changes, which occur during puberty. It gets resolved without treatment within six months to two years in most of the cases.
- **Gynecomastia in adults:** The prevalence is high in the age groups of 50–69 years.

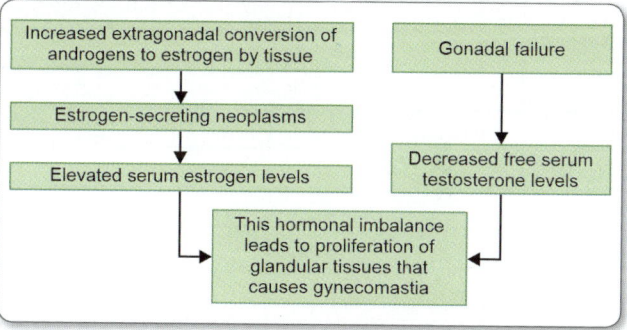

MALE MENOPAUSE

Andropause is commonly known as Male menopause. It occurs because of the age-related hormonal changes, which generally affects the males who are in the age group of 50 years and above. It is also called testosterone deficiency, and late-onset hypogonadism.

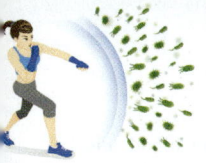

Pathophysiology of Immune System Disorders

INTRODUCTION—IMMUNE SYSTEM

The immune system is a complex system that is responsible for protecting us against infections and foreign substances. The three lines of defense include.

1. **Physical and chemical barriers** to infection: To keep invaders out (through skin, mucus membranes,).

2. **Inflammatory response:** Consists of nonspecific ways to defend against pathogens that have broken through the first line of defense (such as with inflammatory response and fever).

3. **Immune response:** It is aggravated in response to specific pathogens that cause diseases (B cells are responsible for producing antibodies whereas T cells are responsible for killing the infected cells). The immune system is associated to the lymphatic system, and the lymph nodes that contain both B and T lymphocytes.

LYMPHATIC SYSTEM

The lymphatic system consists of primary lymphatic organs and secondary lymphatic organs:

- **Primary lymphatic organs** are the red bone marrow and the thymus.
  - **Red bone marrow** is the soft, spongy, nutrient rich tissue, which is found in the cavities of long bones, and is the site of blood cell production.
  - **Thymus gland** is an important part of the immune system. It primarily functions to maintain the level of lymphocytes, to reject foreign substances and to maintain the response of body to the entry of antigens.
- **Secondary lymphatic organs** are the spleen, lymph nodes, tonsils, Peyer's patches, and the appendix.

- **The spleen** is a ductless gland that stores the blood and destroys the old red blood cells (RBCs).
- **Lymph nodes** act as filters, with an internal honeycomb of connective tissues filled with lymphocytes that collect and destroy bacteria and viruses.
- **Tonsils** are often the first organs to encounter pathogens and antigens that come into the body by mouth or nose.
- **Peyer's patches**, located in the wall of the intestine and the appendix, attached to the cecum of the large intestine, intercept pathogens that come into the body through the intestinal tract.

Functions of lymphatic system is depicted in Figure 1.

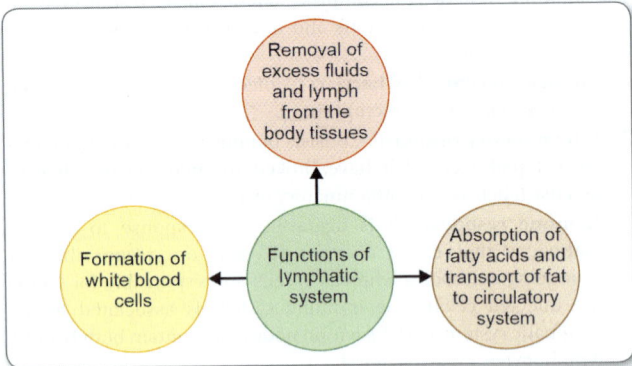

Fig. 1: Functions of lymphatic system

TYPES OF IMMUNITY

- **Humoral immunity:** It is initiated when there is a binding of an antibody to an antigen. This antigen is then absorbed by the B cell, which then forwards this antigen to specialized helper T cell, causing an activation of the B cell. There occurs a rapid growth of activated B cells leading to the production of plasma cells, which release antibodies into the bloodstream, and also to the *memory B cells*. These cells, then store information about the particular pathogen to provide future immunity.
- **Cell-mediated immunity:** The production of antibodies is not alone enough for protecting the body against pathogens. In such circumstances, **cell-mediated immunity** is used by the immune system to destroy infected body cells.

T cells are primarily responsible for cell-mediated immunity. *'Killer T cells' (cytotoxic T cells)* eliminates the infected cells of the body by releasing toxins and promoting 'apoptosis' (programmed cell death). *Helper T cells* activate other cells of immune system.

The pathophysiological changes in disorders related to immune system are discussed here as follows.

HUMAN IMMUNODEFICIENCY VIRUS AND ACQUIRED IMMUNE DEFICIENCY SYNDROME

Viruses are intracellular parasites. Human immunodeficiency virus (HIV) belongs to a group of viruses known as retroviruses. These viruses carry their genetic material in the form of ribonucleic acid (RNA) rather than deoxyribonucleic acid (DNA). HIV consists of a viral core containing the viral RNA surrounded by an envelope consisting of glycoproteins (GP). The fusion of viral envelope with the plasma membrane of the cell is required for allowing entry of HIV to the targeted cell.

There are many steps of life cycle of HIV. At first, there occurs an attachment of HIV GP120 and GP41 to the uninfected CD4 cell receptors and then get fused with the cell membrane. Second, on-coating occurs in which the contents of the viral core are emptied into the host cell. Third, the viral genetic material is copied by HIV enzyme reverse transcriptase into double-stranded DNA from RNA. Next, splitting of double-stranded DNA occurs into the cellular DNA through another HIV enzyme integrase. Fifth, new viral proteins are produced using the integrated DNA. Sixth, slicing of HIV protease occurs into the new proteins (polyproteins). Seventh, the new proteins join the viral RNA into new viral particles. Finally, the process is started all over again by such new viral particles (Fig. 2).

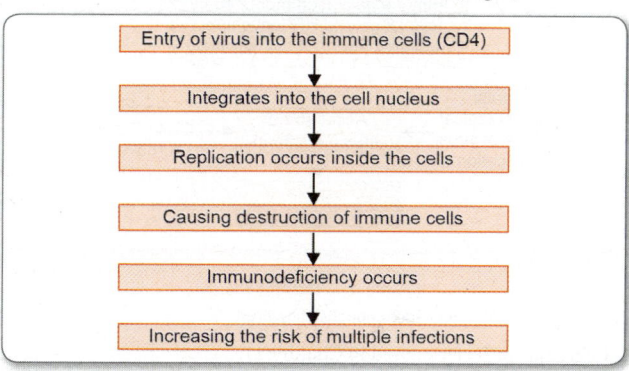

Entry of virus into the immune cells (CD4)
↓
Integrates into the cell nucleus
↓
Replication occurs inside the cells
↓
Causing destruction of immune cells
↓
Immunodeficiency occurs
↓
Increasing the risk of multiple infections

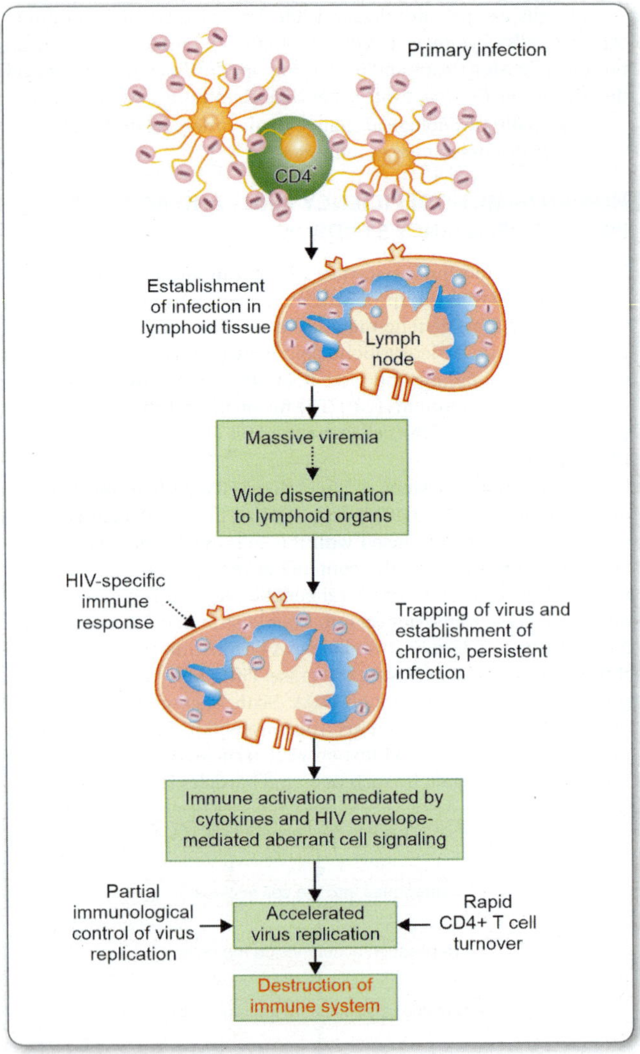

Primary infection

CD4⁺

Establishment of infection in lymphoid tissue

Lymph node

Massive viremia

⋮

Wide dissemination to lymphoid organs

HIV-specific immune response

Trapping of virus and establishment of chronic, persistent infection

Immune activation mediated by cytokines and HIV envelope-mediated aberrant cell signaling

Partial immunological control of virus replication

Accelerated virus replication

Rapid CD4+ T cell turnover

Destruction of immune system

Fig. 2: HIV infection

Abbreviation: HIV, human immunodeficiency virus

Allergic rhinitis: Discussed in Chapter 11.

ANAPHYLAXIS

Anaphylaxis is an acute, systemic hypersensitivity reaction that mainly occurs in already sensitized people when they are re-exposed to the sensitizing agent. The triggering factors may include certain drugs (antibiotics, insulin, streptokinase), food items (nuts, seafood, eggs) and latex. An interaction of antigen with IgE on basophils and mast cells triggers release of histamine, leukotrienes, and other mediators that cause diffuse smooth muscle contraction (resulting in bronchoconstriction, vomiting, or diarrhea) and vasodilation with plasma leakage (resulting in angioedema or urticaria).

Pathophysiological Changes

Pathophysiological changes are given in Figure 3.

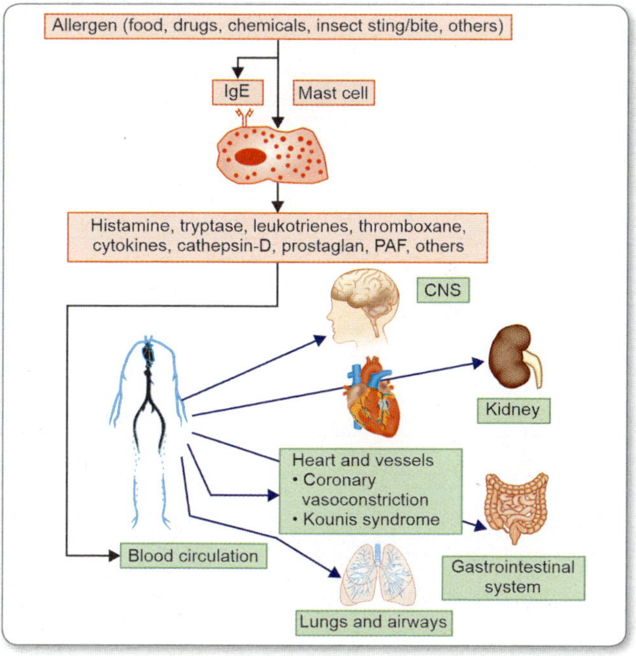

Fig. 3: Pathophysiological changes

Abbreviations: CNS, central nervous system; IgE, immunoglobulin E; PAF, platelet-activating factor

- **Lupus erythematosus:** Discussed in Chapter 12
- **Rheumatoid arthritis:** Discussed in Chapter 9

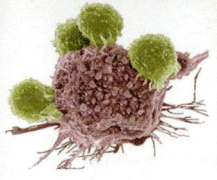

CHAPTER

16

Pathophysiology of Cancer

INTRODUCTION

An uncontrolled growth of abnormal cells anywhere in a body is termed as cancer. The abnormal cells that constitute the cancer tissues are identified by the name of the organ from which these abnormal cells originate like lung cancer, breast cancer, colon cancer. The harm to the body by cancers occurs when there is an uncontrollable division of abnormal cells that forms lumps or masses. This abnormal growth of cells occurs by a chemical change in the structure or function of genes more commonly known as **mutation** (Fig. 1).

Cancer generally takes on the characteristics of cell it mutates and further takes on the characteristics of mutation. Cells are normally having a division limit of 50–60 before disintegration, but this division limit gets override in case of cancerous cells. This leads to disturbance in the growth regulating signals in the cells' surrounding environment causing abnormal cell growth.

Two mainly affected genes by the changes are oncogenes and tumor suppressor genes.

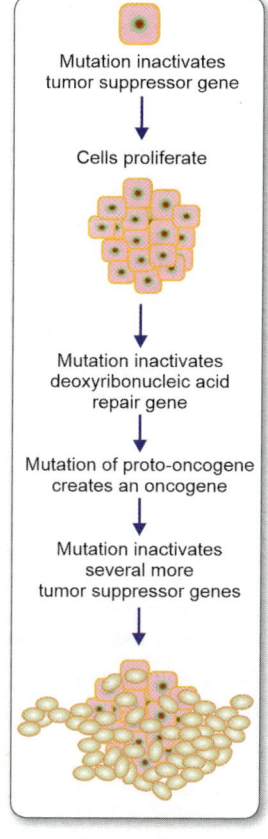

Fig. 1: Mutation

Oncogenes are primarily responsible for division of cells and as they get altered because of mutation, cause abnormally high levels and eventually cancerous changes in the tissues.

Tumor suppressor genes normally inhibit the cell division but in case of cancer, the function of these genes is highly altered.

Other genes that are affected include **suicide genes** (control apoptosis) and **DNA-repair genes** that cause repair of damaged DNA. The progression to cancerous cell formation:

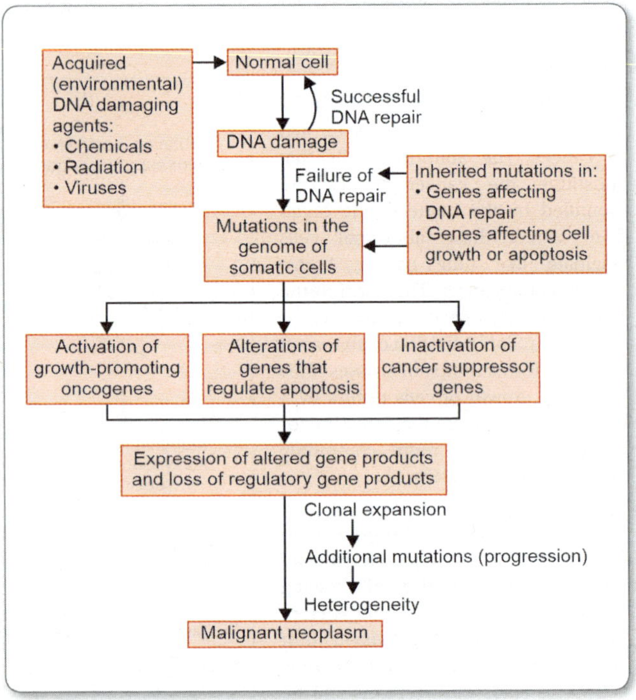

```
Acquired                  →   Normal cell
(environmental)                        ↑  Successful
DNA damaging                           │  DNA repair
agents:                       DNA damage
• Chemicals
• Radiation             Failure of  ←  Inherited mutations in:
• Viruses               DNA repair     • Genes affecting
                                          DNA repair
                        Mutations in the   • Genes affecting cell
                        genome of             growth or apoptosis
                        somatic cells

   Activation of        Alterations of      Inactivation of
   growth-promoting     genes that          cancer suppressor
   oncogenes            regulate apoptosis  genes

          Expression of altered gene products
          and loss of regulatory gene products
                          │  Clonal expansion
                          ↓
                  Additional mutations (progression)
                          ↓
                       Heterogeneity
             Malignant neoplasm
```

Abbreviation: DNA, deoxyribonucleic acid

This chapter highlights the changes that take place in various types of cancers.

CANCER OF THE EYE

Intraocular cancers affect the eye. Primary intraocular cancers are the ones that start in the eye itself whereas cancers spreading from any other area to the eye are known as secondary intraocular cancers.

Types of Eye Cancer

- **Melanoma** is the most common type of primary intraocular cancer that occurs within the eyeball and is also known as uveal melanoma. Iris, choroid and ciliary body are the parts of uvea. Uveal melanomas most commonly occur in choroid or ciliary body followed by iris.
- Other types include Intraocular lymphoma, retinoblastoma and hemangioma (benign tumor of retina and choroid that initiates in the blood vessels).
- Rare types of intraocular cancers include conjunctival melanoma, eyelid carcinoma and lacrimal gland tumor.

ORAL CANCER

These mainly occur due to mutations in the squamous cells causing them to grow uncontrollably.

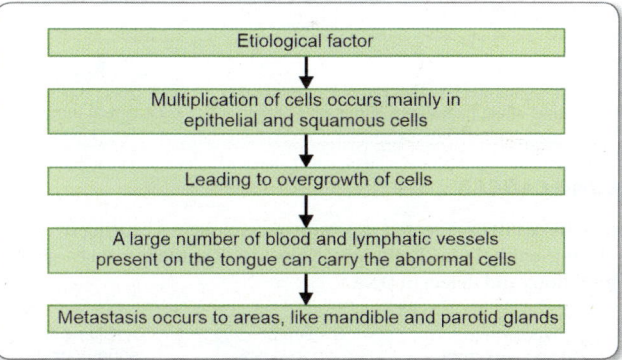

LARYNGEAL CANCER

It occurs in the cells lining the voice-box. As a result of gene mutation, there is a disturbed growth of squamous cells of the larynx leading to the onset of symptoms.

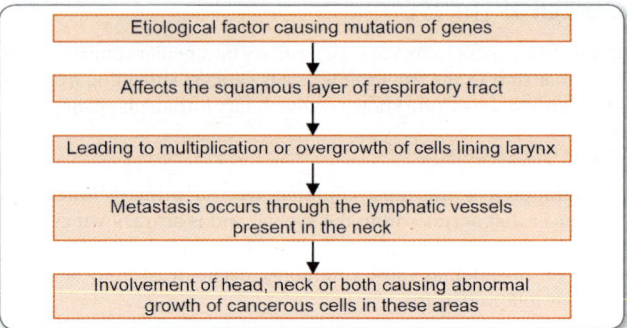

Etiological factor causing mutation of genes

↓

Affects the squamous layer of respiratory tract

↓

Leading to multiplication or overgrowth of cells lining larynx

↓

Metastasis occurs through the lymphatic vessels present in the neck

↓

Involvement of head, neck or both causing abnormal growth of cancerous cells in these areas

BREAST CANCER

It is a type of malignant tumor that starts in the cells of breast. Exposure to estrogen causing damage to DNA and mutations in genes are responsible for an abnormal proliferation of epithelial cells lining the breast.

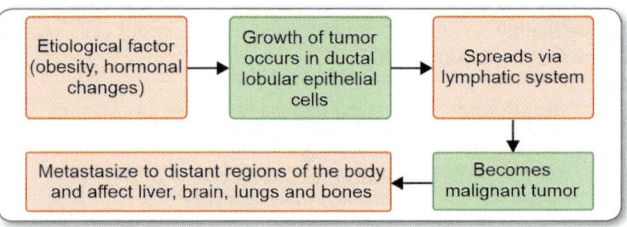

Etiological factor (obesity, hormonal changes) → Growth of tumor occurs in ductal lobular epithelial cells → Spreads via lymphatic system

↓

Metastasize to distant regions of the body and affect liver, brain, lungs and bones ← Becomes malignant tumor

LUNG CANCER

It is the result of repeated exposure to carcinogens causing dysplasia of lung epithelium. Prolonged exposure eventually causes genetic mutations and defect in DNA.

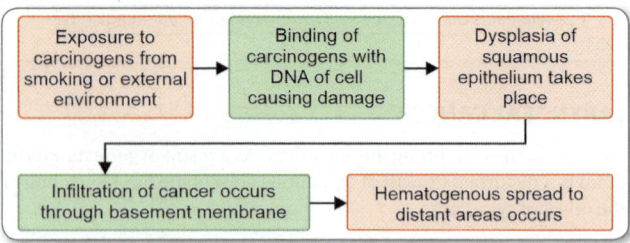

Exposure to carcinogens from smoking or external environment → Binding of carcinogens with DNA of cell causing damage → Dysplasia of squamous epithelium takes place

↓

Infiltration of cancer occurs through basement membrane → Hematogenous spread to distant areas occurs

Abbreviation: DNA, deoxyribonucleic acid

GASTRIC CANCER

Genetic and environmental factors initially cause gastritis further progressing to metaplasia of intestinal mucosa and then dysplasia leading to formation of cancerous mass.

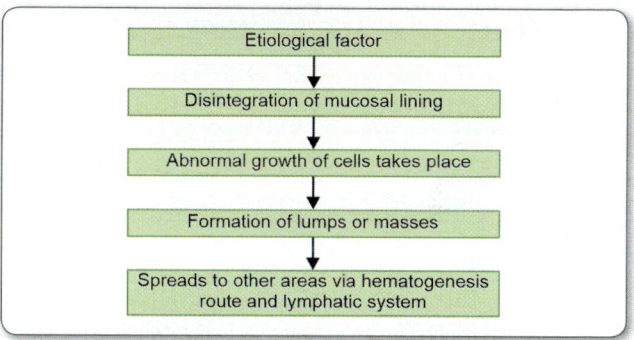

COLORECTAL CANCER

Most commonly referred to as colon cancer and is caused by an uncontrolled growth of cells in colon or rectum.

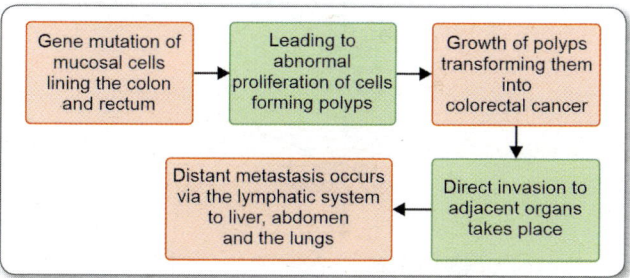

BLADDER CANCER

It is initiated by chronic inflammation causing transformation of normal urothelium to the carcinoma of bladder.

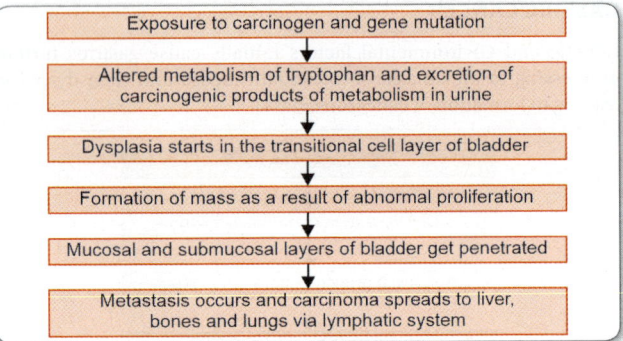

Exposure to carcinogen and gene mutation
Altered metabolism of tryptophan and excretion of carcinogenic products of metabolism in urine
Dysplasia starts in the transitional cell layer of bladder
Formation of mass as a result of abnormal proliferation
Mucosal and submucosal layers of bladder get penetrated
Metastasis occurs and carcinoma spreads to liver, bones and lungs via lymphatic system

LIVER CANCER

Presence of hepatitis B virus (HBV) infection causes increase in turnover of cells leading to the formation of hepatocellular carcinoma (Fig. 2).

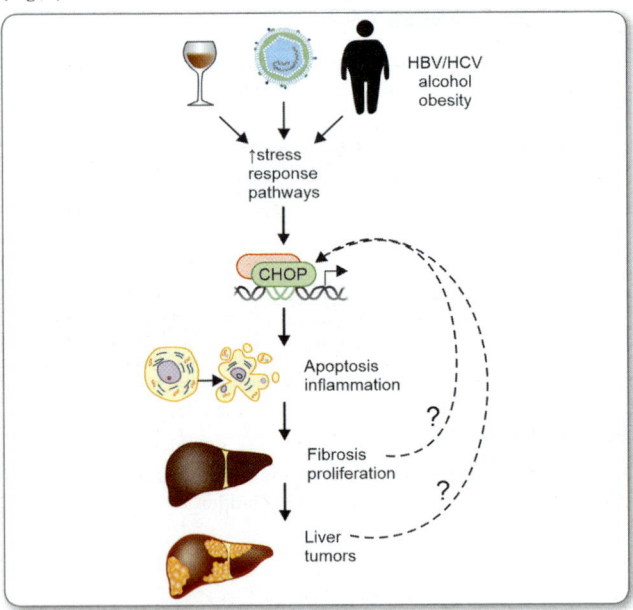

Fig. 2: Liver cancer

Abbreviations: HBV, hepatitis B virus; HCV, hepatitis C virus

Pathophysiology of liver cancer has been displayed in Figure 3.

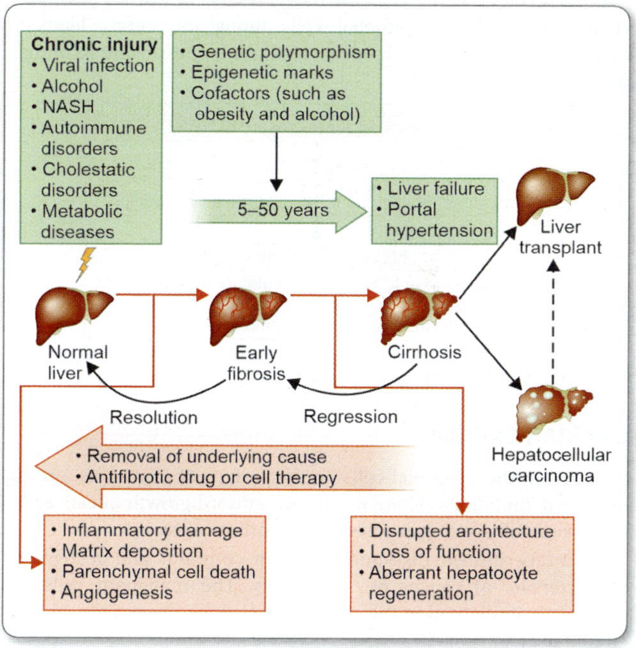

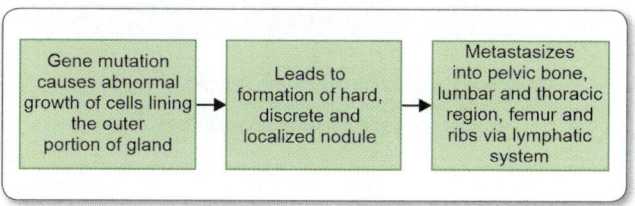

Fig. 3: Pathophysiology of liver cancer

Abbreviation: NASH, nonalcoholic steatohepatitis

PROSTATE CANCER

It is an adenocarcinoma that develops from the mutations in the cells present in the prostate gland. An abnormal multiplication leads to the formation of tumor nodule that surrounds the tissues of prostate gland. The tumor may be localized or there may be an extracapsular extension. Metastasis commonly occurs to bones and lymph nodes.

Gene mutation causes abnormal growth of cells lining the outer portion of gland	Leads to formation of hard, discrete and localized nodule	Metastasizes into pelvic bone, lumbar and thoracic region, femur and ribs via lymphatic system

CERVICAL CANCER

Hypertrophy of intraepithelial cells lining the cervix leads to carcinoma of cervix, which occurs as a result of exposure to human papilloma virus (HPV).

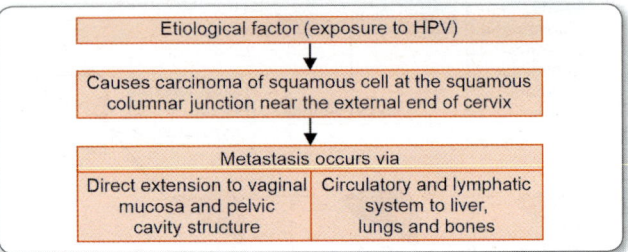

Abbreviation: HPV, human papilloma virus

OVARIAN CANCER

It begins in the epithelial cells on the surface of ovaries as a result of genetic mutations. There occurs an outward growth of cancerous cells eventually getting exposed to the peritoneal cavity.

Intraperitoneal dissemination is a common and recognized characteristic of cancer of the ovaries. The malignant cells are commonly implanted in the sites of stasis along the peritoneal fluid circulation.

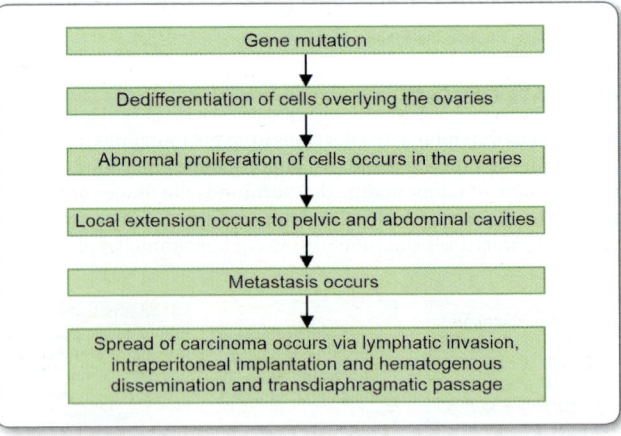

BRAIN TUMOR

Primary brain tumors primarily occur in the tissues of central nervous system and are the result of changes in genes that cause an uncontrolled growth of the cells. Metastatic lesions are also responsible for the formation of tumors in brain (Fig. 4).

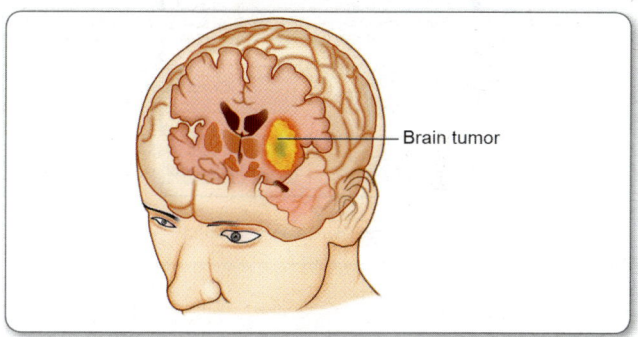

Fig. 4: Brain tumor

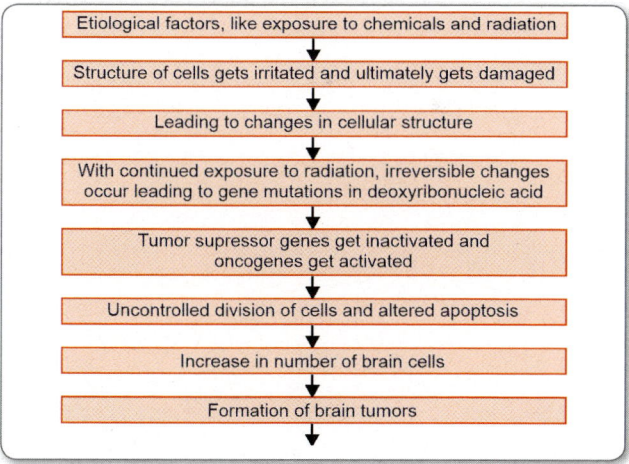

Contd...

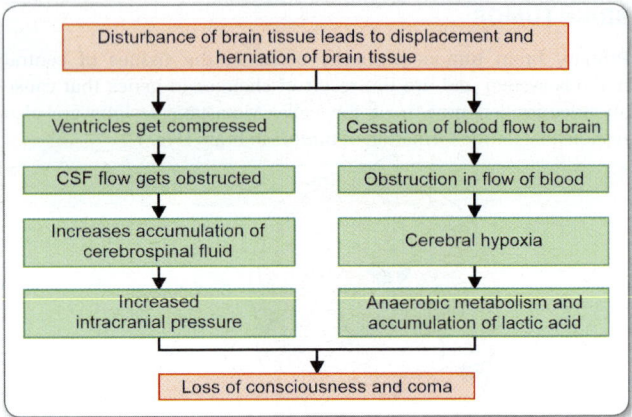

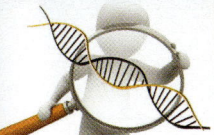

Pathophysiology of Genetic Disorders

INTRODUCTION

Genes are considered to be the building blocks of heredity and are passed on to the children from parents. Genes are also responsible for holding deoxyribonucleic acid (DNA) and facilitating the work of proteins in the cells. The movement of molecules, building of structure and breaking up of toxins are amongst other functions performed by the genes.

Genetic disorders represent mutation or changes in function of the genes or in the structure of chromosomes. A single or polygenic gene trait/s may be involved in the genetic disorder. A mutated gene may be inherited from one or both the parents.

The specific types of genetic disorders are:

SINGLE-GENE DISORDERS

In single-gene disorders, mutation occurs in a single gene, e.g., sickle cell anemia.

These disorders may be dominant or recessive, and genes located on either non-sex or sex chromosomes may be affected.

Autosomal Dominant

These are the disorders that take place in a heterozygous state, when there is one copy of healthy gene and another copy of a relevant gene is mutant in nature. The effects of alleles (mutant version of gene) override the effects of healthy gene, as a result of which the symptoms occur even in the presence of one copy of healthy gene. The spread of dominant genes is vertically down from parents to children. The symptoms occur in a severe form in case there occurs two copies of the mutant gene (homozygous) (Fig. 1).

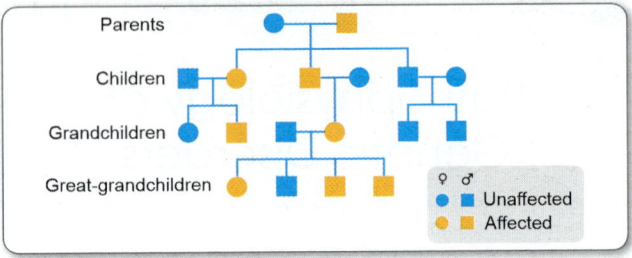

Fig. 1: Inheritance pattern of autosomal dominant disease

Marfan's Syndrome

It is an autosomal disease of connective tissue, which is caused by mutation in FBN1 gene, that encodes Fibrillin 1. Reduced or abnormal fibrillin-1 leads to weakness of tissues, increased beta signaling of transforming growth factor and loss of interactions of the cellular matrix. Marfan syndrome typically affects skeletal, cardiovascular, ocular and neural system and the diagnosis is based on Ghent criteria.

Marfan syndrome-ghent criteria

Cardiovascular system-major criteria	Ocular system-major criterion
• Dilation of ascending aorta • Aortic dissection **Minor criteria** • MVP • Dilation of MPA • Premature mitral annular calcification (<40 years) • Descending thoracic or Abdominal aortic aneurysm (<50 years) CVS involvement: One minor criterion	• Ectopia lentis **Skeletal system-major criteria** Presence of at least four of the following • Pectus carinatum • Pectus excavatum requiring surgery • Reduced US to LS ratio (0.85–0.95) or arm span to height ratio >1.05 • Wrist and thumb signs • Scoliosis >20° or spondylolisthesis • Reduced extension at elbows (<170°) • Medial displacement of medial malleolus causing pes planus • Protusio acetabulae of any degree

Von Willebrand Disease

Von Willebrand disease is a condition that can cause extended or excessive bleeding.

When there is an injury to the blood vessel resulting in bleeding, platelets form a plug at the site of injury along with other clotting factors to control bleeding. Von Willebrand factor (VWF) is the plasma protein that makes the platelets to stick with each other and form a clump and it also carries factor VIII. In case of decrease in plasma levels or a defect in VWF, clotting ability of blood decreases resulting in heavy and continuous bleeding.

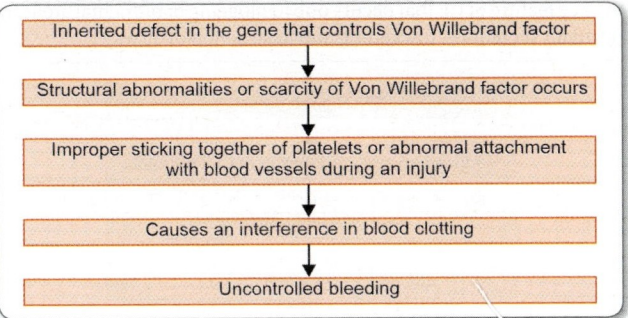

Autosomal Recessive

These are the single gene disorders that take place only in homozygous state, when a person carries two alleles of the relevant gene. Compensation can occur by the healthy allele in response of the effects caused by mutant allele as a result of which the symptoms are not evident in the presence of one healthy and one mutant gene. But if two mutant alleles are inherited by the parent, their effect can be easily exerted resulting in symptoms (Fig. 2).

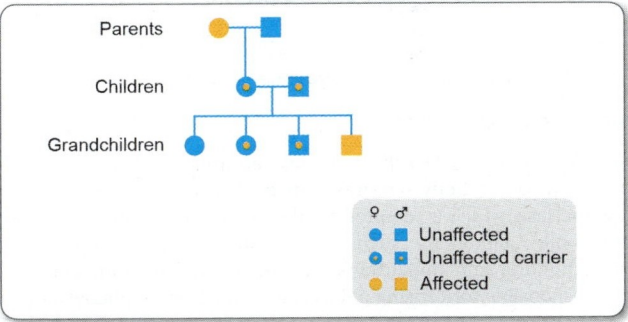

Fig. 2: Inheritance pattern of autosomal recessive disease

Cystic Fibrosis

This disease is caused by mutations in the CF transmembrane conductance regulator (CFTR) protein that regulates the movement of chloride and sodium ions across the cell membrane. The transportation problem related to chloride causes production of thick secretions in the lungs, pancreas, liver, intestine, and reproductive tract. The obstruction in the airflow is considered to be the key feature of CF that occurs due to plugging of bronchial areas by purulent secretions, thickening and destruction of airway.

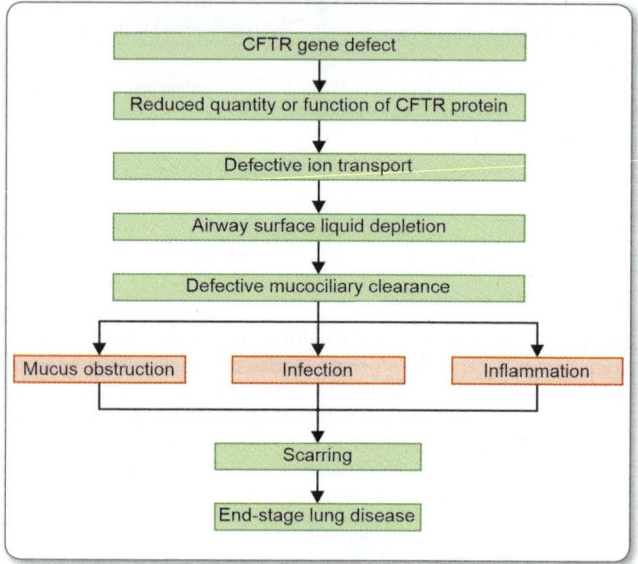

Abbreviation: CFTR, cystic fibrosis transmembrane conductance regulator

Phenylketonuria (PKU)

It is a rare inherited disorder that causes an amino acid phenylalanine to build up in the body. It results from the deficiency of phenylalanine hydroxylase, which is required for the breakdown of phenylalanine. Metabolic alterations such as oxidative stress, dysfunctional mitochondria and impairment in proteins and neurotransmitters are responsible for causing a decrease in the level of phenylalanine hydroxylase.

The severe form of PKU is termed as **Classic PKU** in which the enzyme needed to convert phenylalanine is either missing or severely reduced, that results in excessively higher levels of phenylalanine and brain damage that is severe in nature. In mild to moderate forms of the disease, there is retention of some enzymatic function, thus, the levels of phenylalanine are not as high leading to less severity of brain damage.

Sickle Cell Disease (Fig. 3)

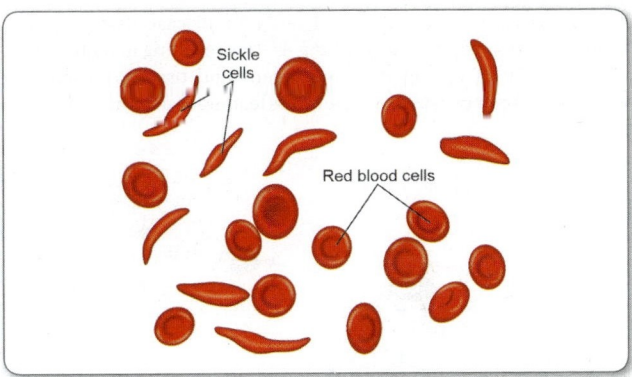

Fig. 3: Sickle cell disease

It is caused by mutation in the beta globin chain in the hemoglobin molecule that helps in producing the iron-rich compound making the blood red and also enables the RBCs to carry oxygen from the lungs. The presence of abnormal hemoglobin makes the RBCs to become sticky, rigid and out of shape.

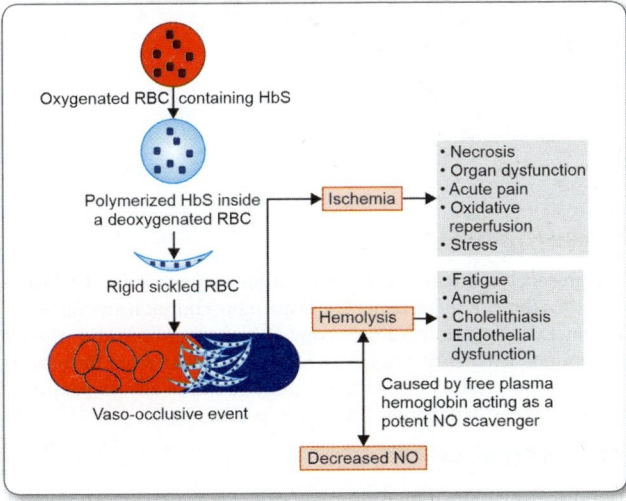

Fig. 4: Pathophysiology of sickle cell disease

Abbreviations: HbS, hemoglobins; NO, nitric oxide; RBC, red blood cell

Wilson's Disease

Wilson's disease is an autosomal recessive disease that originates from a defect in copper transporting ATPase resulting in pathological accumulation of copper in many organs and tissues. Presence of excessive copper causes oxidative stress leading to destruction of cells (Fig. 5).

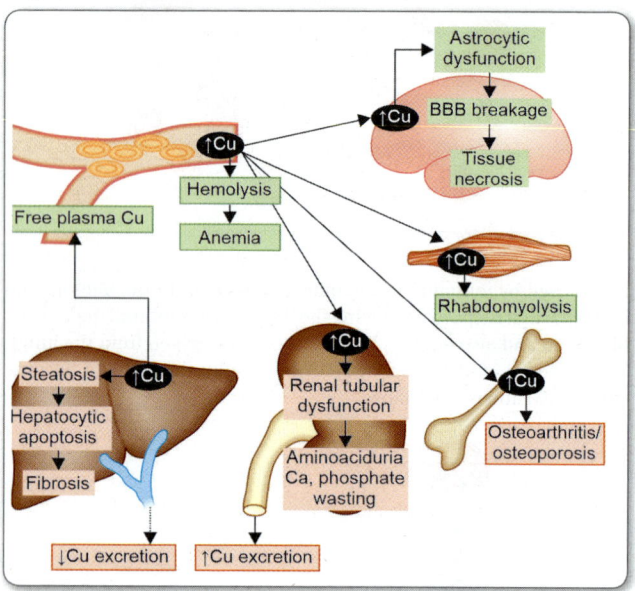

Fig. 5: Wilson's disease

X-linked Diseases

The presence of mutated gene on X chromosomes results in X-linked disorders that are single gene. These are more common among males as they (XY) have only a single copy of X-chromosome and when it gets mutated, males do not have a healthy copy to restore the normal function. According to inheritance pattern, males always pass their X chromosome to daughters but never to sons (Fig. 6).

X-linked Recessive

The disease is transmitted from a carrier mother, who inherits the copy of mutant gene from her father, which is known as "Knight's Move".

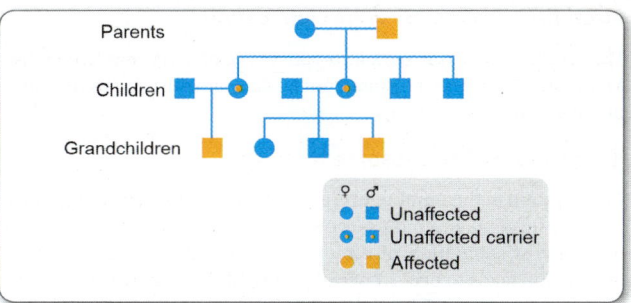

Fig. 6: Inheritance pattern of X-linked disease

Males pass their X chromosome to the daughters and never to the sons, the daughters are then called as 'Obligate carriers' and no symptoms are evident since they also have a healthy copy of genes (Fig. 7).

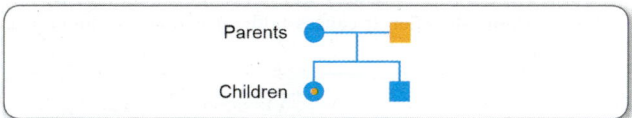

Fig. 7: Inheritance pattern of X-linked mutant gene from father to daughter

Female carriers pass the defective X chromosome to half of their daughters (carriers) and half to their sons (affected). The other children receive healthy copy of gene (Fig. 8).

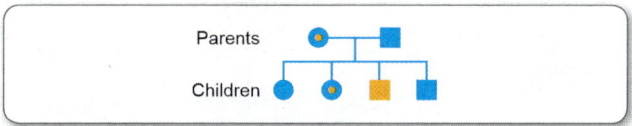

Fig. 8: Inheritance pattern of X-linked mutant gene from a carrier mother

X-linked Dominant

These are very uncommon and their frequency of occurrence is same in males and females. X-linked dominant diseases cannot be transmitted from fathers to sons as they do not pass the X chromosomes to their sons.

CHROMOSOMAL DISORDERS

They occur when the chromosomes or parts of chromosomes are changed or missing, e.g., Down's syndrome.

Alterations in Chromosome Duplication

The presence of distinctive karyotypes of two or more cells is known as Mosaicism. This defect results from an accident during chromosomal duplication.

Alterations in Chromosome Number

An alteration in the number of chromosomes is called as **Aneuploidy.** The cause of aneuploidy is non-disjunction that occurs because of failure of separation of the chromosomes during genesis. Non-disjunction leads to occurrence of germ cells having an even number of chromosomes (22 or 24), but the products of conception formed will have an uneven number of chromosomes (45 or 47). Monosomy refers to the presence of only one member of a pair of chromosomes, whereas Polysomy occurs when a germ cell having more than 23 chromosomes is involved in the conception.

- **Down's syndrome (Trisomy 21)** is the most common type of chromosome disorder. It causes both structural and functional defects.

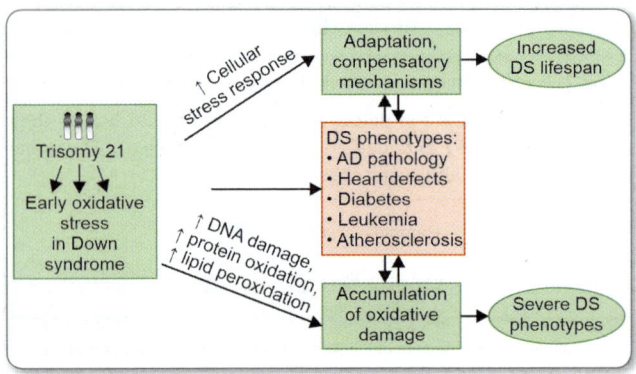

Abbreviation: DS, Down syndrome

- **Turner's syndrome (Monosomy X)** is the monosomy of X chromosome with an absence of ovaries.

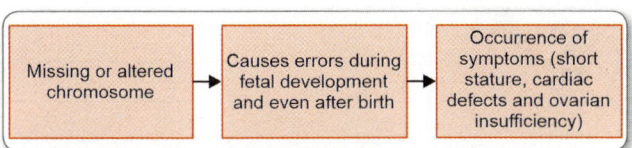

- **Klinefelter's syndrome (Polysomy X)** is mainly characterized by an X-chromatin positive male and is associated with dysfunction of testes. Rarely, there may be more than one extra X chromosome. It can be caused by either one extra copy of X chromosome in each cell (XXY) or an extra X chromosome in few cells.

  The consequences of an extra X chromosome include hypogonadism, gynecomastia and psychosocial concerns.

Alterations in Chromosome's Structure

These mainly result from a break in one or more chromosomes followed by rearrangement of the parts of chromosomes. The factors responsible for causing breakage involve exposure to X-rays, chemical, viral infections and changes in the cellular environment.

COMPLEX DISORDERS

Mutations are present in two or more genes, e.g., colon cancer.

INDEX

Refer 'f' for figure and 't' for table, respectively.

T

U

V

W